M000209366

VETERINARY
ONCOLOGY
SECRETS

VETERINARY ONCOLOGY SECRETS

ROBERT C. ROSENTHAL, DVM, PhD, Dipl ACVIM, Dipl ACVR

Head of Medicine
Veterinary Specialists of Rochester
and Adjunct Assistant Professor
Department of Radiation Oncology
University of Rochester
   School of Medicine and Denistry
Rochester, New York

Publisher: HANLEY & BELFUS, INC.
                  Medical Publishers
                  210 South 13th Street
                  Philadelphia, PA 19107
                  (215) 546-7293; 800-962-1892
                  FAX (215) 790-9330
                  Web site: http://www.hanleyandbelfus.com

Note to the reader: Although the information in this book has been carefully reviewed for correctness of dosage and indications, neither the authors nor the editor nor the publisher can accept any legal responsibility for any errors or omissions that may be made. Neither the publisher nor the editor makes any warranty, expressed or implied, with respect to the material contained herein. Before prescribing any drug, the reader must review the manufacturer's current product information (package inserts) for accepted indications, absolute dosage recommendations, and other information pertinent to the safe and effective use of the product described.

Library of Congress Cataloging-in-Publication Data

Veterinary Oncology Secrets / edited by Robert C. Rosenthal.
     p. ; cm. — (The Secrets Series®)
  Includes index.
  ISBN 1-56053-416-8 (alk. paper)
     1. Veterinary oncology—Examinations, questions, etc. I. Rosenthal, Robert C., 1945–
II. Series.
  [DNLM: 1. Neoplasma—veterinary—Examination Questions. SF 910.T8 V5865 2000]
SF910.T8 V48 2001
636.089'6992'076—dc21

                                                                    00-061393

VETERINARY ONCOLOGY SECRETS   ISBN 1-56053-416-8

© 2001 by Hanley & Belfus, Inc. All rights reserved. No part of this book may be reproduced, reused, republished, or transmitted in any form, or stored in a data base or retrieval system, without written permission of the publisher.

Last digit is the print number: 9   8   7   6   5   4   3   2   1

Dedication

To Bobbie—of course, who else?

To Dr. Erwin Small—the model of service and caring

To Betsy and Irene—the work doesn't get done without them

To all the VSR interns—the future

CONTENTS

CONTRIBUTORS

Laura J. Armbrust, DVM
Resident in Radiology, Department of Clinical Sciences, Kansas State University, Manhattan, Kansas

Philip J. Bergman DVM, MS, PhD, Dipl ACVIM
Head, Donaldson-Atwood Cancer Clinic, The Animal Medical Center, New York; Research Associate, Memorial Sloan-Kettering Cancer Center, New York, New York

David S. Biller, DVM, Dipl ACVR
Professor of Radiology, Department of Clinical Sciences, Kansas State University, Manhattan, Kansas

Ruthanne Chun, DVM, Dipl ACVIM
Assistant Professor of Oncology, Department of Veterinary Clinical Sciences, Kansas State University, Manhattan, Kansas

Steven I. Cooper, MSW, CSW-R, BCD
Social Worker, Rochester, New York

Rick L. Cowell, DVM, Dipl ACVP
Director, Clinical Pathology Laboratory; Professor, Clinical Pathology, Department of Pathobiology, Oklahoma State University, College of Veterinary Medicine, Stillwater, Oklahoma

Steven E. Crow, DVM, Dipl ACVIM
Sacramento Animal Medical Group, Inc., Carmichael, California

Karen E. Dorsey, DVM
Senior Resident, Veterinary Clinical Pathology, Department of Pathobiology, Oklahoma State University, College of Veterinary Medicine, Stillwater, Oklahoma

Linda S. Fineman, DVM, Dipl ACVIM
Pacific Veterinary Specialists, Capitola; South Bay Veterinary Specialists, San Jose, California

James A. Flanders, DVM, Dipl ACVS
Associate Professor, Department of Clinical Sciences, Cornell University, Ithaca, New York

Kevin A. Hahn, DVM, PhD, Dipl ACVIM
Medical Oncologist, Gulf Coast Veterinary Oncology, Houston, Texas

Alan S. Hammer, DVM, Dipl ACVIM
North Coast Veterinary Specialists, Madison, Ohio

Carolyn J. Henry, DVM, MS, Dipl ACVIM
Assistant Professor of Oncology, Department of Veterinary Medicine and Surgery, University of Missouri, Columbia, Missouri

Mary Lynn Higginbotham, DVM
Oncology Resident, Department of Small Animal Medicine and Surgery, University of Missouri, Columbia, Missouri

Dennis W. Macy, DVM, Dipl ACVIM
Professor, Department of Clinical Sciences, Colorado State University College of Veterinary Medicine, Fort Collins, Colorado

Glenna E. Mauldin, DVM, MS, Dipl ACVIM
Assistant Professor of Oncology, Department of Veterinary Clinical Services, Louisiana State University School of Veterinary Medicine, Baton Rouge, Louisiana

G. Neal Mauldin, DVM, Dipl ACVIM, Dipl ACVR
Assistant Professor of Oncology, Department of Veterinary Clinical Services, Louisiana State University School of Veterinary Medicine, Baton Rouge, Louisiana

Dudley McCaw, DVM, Dipl ACVIM
Associate Professor, Department of Veterinary Medicine and Surgery, University of Missouri, Columbia, Missouri

Karelle A. Meleo, DVM, Dipl ACVIM, Dipl ACVR
Veterinary Oncology Services, Edmonds, Washington

Barbara Norton, MSW, CSW-R
Social Worker, Webster, New York

Greg Ogilvie, DVM, Dipl ACVIM
Professor, Department of Clinical Sciences, Colorado State University College of Veterinary Medicine, Fort Collins, Colorado

Jeffrey C. Philibert, DVM
Staff Veterinarian, Cancer Care Center, Angell Memorial Animal Hospital, Boston, Massachusetts

Robert C. Rosenthal, DVM, PhD, Dipl ACVIM, Dipl ACVR
Head of Medicine, Veterinary Specialists of Rochester, Rochester; Adjunct Assistant Professor, Department of Radiation Oncology, University of Rochester School of Medicine and Dentistry, Rochester, New York

Peter H. Rowland, DVM, Dipl ACVP
Histopathology Consulting, Waterford, New York

Stacy B. Smith, DVM
Resident in Clinical Pathology, Oklahoma State University, College of Veterinary Medicine, Stillwater, Oklahoma

John Speciale, DVM, Dipl ACVIM
Staff Neurologist, Veterinary Specialists of Rochester, Rochester, New York

Kimberly M. Stanz, DVM, Dipl ACVO
Veterinary Specialists of Western New York, Buffalo, New York

Steven J. Susaneck, DVM, Dipl ACVIM
Greater Houston Veterinary Specialists, Houston, Texas

Richard E. Weller, DVM, Dipl ACVIM
Senior Program Manager, Molecular Biosciences Department, Pacific Northwest National Laboratory, Richland, Washington

John Paul Woods, DVM, Dipl ACVIM
Associate Professor, Department of Clinical Studies, Ontario Veterinary College, University of Guelph, Guelph, Ontario, Canada

PREFACE

Veterinary oncology has seen tremendous growth since the first textbook devoted to the subject in the late 1970s. Cancer is usually at the top of the list when owners are asked about health concerns for their pets (and it remains a leading cause of death among dogs and cats). A casual perusal of the literature reveals the extent to which both basic oncologic science and clinical medicine attempt to deal with the expanding knowledge—and the increasing number of questions that new information naturally brings. This volume, *Veterinary Oncology Secrets*, joins others in this series by presenting in question and answer format the type of information so important to veterinary students, interns and residents, general practitioners, and specialists in a number of clinical fields. For the most part, these questions are among those asked every day; the answers provide concise practical responses, with key data in a highly understandable format. Beyond the "simple answer" lies the challenge of asking the next pointed question and seeking the next level of understanding. I am certain that the readers of this volume will find its contents both helpful in their busy day-to-day work and a stimulus to pursue the exciting field of veterinary oncology more fully.

The contributing authors were chosen for their practical knowledge and pertinent experience. Each was free to explore the topic in question with minimal restrictions (there was, however, a limit to the size of the book!). The reader will notice that to some extent the style varies from chapter to chapter. Some authors have tended toward quite simple responses; some have provided more complex answers. Some authors have written in a conversational style; some have taken a more Aristotelian, list-making approach. Every chapter reflects its author, and the overall picture is a glimpse of the very large, complex, and evolving field of veterinary oncology. The reader is invited to use this work as an aid to everyday work and a doorway to greater insight.

Robert C. Rosenthal, DVM, PhD

1. EPIDEMIOLOGY, ETIOLOGY, AND PUBLIC HEALTH

Richard Weller, DVM, Dipl ACVIM

1. Why should I be interested in veterinary cancer epidemiology?

Data from epidemiological studies of animals have been used to gain information on the prevalence of various animal diseases compiled according to age, breed, sex, or environment. This can point toward emergent or significant diseases in veterinary medicine and identify the risk factors for those diseases. The results can influence research agendas, product development, and the practice of veterinary medicine itself.

2. Where does the information come from for these studies?

Most are retrospective studies that use hospital records, interviews with pet owners and veterinarians, questionnaires and surveys, necropsy reports, Internet subscribers, pet insurance registries, or veterinary cancer registries as data sources.

3. What is the typical design for these studies?

Most are case-control studies or retrospective surveys.

4. Describe a case-control study.

In case-control studies, risk factors in a population with the disease (cases) are compared with risk factors in a sample without the disease (controls). This is the best study design for studying rare diseases and gives an odds ratio (close predictor of relative risk).

5. What are the relative advantages and disadvantages of case-control studies?

ADVANTAGES	DISADVANTAGES
Best study for rare diseases	Increased bias potential because of sampling of two populations
Relatively inexpensive	Increased bias because the study is retrospective; increased differences between cases and controls
Short duration	Does not address sequence of events (weaker proof of causality)
Relatively small	Can only measure one disease variable Does not give information about prevalence or incidence

6. What has been learned from the results of these studies regarding cancer in companion animals?

Cancer is an important cause of death or euthanasia in companion animals. Nearly 16% to 24% of deaths were attributed to cancer. Age, breed, sex, neutering, environment, and organ system influence relative frequencies and relative risks of cancer.

7. What causes cancer in companion animals?

Cancer generally shows multifactorial etiology. The etiology of cancer is usually divided into environmental (exogenous) and internal (endogenous) factors. Environmental factors can include ionizing radiation, chemical carcinogens, and viruses, while internal genetic factors also play a role.

8. Give some specific examples of environmental factors associated with cancer in companion animals?

FACTOR	NEOPLASM
Ionizing radiation (ultraviolet light)	Skin cancer in dogs and cats
RNA-containing retroviruses	Malignant lymphoma in cats
Secondary tobacco smoke	Nasal cancer in dogs
Herbicides	Malignant lymphoma in dogs
Clinical use of medroxyprogesterone acetate	Mammary cancer in bitches

9. Isn't the risk of nasal cancer in dogs a simple function of skull type?
No. While skull type plays a role, the results of a retrospective study of carcinoma of the nasal cavity and paranasal sinuses in dogs showed that mongrel dogs, often at low risk for other types of cancer, displayed the same risk as all breeds combined, suggesting the influence of environmental factors such as secondary tobacco smoke.

10. What are some of the internal genetic factors that cause cancer in companion animals?
At present, it is difficult to point to specific genetic factors that might predispose companion animals to cancer. Although the hereditary cancers of humans have been reported to number between 50 and 200, similar diseases are largely undocumented in animals. Immune senescence is also thought to be causally related to the increased incidence of tumors observed in aging populations. Immunologic assays conducted on a number of species have shown significant declines in cellular immune function with age.

11. In addition to their effect(s) on the immune system, in what other ways do age and genetic factors influence relative risks of cancer?
Breed– and body weight–specific differences in life span and cancer incidence among dogs may be controlled by genetic factors influencing senescence. For example, the ex vivo proliferative capacity of skin fibroblasts and life span in small- and large-breed dogs was inversely correlated to the frame size of the breeds. Cellular growth potential was also inversely proportional to body size and age.

12. How do genetic factors impact the etiology of cancer?
Genetic factors play a role in pathogenesis, as evidenced by breed and family-related aggregates of neoplastic diseases.

13. Give an example of genetic factors impacting the etiology of cancer.
Among all breeds, the boxer dog has the highest relative risk for all types of cancer, and aggregates of canine osteosarcoma have been described in families of Saint Bernard dogs.

14. Do we know the genetic basis for these observations?
Not yet, but a multicenter effort is underway to develop a comprehensive genetic linkage map of the dog.

15. Why should we genetically map the dog and not other animal species?
Purebred strains, pronounced phenotypic variation, and a high incidence of heritable disease make the dog a unique resource for dissecting the molecular basis of simple and complex genetic diseases and traits. The dog is also uniquely suited to complement genetic analyses in humans.

16. How will that help in the search for the genetic factors that influence the development of cancer in the dog?

Cancer susceptibility genes may be more effectively studied in appropriate animal models such as the dog.

17. Doesn't that assume some similarity in cancer susceptibility genes among species?

Yes it does, but one study has already shown greater than 80% homology between the canine BRCA-1 gene and the human BRCA-1 gene. If the biologic function of BRCA-1 and factors affecting expressivity, such as gene-environment and gene-gene interactions, are also similar among species, this could eventually point to a role for BRCA-1 in the etiology of some canine mammary cancers.

18. Why is the dog a good model for studying cancer susceptibility genes?

Because of the genetic diversity between breeds, the dog is a suitable species for differentiation between genetically determined predisposition and environmental influences in the etiology of cancer. Epidemiologic surveillance of cancer morbidity in dogs may be a useful instrument for tracing carcinogens.

19. What role, if any, can veterinary cancer epidemiology play in cancer prevention?

Epidemiology may provide a means to prevent cancer by, for example, pointing to withdrawal of hormones (mammary cancer) or isolation of tumor-virus–positive animals (malignant lymphoma). The epidemiologic study of naturally occurring environmental diseases in animals, regarded as "sentinel" health events, can also provide valuable information on agents thought to cause cancer in humans as well.

CONTROVERSIES

20. Does feline leukemia virus cause vaccine-associated feline sarcomas?

Despite the strong association reported between feline leukemia virus vaccination and fibrosarcoma tumorigenesis in cats, the results of two epidemiologic retrospective studies suggest that feline leukemia virus and, therefore, feline sarcoma virus do not have a role in the pathogenesis of vaccine-associated feline sarcomas.

21. Should tumor-virus–positive (feline leukemia virus, bovine leukemia virus) animals be kept away from humans?

No. Although some viruses can, under difficult experimental conditions, cross the species barrier, there is no evidence for a public health hazard for humans. They should, however, be isolated from tumor-virus–negative animals of the same species.

BIBLIOGRAPHY

1. Arnesen K, Gamlem H, Glattre E, et al: Registration of canine cancer. Tidsskr Nor Laegeforen 115:714–717, 1995.
2. Kass PH, Barnes WG Jr, Spangler WL, et al: Epidemiologic evidence for a causal relation between vaccination and fibrosarcoma tumorigenesis in cats. J Am Vet Med Assoc 203:396–405, 1993.
3. Li Y, Deeb B, Pendergrass W, Wolf N: Cellular proliferative capacity and life span in small and large dogs. J Gerontol A Biol Sci Med Sci 51:B403–B408, 1996.
4. Misdorp W: Veterinary cancer epidemiology. Vet Q 18:32–36, 1996.
5. Neff MW, Broman KW, Mellersh CS, et al: A second-generation linkage map of the domestic dog, Canis familiaris. Genetics 151:803–820, 1999.
6. Reif JS, Bruns C, Lower KS: Cancer of the nasal cavity and paranasal sinuses and exposure to environmental tobacco smoke in pet dogs. Am J Epidemiol 147:488–492, 1998.
7. Szabo CI, Wagner LA, Francisco LV, et al: Human, canine and murine BRCA1 genes: sequence comparison among species. Hum Mol Genet 5:1289–1298, 1996.

2. CANCER BIOLOGY, METASTASIS, AND PARANEOPLASIA

Philip J. Bergman, DVM, MS, PhD, *Dipl* ACVIM

1. Why does a clinician need to understand cancer biology, metastasis, and paraneoplasia?

Over the past 40–50 years, progress in the basic understanding of cancer biology has significantly helped cancer clinicians in the diagnosis, prognosis, and treatment of clinically relevant cancers. Therefore, it can be strongly argued that future advancements in the diagnosis, prognosis, and treatment of cancers will be closely tied to advancements in the understanding of cancer biology. The old adage "Know what you are treating before you treat" holds true for diagnosis, prognosis, and therapy. Obtaining the most advanced knowledge possible about the basic biology of cancer affords the best chance of making major advances in the war against cancer.

Many cancer researchers and clinicians are predicting that the next 10–20 years will be the most exciting in the history of cancer. The tools of molecular biology are allowing investigators to open windows into the cancer cell and explore its proteins and genetics. (See the bibliography at the end of this chapter for additional information.)

2. Do I really have to understand all the cancer biology-related terms (e.g., proto-oncogene, chemical carcinogenesis, apoptosis)?

Yes, yes, yes! As discussed above, a greater understanding of the basics of cancer biology has consistently translated into advancements in the diagnosis, prognosis, and treatment of clinically relevant cancers. Therefore, the astute cancer clinician will recognize that one must first understand the components and terms used in cancer biology before being able to move toward making advances in the clinic.

3. What is the difference between a proto-oncogene and oncogene?

The process of how a normal cell transforms into a malignant cell is beginning to be better understood. A major genetic change in transformed cells is the conversion of proto-oncogenes to oncogenes. A *proto-oncogene* is a normal gene (i.e., sequence of DNA) that regulates the growth and differentiation of a cell. Proto-oncogene products (proteins) are exquisitely regulated in normal cells to allow for continuing cellular homeostasis. *Oncogenes* are altered proto-oncogenes (altered genes or expression of the gene product) that have allowed the cell to potentially undergo malignant transformation.

4. What is a tumor suppressor gene? Describe the impact of the loss of a tumor suppressor gene.

Another major genetic change in transformed cells is the loss of tumor suppressor genes. A tumor suppressor gene (TSG) is a gene that encodes for a protein that acts as an anti-oncogene by inhibiting or restricting cellular proliferation. Genetic loss or loss of function of a TSG can allow the cell to divide uncontrollably, which may lead to the development of a cancer.

5. How are mutations in oncogenes and TSGs usually obtained?

Mutations may occur by somatic means or may be passed on through the germline. Mutations in oncogenes are most commonly derived through somatic means. Mutations in TSGs can be obtained through somatic means, or may be passed down to progeny through the germline.

6. Can a single mutation typically lead to the development of a cancer?

In the vast majority of malignancies examined to date, two or more genetic mutations in oncogenes and/or TSGs are required. A single oncogene or TSG mutation is generally considered "necessary but not sufficient" for the development of a malignancy.

7. What are some of the general classes of proto-oncogenes or proto-oncogene products?

As mentioned, oncogenes are derived from proto-oncogenes, which invariably have integral roles in the growth and differentiation of cells. Some classes of proto-oncogenes are:

- Growth factor receptors (e.g., epidermal growth factor receptor)
- Growth factors (e.g., epidermal growth factor, transforming growth factor-α)
- Nuclear proteins (e.g., myc, fos/jun)
- Nucleotide binding (e.g., ras)
- Cytoplasmic growth factor/growth factor receptor (e.g., src, fyn, fak)
- Kinases (protein tyrosine kinases, serine-threonine kinases)

8. What are the four stages of the cell cycle?

Cancer is classically thought of as a disorder of uncontrolled cell growth. Great strides have been made recently in understanding the various components of cell growth. Normal cells and cancer cells grow in number by dividing. The four stages are:

G1 (growth 1)/**G0** (growth—resting stage)
S (synthesis)
G2 (growth 2)
M (mitosis)

9. How is the rate of tumor growth generally categorized?

The rate of tumor cell growth can be extremely variable across and within tumor cell types. However, there are three general categories:

Potential doubling time (Tpot)—time for doubling in size if no cell loss occurred
Volume doubling time (Tvol)—time for doubling in volume (assuming cell loss is ongoing)
Cell cycle time (Tc)—time the cancer cell takes to traverse the four stages of the cell cycle

10. What is apoptosis?

Cancer is generally thought of as a disease of uncontrolled cell growth. An often forgotten potential cause of an increased number of cells (i.e., a possible tumor) is dysregulation of cell death. Tumor cells can die a necrotic death; however, most die by apoptosis when treated with chemotherapy and/or radiation therapy.

Apoptosis is the physiologic (necrosis is pathologic) death and subsequent removal of cells by **programmed cell death**. It is a process that is evolutionarily conserved, and all nucleated cells are able to undergo apoptosis with the correct set of stimuli or lack of inhibition. Apoptosis is tightly regulated in the normal organism as a mechanism of checks and balances to ensure **cellular homeostasis**.

11. What are examples of important normal apoptotic processes?

- Prostatic involution after castration in humans or dogs
- Regression of mammary tissue after lactation has completed
- Death of intestinal epithelial cells as they move up the crypt
- Deletion of auto-reactive T-cells
- Loss of interdigital cells in-utero to form the hand or the paw
- Shedding of a tadpole's tail

12. Why is it important that we understand the function of apoptosis?

Apoptosis is the "default death pathway," meaning that if the correct survival signals are not present, the cell will undergo programmed cell death and die an apoptotic death. Chemotherapy agents and radiation therapy kill cancer cells via apoptosis. Since apoptosis is a tightly regulated methodology for physiologic cell removal of potentially all nucleated cells, it is important to obtain additional knowledge about the molecular processes governing this incredibly important process. Such additional information may then allow investigators to develop novel and possibly specific therapies to use singly or in combination with standardized anti-cancer agents. In addition, because apoptosis is one of the final steps in the death of a cell, mechanisms that block apoptosis are know known to be critical mechanisms of drug and radiation resistance.

13. What are the three steps of carcinogenesis? Is each step reversible or irreversible?

The development of a cancer is generally a multi-step process, and therefore termed "multistep carcinogenesis."

1. Initiation is irreversible (i.e., genetic).
2. Promotion is reversible (i.e., epi-genetic).
3. Progression is irreversible (i.e., multiple genetic changes).

14. At which step can the multi-step carcinogenesis cascade no longer be reversed to prevent a malignancy from occurring?

Once a tumor begins to proceed through the progression phase, it can no longer be reversed.

15. What are the five pathways through which multi-step carcinogenesis can occur? Give two examples for each pathway.

- Chemical carcinogenesis; benzene, polychlorobiphenyls
- Physical carcinogenesis; ionizing radiation, various fibers, ultraviolet radiation
- Biological carcinogenesis; hormones (diethylstilbesterol, others), parasites (e.g., *Spirocerca lupi*) and viruses (e.g., FeLV, Rous sarcoma virus, human papilloma virus)
- Heritable carcinogenesis; retinoblastoma, Von Hippel Lindau
- Passive carcinogenesis; multiple genetic mutations accumulated over time leading to a variety of spontaneous malignancies

16. Is metastasis an active or a random process, and why?

The majority of cancer-related deaths in veterinary and human oncology are due to metastasis. Unfortunately, the advances made in the treatment of primary tumors (surgery, radiation, and possibly chemotherapy) have not been made in the treatment of metastatic disease.

Metastasis is an active, complex, and multi-step process. A 1-cm tumor is composed of approximately one billion cells. A tumor of this size routinely sheds approximately 1 million cells into the systemic circulation each day. However, the vast majority of these circulating cells do not metastasize because they do not have the capability to traverse all steps of the metastatic cascade.

17. What are the steps of the metastatic cascade mentioned in Question 16?

- Tumor proliferation (via initiation, promotion, and progression)
- Primary tumor angiogenesis
- Detachment
- Invasion of local tissues
- Intravasation
- Circulation, arrest, and interaction with local tissues
- Attachment
- Extravasation
- Invasion of local tissues

- Secondary tumor angiogenesis
- Cycle repeats again ("metastases of a metastasis")

18. Explain the "seed and soil hypothesis" and the vascular entrapment hypothesis.

The *seed and soil hypothesis*, a leading theory of metastasis developed by Paget and promoted by Fidler, revolves around interactions between the cancer cell (the "seed") and the host target organ (the "soil") that can potentially possess favorable or less favorable conditions for metastasis. Cancers seen in veterinary medicine that support this theory include the predilection of renal lymphoma cells for the development of CNS metastases. Cancers seen in human medicine that support this theory include skin melanoma metastasizing to brain, and colon carcinoma metastasizing to liver.

The *vascular entrapment hypothesis* predicts that metastasis may be seen at certain organs due to vascular connections with the primary tumor via entrapment in capillary beds distal to the tumor. Some investigators believe that this explains the preponderance of pulmonary metastases and the occurrence of metastases in distal limbs.

19. Are these two hypotheses mutually exclusive?

No. The vascular entrapment hypothesis is extremely controversial, as recent evidence suggests that the "soil" of the pulmonary parenchyma may provide a highly desirable locale for the development of subsequent metastases, further supporting the seed and soil hypothesis. That said, recent work using ultravideomicroscopy has shown that vascular entrapment may aid in allowing the necessary communication between a circulating cancer cell and its respective preferential soil for the subsequent development of a metastasis.

20. True or false: The performance of a biopsy increases the chance of metastasis.

False. A multitude of research studies over the last 40 years have not been able to support this statement. It is true that there are an increased number of circulating cancer cells present in the systemic circulation of a patient undergoing a biopsy. However, remember that metastasis is an active and highly selective process. Tumor cells released into the circulation due to the biopsy are not capable of traversing the multiple steps necessary for the formation of a metastasis.

Note that fine-needle aspiration and/or biopsy of certain cancers (e.g., transitional cell carcinoma of the urinary bladder via trans-abdominal aspiration/biopsy) can lead to aspiration/biopsy tract tumors. This *not* a metastatic event and should be considered a direct extension of the tumor.

21. What are paraneoplastic syndromes?

Paraneoplastic syndromes (PNS) are neoplasm-associated alterations in bodily structure and/or function that occur distant to the tumor.

22. What causes paraneoplastic syndromes?

The cause of most PNS is unknown, and most are systemic by nature.

23. Why is it so important to know about paraneoplastic syndromes?

- PNS often result in more morbidity than the primary malignancy.
- PNS are commonly underestimated in importance to diagnosis, treatment, and prognosis.
- PNS may be the first sign of a malignancy.
- The persistence of a PNS after therapy may signify metastasis and/or ineffective therapy.

24. Name a variety of PNS seen in veterinary patients.

Humoral hypercalcemia of malignancy
Hypoglycemia
Hyperhistaminemia

Cachexia/anorexia complex
Hypertrophic osteopathy
Fever
Inappropriate secretion of antidiuretic hormone
Hyperviscosity
Others (anemia, thrombocytopenia, thrombocytosis, DIC, neutropenia, neutrophilia, neuromuscular)

25. **Name the most common neoplasms associated with paraneoplastic hypercalcemia.**
    Lymphoma
    Anal sac apocrine gland adenocarcinoma
    Parathyroid neoplasia
    Nasal neoplasia
    Multiple myeloma
    Primary and secondary bone tumors
    Thymoma
    Almost any other tumor

26. **What is the pathophysiologic etiology of paraneoplastic hypercalcemia?**
    • There are a number of pathways involved that may work in tandem or seperately.
    • Ectopic production of PTH (PTH-rp; parathryroid hormone–related protein)
    • Prostaglandin-induced osteolysis
    • Ectopic production of osteoclast-activating factor
    • Direct tumor osteolysis
    • Others (e.g., 1,25 dihydroxyvitamin D)

27. **List the possible clinical signs of paraneoplastic hypercalcemia.**

Anorexia/weight loss	Lethargy/dehydration
Vomiting	Bradycardia
Constipation	Other cardiac dysrhythmias
Generalized muscle weakness	Hypertension
Polyuria/polydipsia	Coma and/or seizures

28. **What are the treatments available for paraneoplastic hypercalcemia?**
    • Rapid diagnosis and then treatment of the underlying neoplasm
    • Saline diuresis
    • Furosemide
    • Prednisone (*Note:* Only use if patient already has diagnosis of cause of PNS hypercalcemia)
    • Others (calcitonin, mithramycin, bisphosphonates, gallium nitrate)

29. **Name the two major categories of paraneoplastic hypoglycemia. Give an example of each.**
    Pancreatic tumor hypoglycemia; insulinoma (increased production of insulin)
    Extra-pancreatic tumor hypoglycemia; intra-abdominal neoplasia such as hepatocellular carcinoma or leiomyoma/leiomyosarcoma (increased production of insulin or insulin-like substances such as IGF-I or IGF-II)

30. **List the clinical signs of paraneoplastic hypoglycemia.**
    Disorientation and weakness
    Nervousness or collapse
    Hunger or anorexia
    Focal neurologic abnormalities
    Seizures and/or coma
    Tachycardia, vomiting, and/or restlessness due to compensatory adrenergic effects

31. Fever of unknown origin can be a common presenting sign in dogs and cats with neoplastic disease. What are some of the tumors associated with PNS fever?

Lymphoma, especially hepatic
Multiple myeloma
Various leukemias and myeloproliferative disorders
Mast cell tumor
Intracranial tumors
Hepatic tumors
Any tumor

32. What are some of the diagnostic tests that should be performed when you suspect a case of paraneoplastic fever?

- Complete history and physical exam pursuing a diagnosis of neoplasia
- Body temperature measurement every 8-12 hours to document persistence of the fever
- Routine diagnostic tests (CBC/platelet count/biochem profile/urinalysis)
- Thoracic (three views of chest) and abdominal radiography
- Neoplasm-specific studies (e.g., FNA/cytology, bone marrow, exploratory surgery)
- Rule out other causes of fever via:
    Blood cultures (aerobic/anaerobic)
    Serologic testing (e.g., rickettsial, immune-mediated, mycoses, bacterial, viral)
    Abdominal ultrasonography
    Arthrocentesis
    ECG and echocardiogram
    GI contrast studies
    Skeletal radiographic studies

33. Name the most common causes of paraneoplastic hyperviscosity.

Multiple myeloma
Polycythemia vera
Hyperleukocytic leukemias
Lymphoma
Various dysproteinemias
Primary macroglobulinemia
Various solid tumors

BIBLIOGRAPHY

1. Chambers AF, MacDonald IC, Schmidt EE, et al: Clinical targets for anti-metastasis therapy. Adv Cancer Res 79:91–121;2000.
2. Bergman PJ.: Paraneoplastic syndromes. In Morgan R (ed): Handbook of Small Animal Practice, 3rd ed. Philadelphia, WB Saunders Inc., 1997.
3. Bergman PJ: Paraneoplastic syndromes. In Withrow SJ, MacEwen EG (eds): Small Animal Clinical Oncology, 3rd ed. Philadelphia, WB Saunders Inc., 2000, in press.
4. Fidler IJ: Angiogenesis and cancer metastasis. Cancer J Sci Am 6 Suppl 2:S134–141; 2000.
5. Fidler IJ: Modulation of the organ microenvironment for treatment of cancer metastasis. J Natl Cancer Inst 87:1588–1592; 1995.
6. Rudin CM, Thompson CB. Apoptosis and disease: regulation and clinical relevance of programmed cell death. Annu Rev Med 48:267–281;1997.
7. Sager R. Tumor suppressor genes: the puzzle and the promise. Science 246:1406–1412; 1989.
8. Soussi T. The p53 tumor suppressor gene: from molecular biology to clinical investigation. Ann N Y Acad Sci 910:121–37; 2000.
9. Weller RE: Paraneoplastic disorders in dogs with hematopoietic tumors. Vet Clin North Am Small Anim Pract 15:805–816; 1985.

3. CLINICAL TRIALS, STATISTICS, AND EVIDENCE-BASED MEDICINE

Robert C. Rosenthal, DVM, PhD, Dipl ACVIM, Dipl ACVR

1. Why do oncologists always talk about clinical trials?

It is through a system of clinical trials that new drugs have been brought to bear in the fight against cancer. Studies in clinical patients are the ultimate test of a drug's efficacy and usefulness, and over the years a series of phased clinical trials have led to the introduction of new drugs. Of course, properly constructed trials can evaluate other modalities as well, such as surgery, radiotherapy, and multimodality approaches. The concept of a controlled trial from which meaningful clinical data is derived has been important in the growth of oncologic practice.

2. What is the purpose of a phase I study?

A phase I study is designed to determine the maximum tolerated dose of a new agent and to assess toxicity. It is restricted to patients with malignancies for which no standard treatment is effective. Typically, a starting dose based on prior animal studies is selected, and dose escalations are evaluated as patients are entered and experience is gained with any dose level. Because the primary intent of these studies is to establish a tolerable dose schedule, measurable disease in the patient is not a requirement.

3. What is the purpose of a phase II study?

A phase II study is designed to answer the question of whether the drug has sufficient anti-tumor activity to warrant further clinical evaluation. Typically, patients with a number of different tumor types are entered and evaluated as part of the phase II trial to determine which tumor types may or may not be responsive to the drug. Phase II trials provide a transition from a modality-oriented to a disease-oriented study focus.

4. What is the purpose of a phase III study?

Phase III studies are intended to establish the value of a new therapy in relation to the current standard therapy. Again, the study is disease-oriented, but each phase III study focuses on a single disease rather than a spectrum of diseases.

5. What is a phase IV study?

When a new therapy has been statistically shown to offer an improvement over prior treatment for a specific disease, site, and stage, it becomes standard care. The phrase "phase IV clinical trial" is used by some to connote the ongoing evaluation of even accepted approaches.

6. Why should a clinician be concerned about statistics?

Statistics has been described as a group of methods and concepts for learning from experience. The experience in question is usually gathered as counts or measurements of separate incidents showing individual variation. Clinical research employs statistical approaches, and it is important that the clinician be a critical reader with sufficient understanding of statistics to interpret the clinical literature in a meaningful way.

7. Define descriptive statistics.

Descriptive statistics are numerical summaries of data. Simply, descriptive statistics help point out three critical features of a data set: **central tendency**, **variability**, and **frequency**

distribution. Indicators of central tendency include the mean, median, and mode. Variation is indicated by the range and variance. Frequency distribution is indicated by a representation of occurrences (frequencies) within intervals, often graphically shown as histograms.

8. Why do oncologists usually talk more about medians than means?

Both the median and the mean point to the center of the data. (The third indicator of central tendency, the mode, merely indicates which number in a set appears the most often.) However, particularly when considering outcome data (remission time, disease-free interval, progression-free interval, survival) the *median*, the number at the middle of an ordered list of all the individual results, generally offers a more meaningful picture. A very few patients with exceptional outcomes (e.g., very long survival) will increase the *mean*, the numerical average, without changing the median. Reporting the mean at the exclusion of the median would most likely skew the data in a positive, but perhaps not accurate, direction.

9. How many statistical tests does a clinician need to understand to grasp the clinical literature?

The field of statistics is large and replete with both options and opinions. Learning statistics has been compared to learning a foreign language (and sometimes this comparison has been considered unfair to even the most foreign of foreign languages!). Fortunately, the clinician can understand most of the reported statistical analyses with a good grasp of a relatively small number of basic concepts and individual testing methods. A survey has pointed out that the statistical reporting in 90% of veterinary medical literature could be understood with comprehension of only five categories of statistical methods: ANOVA, *t*-test, contingency tables, nonparametric tests, and simple linear regression.

10. What is a P value? How should a P value be interpreted?

A P value is a probability, usually the probability of obtaining a result as extreme as or more extreme than the one observed if the difference is due entirely to random variation in measurements, or, more simply, if the result is due to chance alone, not to any real difference in the groups studied. The investigator sets the P value before the study is done.

In biological experiments the P value usually is set at 0.05. Therefore, if the P value is < 0.05, the result is statistically significant (although not necessarily clinically significant); if the P value is > 0.05, the difference in groups is not statistically significant. If the P value is declared as 0.05, a resultant P value of 0.01 is no more significant than one of 0.03, as each is less than the declared value. Similarly, if the resultant P value is 0.10 or 0.06, the interpretation is the same—there is no significant difference in the groups. Some authors have used the term "trend toward significance" when a single P value is slightly higher than 0.05, but such usage should be discouraged among investigators and interpreted with great skepticism by readers.

In some cases, the investigator does not declare a P value, but reports the P values of each of the statistical tests performed as decided at the time the study was designed. In that case, the reader is free to interpret whether the result carries enough weight to be considered significant and to what extent.

11. What is meant by the power of a statistical test? What about the size of a study?

The power of a statistical test is the probability of rejecting the null hypothesis (that is, the hypothesis to be tested) when it is false. Many factors influence the power of a test. Sample size, declared significance level, the statistical procedure, and the magnitude of the difference between the hypothesized and actual values of a population quantity all affect power. The investigator can control some of these factors.

Limited sample size is often cited as a drawback of published clinical trials and other reports in veterinary medicine. Large sample sizes are preferable because they allow the detection of small differences between groups. On issues of power and sample size needed for a meaningful study, a statistician should be consulted as the study is being designed—before, not after, the study is done.

12. What is a survival curve? How should a survival curve be interpreted?

A survival curve is a plot of the percent of animals still alive (or in remission in some instances) at any time from the beginning of the evaluation. It is possible to read a median time from such curves, but if the curves of two groups are presented on the same diagram, it is not possible to tell by inspection alone whether there is a statistical difference. For that determination, the reader must find in either the legend or the text both the means used to generate the survival curve and the resultant P value from the comparison of curves. Different methods emphasize the importance of different portions of the curve, so some care is needed in interpretation.

13. What is the difference between randomization and stratification?

Randomization and stratification are both important in the design of good studies. Patients are randomized to treatment groups by a number of different schemes to eliminate investigator bias. Randomization *precedes* stratification, which is the separation of patients into groups based on known prognostic factors to account for the differences those factors imply.

14. Why do investigators report confidence intervals?

Confidence intervals allow numerical estimations that may be of more clinical importance than the statistical significance offered by P values. The confidence interval is used to estimate a population quantity, most often population percentages; population means difference between population percentages; or differences between population means. It is calculated based on a confidence level, but these must be somewhat limited (e.g., 95% vs. 99%) as the very wide confidence intervals associated with very high confidence levels may preclude meaningful estimates due to their very width.

15. Define evidence-based medicine.

Evidence-based medicine (EBM) was first defined as the conscientious, explicit, and judicious use of current best evidence in making decisions about the care of individual patients. A recently updated definition states that EBM is the integration of best research evidence with clinical expertise and patient values. For veterinarians, the explicit inclusion of patient values is particularly appropriate. Although the need to state this philosophy so blatantly may seem like overkill to practicing veterinarians, researchers observing physicians (there are none specifically regarding veterinarians) point out that there are often gaps between perceived needs and actions and reality in terms of information pertinent to patients.

16. What is involved in an EBM practice?

EBM is an ongoing process in which clinical questions raised by work with patients generate answerable clinical questions. Careful, accurate searching for the best current evidence and the evaluation of that evidence are critical components of EBM. The application of these results to individual patients and the subsequent assessment of personal performance round out the basic tenets of EBM.

17. How does one ask an answerable clinical question as defined by EBM?

A well-formulated clinical question arises out of clinical work. Most of the questions involve treatment, diagnosis, or prognosis, but other areas may be subject to such questions as well. A well-formulated clinical question regarding therapy has four parts: (1) a description of the patient or problem, (2) a description of the proposed intervention, (3) a comparison intervention, and (4) a defined outcome of interest. For example, "In a dog with a solitary, resected, grade II mast cell tumor with microscopic residual disease but no disseminated disease (the patient/problem), is adjuvant radiotherapy (the intervention) better than a second surgery (the alternate intervention) in prolonging survival time (the outcome)?"

18. What is meant by "best current evidence"?

Strictly speaking, properly designed and conducted blind, randomized clinical trails provide the best evidence, but unfortunately these are difficult to come by in veterinary medicine. Although considered of lesser quality, evidence can also be gathered from un-randomized but well-designed clinical trials, from controlled experimental studies, from cohort or case-control studies, or from dramatic results in uncontrolled studies. At an even lower level of quality are the opinions of experts on the basis of experience, descriptive studies, findings in other species, or a pathophysiologic rationale.

19. Is it practical to apply EBM principles to veterinary oncologic cases?

Absolutely! Although the standard is high, it is well worth striving toward. In veterinary medicine, the field of oncology is rapidly changing, and there will be new answers to questions in many areas. Asking and answering well-formulated clinical questions, applying the new information to direct patient care, and reflecting on the entire process will benefit patients and enrich and enliven the practice of veterinary oncology. There are easily accessible and understandable texts available that further describe the process, and the reader is encouraged to pursue them.

BIBLIOGRAPHY

1. Bellair III JC, Mosteller F: Medical Uses of Statistics, 2nd ed. Boston, NEJM Books, 1992.
2. Meldrum ML: A brief history of the randomized controlled trial: From oranges and lemons to the gold standard. Hematol Oncol Clin North Am 14(1):745–760, 2000.
3. Meyerson LJ, Wiens BL, LaVange LM, et al: Quality control of oncology clinical trials. Hematol Oncol Clin North Am 14(1):953–972, 2000
4. Sackett DL, Straus SE, Richardson WS, et al: Evidence-Based Medicine: How to Practice and Teach EBM, 2nd ed. Edinburgh, Churchill Livingstone, 2000.
5. Schott S: Statistics for Health Professionals. Philadelphia, W.B. Saunders, 1990.
6. Rosenthal RC: Evidence-based medicine concepts. Proc ACVIM 18:348–350, 2000.
7. Woolf SH, George JN: Evidence-based medicine: Interpreting studies and setting policy. Hematol Oncol Clin North Am 14(1):761–784, 2000.

4. PSYCHOSOCIAL ISSUES

Barbara J. Norton, MSW, CSW-R, and Steven I. Cooper, MSW, CSW-R, BCD

1. Having been told their pet is seriously ill, what other things might owners need to hear from their veterinarian?

Owners will need both information and comfort. Thus, owners benefit by being given information such as details of the problem, prognosis, and proposed treatment. Additionally, a concerned and supportive demeanor by the veterinarian is helpful in this situation.

2. What kinds of reactions can you expect from an owner who was just told that his pet is very ill?

People react to loss in various ways. Common reactions include anger, disbelief or denial, shock, guilt, fear, and tearfulness. These responses are expected when a person is confronted with significant emotional stress.

3. What do you say to the person who reacts with anger?

It is important to not get angry yourself or at least not to show it. Speak in a rational, calm manner. Understand that anger expressed is often fear and sadness disguised. Speak to those emotions, and you will be of the most help. Sometimes angry owners may need to leave and return later.

4. What do you say to the person who responds with hysterical grief?

Keep a firm, compassionate tone. Make gentle, soothing comments that reflect your understanding. Give encouragement and, if able, assist in contacting supportive family and friends. Follow-up with a phone call to inquire about the owner's well-being can be very helpful.

5. What do you say to the person who reacts with denial?

One of the most difficult reactions to respond to is an owner's denial. Denial is a psychological defense mechanism. Denial occurs when a person's emotional well-being is threatened and he "blocks out" the upsetting information. For example, denial can be expressed when an owner appears to have stopped listening or, after having been given negative medical information about the pet, the owner responds by saying, "You're wrong, you're mistaken, and my animal is fine." Some helpful approaches you may consider include gently restating the information, offering to review it in a day or two when the denial may be less, and having a supportive family member present who is not in denial.

6. What are some considerations in regard to discussing the imminent death of an owner's beloved pet?

This discussion should be held in a private atmosphere. The more comfortable the surroundings are, the better. Avoid interruptions such as the telephone ringing or other staff demands. After receiving the news, some people may appreciate some time alone for reflection.

7. How can the veterinarian help an owner make end-of-life decisions as the pet's health begins to fail?

People need an honest, gentle description of their pet's condition. Following this, a complete review of treatment can set the stage for future decisions. Encouraging questions such as, "Was everything done that could be done?" can help the owner begin a normal grief process. If clinically appropriate, the subject of euthanasia can be introduced at this time.

8. After an owner decides to euthanize his pet, what do you say when he asks, "Should I be there?"

Most people know what they want to do before they ask this question. You can help them by supporting either option and asking questions that clarify their real feelings.

9. What advice can you give to parents to help them help their children who are grieving the loss of a pet?

Tell parents not to hide their own grief. Children need to know loss and grief are a natural part of life. It is advisable to let children say good-bye to a beloved pet, which sometimes means allowing them to view the dead body. Encourage rituals, memorial, and burials. Always be honest. Avoid phrases such as "put to sleep" or "gone away" when referring to the death. Don't be afraid of the words "killed" and "dead."

10. When asking about euthanasia, what do you tell an owner who asks, "Will my pet suffer?"

Reviewing the procedure beforehand enables pet owners to know what to expect. This can lead to a lessening of anxiety, which helps to alleviate some of the acute pain from the loss. Reassure the owner that euthanasia is a loving decision to relieve the pet's pain and suffering.

11. How do you help the owner who feels guilt over the decision to euthanize if it is, in part, due to money concerns?

Recognition of the owner's love and caring for the pet as primary reasons for choosing euthanasia should be expressed. It is helpful for the veterinarian to convey an understanding of the reality of finite resources for medical care in this day and age.

12. What do you tell a multiple pet owner who is concerned about how the other animals will react to the loss of a pet?

An owner might see increased vocalization, for example, excessive crying or whining; decreased appetite; pacing; "searching behaviors"; and sleeplessness.

13. What do you say to an owner who has questions about when to get another pet?

After the acute period of grief has eased, better consideration by owners can be given to getting another pet. There is no reason to preclude getting another pet soon after the death of one. There is much need for good homes for pets, and grieving pet owners have proven they can love an animal.

14. What can you do if you become concerned about an owner who is not coping well with the loss of a pet?

The owner may have unresolved feelings about the pet's death. This loss may elicit many different meanings for owners, depending on their own psychological makeup. Depression and anxiety are frequently preceded by significant losses. A referral to a counselor or therapist in such a case usually is appropriate.

15. What are some of the warning signs of burn-out among animal care professionals?

Irritability, anger, poor sleep, poor appetite, impatience, poor concentration, indifference, apathy, fatigue, substance abuse, and withdrawal.

16. What can you do if you or a colleague display symptoms of burn-out?

- Take advantage of vacation days.
- Encourage ventilation of feelings with supportive friends, family, and colleagues.
- Take quiet time alone for self-examination.
- Exercise.
- Remember that no one is perfect. Respect your own limits.
- Sometimes talking to a mental health professional can help.

17. How do children of different developmental stages think about death, and how can a veterinarian talk with them when they are facing the loss of a pet?

Children at different developmental stages have different capacities to understand death and react differently when it occurs.

Infants sense increased stress levels in their environment and can react by more frequent crying, whining, clinging, or withdrawing. They can be reassured by being held, rocked, and cuddled. It is important to them to keep routines at this time.

Toddlers are able to understand the loss of a pet is important, but they do not know death is a permanent condition. They should be encouraged to express their grief through positive vehicles such as artwork, play, and utilization of developing verbal skills by talking.

For **younger school-age children**, attachment to a pet and its subsequent loss becomes more real. They understand the permanency of loss. They may also blame themselves because they feel the world revolves around them and is in their control. It is very important to talk with children in this age group about the death of their pet and death in general.

Older school-age children know death is permanent. Their cognitive capacities are more developed, as is their ability to feel loss more intensely. Preoccupation with the morbid details of death is likely and normal. With this age group, frank answers about death will assist them to resolve their feelings. Involvement more directly in after-death arrangements can help them work through their feelings of grief more effectively.

Adolescents are developmentally practicing independence. In the zeal to be independent, they may feign indifference to the loss of a pet. It is easy to mistake this behavior for lack of grief on their part. Spending time, trying to share feelings, and answering questions when they are more amenable serves to help them through this difficult period.

18. Is it safe emotionally for a child to be present for his beloved pet's euthanasia?

This is an extremely difficult question to answer. This decision revolves around the parents' judgment with regard to their child's ability to tolerate the experience in a relatively constructive way. If a child lacks a certain maturity, the experience can become more traumatic and, thus, a destructive event. On the other hand, it can be a healing albeit agonizing moment leading to acceptance of the loss and a more profound understanding of death and life. If a decision is made to have the child present, a veterinarian can help prepare the child by:

- Meeting with the family beforehand to clarify what *exactly* will be happening step by step.
- Before beginning, allowing the child to say good-bye by spending time with the animal.
- After death, allowing the child to spend as much time as needed with the body.
- Encouraging some form of memorial or funeral ceremony.

19. How can an owner's responses change during their ailing pet's cancer treatment?

As cancer treatment proceeds, both the veterinarian and the owner are faced with changing degrees and qualities of uncertainty and anxiety. In the prediagnostic phase of cancer care, one does not know the nature of the problem. Anxieties are associated with fears that a serious condition exists, and owners have corresponding mental images of disability and suffering. Trying to encourage owners not to "think the worst" and assuring that you will work closely with them to obtain the needed information can be helpful. As the treatment enters the diagnostic phase, more information about the condition, treatment options, and prognosis is available. Owners will be confronted with anxieties and conflicts about their pet's pain level, cost versus benefits, treatment decisions, and informing their children. Owners should be given an informed, compassionate review of the options and support to reach the best decision. Uncertainties and fears can be validated and shared between the veterinarian and the owner. As treatment decisions have been made and the case moves into the therapeutic phase, owners will be hoping for good news, have "miracle" fantasies, and worry about adverse effects. Although frequent calls from owners to vets can be demanding, it would be important here to make good on your earlier promise to work together and to be able to provide ongoing dialogue about the pet's condition and progress. If possible, invite owners to visit their pet, and even offer them a few minutes of your time when they arrive. For pets that remit from their illness and go home with hopeful owners, the relapse phase of treatment can be particularly stressful and saddening. During the relapse stage of illness, any hopes or denied fantasies of miracle cures the owner had are badly threatened. Owners once again need to confront treatment and prognosis decisions, but they also imagine their pets are sadly slipping away from them toward death. Comfort around any hope for additional remissions can be helpful here. After the pet enters the phase of terminal care, issues around death and dying become relevant.

CONTROVERSY

20. Working with dying or injured animals; needing to participate in euthanasia; and interacting with bereft pet owners can create a "vicarious traumatization" in veterinary health care professionals. Does this phenomenon really exist?

Con: Vicarious traumatization does not really exist. Over time, veterinary health care professionals learn to cope with their situations and develop skills that serve in self-protective ways.

Pro: Vicarious traumatization exists but is often denied, leading sometimes to greater emotional problems, such as negativity, burn-out, indifference, and depression.

BIBLIOGRAPHY

1. Bowlby J: Attachment and Loss, Vol 1. New York, Basic Books, 1969.
2. Maeder T: Wounded healers. Atlantic Monthly 1:37–47, 1998.
3. Pearlman L, et al: Trauma and the Therapist: Countertransference and Vicarious Traumatization in Psychotherapy with Incest Survivors. New York, WW Norton and Company, 1995.
4. Stern M, Cropper S: Loving and Losing a Pet. New Jersey, Jason Aronson Inc, 1998.

5. HISTORY, PHYSICAL EXAMINATION, AND DIAGNOSTIC TESTING

Robert C. Rosenthal, DVM, PhD, Dipl ACVIM, Dipl ACVR

1. How does a clinician make a diagnosis?

There are several recognized ways of arriving at a diagnosis, which is simply the doctor's opinion of the best explanation of the patient's problems. Experienced clinicians usually arrive at a diagnosis through a hypothetical-deductive method.

2. In what other ways are diagnoses made?

Other methods of diagnosis include (*a*) exhaustion, (*b*) pattern recognition, and (*c*) algorithm. Exhaustion, considered the approach of the novice, involves asking every possible question and sifting through all the data for clues. Pattern recognition (also called "Aunt Minnie" or gestalt) is knowing the diagosis at first sight, from previous experience with the overall appearance of a patient with a given condition. Experienced clinicians also employ pattern recognition in diagnosis. Diagnosis by algorithm involves answering a series of inclusionary/exclusionary questions and has been considered a useful approach even by those with relatively limited training or experience (if the algorithm asks the right questions!).

3. Why are the history and physical examination called "the pillars of diagnosis"?

Despite the plethora of tests available to support a clinician's diagnosis or to rule out diagnostic possibilities, it remains true that most clinical presentations are "solved" by simply listening to what the owner says about the patient and performing a good physical examination.

4. What questions are included in the complete medical history? What specific questions should be asked in taking a history of a cancer patient?

There is no such thing as "*the* complete medical history." Each patient's history is unique, and there is no way that all the information on any patient could be compiled. It is always important, however, to ask at least a few basic questions of all owners and to follow with questions germane to the presentation at hand (although these, too, will vary from patient to patient).

5. What are the most important questions about a patient's history?

It is most important to establish why the owner has brought the patient for examination. The initial encapsulation of the patient's problem often discloses critical information for the clinician. Simply asking, "Why did you bring Tillie in today?" will provide a good deal of information. Other important questions include inquiries about general attitude, diet and appetite, water consumption, and patterns of urination and defecation.

6. Do all questions serve the same purpose?

No. In fact, clinicians ask different types of questions as the history-taking process continues depending on their understanding of the case at any time. *Searching* questions are asked to support, strengthen, or rule out hypotheses. *Scanning* questions are broader in scope and are asked to expose new clues or explore new leads.

7. What is the best approach to the physical examination of a cancer patient?

Every pet presented for reasons of illness (or even for routine wellness examination and vaccination) deserves a complete physical examination. There are several approaches to physical examination. Some clinicians prefer to examine patients on a regional basis; others prefer a systems approach. There is no absolute right or wrong approach. In all instances, however, the clinician should establish and follow a pattern that assures completeness.

8. What is meant by the dictum "work toward the obvious"?

Although it is important to have a consistent pattern of examination, it is perhaps even more important not to miss potentially critical findings by being distracted by the outstanding clinical sign. Thus, the clinician should reserve the detailed examination of the system seemingly involved in the presenting complaint for last.

9. Why do some clinicians always perform thoracic (cardiac and pulmonary) auscultation as the final part of the physical examination?

Although experienced clinicians usually have arrived at a tentative (working) diagnosis or have a short differential list, treatment plan, or diagnostic plan in mind early in the clinical encounter, it is useful near the end of the physical examination to take some time to think about the findings and to organize the impending discussion with the owner. Because putting on a stethoscope is a powerful nonverbal signal that quiet is in order (so the doctor can hear), the clinician has the opportunity not to be distracted by an owner's comments or questions.

10. What is the minimal database for a cancer patient?

The expression "the minimal data base" is a misnomer. No single database is appropriate for all patients, even for all cancer patients. A minimal database is problem-defined and will, therefore, vary from patient to patient. With some fairly simple reasoning, however, the clinician can certainly rationalize the need for the inclusion of at least a complete blood count, profile biochemical screen, and urinalysis for almost any sick patient. These tests provide a wealth of important information. Beyond those, diagnostic tests are selected based on such factors as the signalment, prior medical history, current history, and putative diagnosis.

11. How is a definitive diagnosis made?

In oncologic practice, the gold standard of diagnosis is histopathologic evaluation of appropriate biopsy material. Advanced imaging and cytology, in addition to routine laboratory tests, radiographs, and selected specific tests depending on the presentation, are helpful and should be employed where appropriate.

12. What is the most common diagnostic oversight that veterinarians make?

The single test that veterinarians seem most often to overlook is the urinalysis. Urinalysis is simply performed in the clinic and provides important information for almost every case. Whole volumes have been written about it, and it should not be left out of any thorough diagnostic workup.

6. CYTOLOGIC EVALUATION OF NEOPLASIA

Karen E. Dorsey, DVM, Rick L. Cowell, DVM, Dipl ACVP,
and Stacy B. Smith, DVM

1. Why do a fine-needle aspiration biopsy?

A fine-needle aspiration biopsy (FNAB) is an easy procedure that can be performed on an outpatient basis. The primary utility of FNAB is to differentiate inflammation from neoplasia. As such, it is very useful in the assessment of suspected cancer patients. Anesthesia is generally not required. Special equipment is not needed, and an answer can be given while the client waits. The question should not be why do an FNAB, but why not?

2. How do I perform an FNAB?

Most organs and masses can be aspirated if they can be isolated and immobilized. Ultrasound is often used for aspirates of internal organs. An FNAB of an external mass will be described here. Materials needed are a 22-gauge needle, 6- to 12-ml syringe, and glass slides. The mass is stabilized with one hand while the needle with the syringe attached is then placed into the mass. For the aspiration technique, the plunger is pulled back multiple times, allowing negative pressure to pull cells from the lesion into the needle. The negative pressure is released, and the needle is removed from the mass. The needle is then detached from the syringe. Air is placed into the syringe, and the needle is reattached. The air is then used to expel the cells in the needle onto a glass slide. Multiple aspirates should be attempted from different sites in the lesion.

3. What is the nonaspiration technique?

Unlike the aspiration technique that uses negative pressure to remove cells from a lesion, the nonaspiration technique uses a stabbing method to remove cells and creates a cell-blood slurry that is collected in the bore of the needle. The same materials are used for this technique as for an aspiration technique. Prior to placing the needle in the lesion or mass, however, the syringe is filled with air. The mass is then stabilized, and the needle (which is attached to the syringe) is placed into the lesion. The needle is then quickly pulled back and reinserted along the same plane several times without leaving the mass (e.g., a rapid stabbing motion). The air in the syringe is used to expel the cells in the needle onto a glass slide. Because only one site is sampled with each collection, the mass must be sampled multiple times at multiple sites.

4. What are ways I can use to smear the sample?

After cells are collected and placed on a glass slide, various methods can be employed to spread the cells. Most of these methods use a spreader slide, which is a second glass slide used to smear the cells. In the squash prep method, the spreader slide is placed gently onto the sample and at a right angle to the sample slide. Downward pressure should not be applied to the spreader slide. The spreader slide is then pushed smoothly along the sample slide. Similar to pushing the spreader slide, it can also be twisted or turned, causing the sample to be smeared. The blood smear technique is another method that uses a spreader slide. The spreader slide is placed at a 30-degree angle to the sample slide. It is then moved over the sample, allowing the sample to be spread by capillary action along its width. The spreader slide is then pushed along the length of the sample slide. Other methods are available, and any method that adequately spreads the sample without causing excessive cell rupturing is adequate. Without proper spreading, most samples are too thick and, thus, not diagnostic. After smearing, the sample is allowed to air-dry.

5. When should I make a line smear?

Line smears are best made with fluid samples of low to moderate cell counts. A line smear is another technique that uses a spreader slide, and the blood smear technique is used. Instead of taking the spreader slide the entire length of the sample slide, it is removed and pulled straight up from the sample slide approximately halfway down the length of the sample slide. This allows the cells to be concentrated at that point.

6. How do I prevent excessive cell rupture?

Excessive cell rupture is a common problem in cytology that can be generally avoided with proper sample collection technique. Some cells are very fragile (e.g., lymphoblasts) and will rupture if not handled gently. Several points in slide preparation should be considered if excessive cellular rupture is a problem. First is the technique employed. The aspiration technique generates negative pressure, and even this small amount of pressure—especially if larger syringes are used—can lead to cell rupturing. The nonaspiration, or stabbing, technique can be used if this is a concern. The second potential problem can come when creating the smear. When using the spreader slide, no downward pressure should be applied to the sample slide. The spreader slide should be gently placed onto the sample slide. Even a minimal amount of downward pressure can rupture cells. To lessen the chance of rupturing cells, a cover slip may be used as a spreader.

7. What can lead to lack of an adequate sample?

Several problems can occur that lead to a lack of an adequate sample. Isolation of the lesion is essential in preventing this problem. Because obesity is a major problem in small animal practice today, the lesion or mass may be hard to isolate because of excessive fat. Multiple collections from the lesion will decrease the chance of a sample being nondiagnostic. A diagnosis is more likely to be achieved when viewing multiple smears. Less aggressive attempts at collecting the sample can lead to a low number of cells being present. Adequate aspirations or adequate stabbing is needed to collect any sample. Some masses, especially mesenchymal tumors, do not exfoliate cells well. In this event, biopsy with histopathology would need to be performed. Excessive blood can also be a problem, leading to hemodilution of the sample. If blood is seen in the hub of the needle when performing an FNAB, negative pressure should be immediately released, the needle withdrawn, and smears made. Continued aspiration in that site will only result in more blood being collected and further dilution of the sample. Another site on the lesion should then be aspirated or another collection technique employed. Some masses, however, will have excessive blood regardless of the technique used.

8. Which stains should I use?

After air-drying, the smears are ready for staining. Many products are available for staining, and most are Wright's-type stains. Wright's stain gives adequate nuclear detail and stains the cytoplasm well. Diff-Quik and DipStat are commercially available stains that can be used for both hematology and cytology. Both of these stains are easy to use and are very adaptable to the thickness of the sample. For instance, a longer staining time is needed for thicker samples than for samples of low cellularity. Limitations are seen with Diff-Quik: It does not stain polychromasia well when used on blood smears, and it will intermittently not stain mast cell granules. However, this is a quick and easy-to-use stain that works well in most situations.

9. Cytologically, what are the differences between cell types?

When viewing a smear, certain questions need to be asked, such as what is the cell distribution or pattern, and what are the cells that are present? In cytology, neoplasias are divided into three main groups or types: (1) epithelial, (2) mesenchymal, and (3) round or discrete cell tumors. Each of these tumor types has a different cell distribution and cytologic appearance. Epithelial tumors tend to exfoliate in clusters or groups and typically consist of fairly large cells, whereas round cell tumors are small individual cells. Both of these tumor types have cells with distinct cytoplasmic borders. Mesenchymal tumors fall in-between epithelial and round cell tumors in cell size. The characteristic feature of mesenchymal (connective tissue) tumors is their spindle appearance and indistinct cytoplasmic borders. Sometimes, cell type cannot be determined. When this is the case, the smears should be sent to an experienced clinical pathologist or cytologist for examination. When determination of the cell type is made, criteria of malignancy need to be evaluated.

10. What are the criteria of malignancy, and why are they important?

Criteria of malignancy are cellular changes that are seen in malignant neoplasms. These changes can be broken into two groups: general cellular changes and nuclear changes. Nuclear changes are more specific for malignant neoplasia. In most cells, at least three of the nuclear changes need to be present to classify a tumor as malignant. Criteria of malignancy apply mostly to epithelial and mesenchymal tumors. Round cell tumors are generally determined by the presence of a certain cell type, which will be discussed later. Nuclear criteria of malignancy include anisokaryosis, macrokaryosis, multinucleation, abnormal mitotic figures, macronucleoli, angular or other bizarre shaped nucleoli, increased nuclear-to-cytoplasmic ratio, a course chromatic pattern, and nuclear molding. General cellular changes include anisocytosis, macrocytosis, and cellular pleomorphism (Fig. 1).

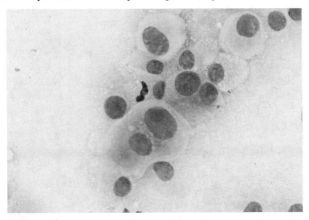

FIGURE 1.   Transitional cell carcinoma. Epithelial cells show marked criteria of malignancy, including anisocytosis, anisokaryosis, macronucleoli, and multinucleation. (Wright's-Giemsa stain, original magnification 500×.)

11. What is dysplasia?

Dysplasia is abnormal or disorderly proliferation of cells secondary to inflammation or irritation. Dysplasia is seen in both epithelial and mesenchymal cells. Differentiation between malignant and dysplastic changes can be difficult. If uncertainty exists when viewing a smear, several options can be considered. Removal of the irritant or treatment of the inflammatory process can be tried with reaspiration at a later date. Another course of action would be to biopsy the lesion for histopathologic review.

12. Why is granulation tissue so difficult to differentiate from a spindle cell tumor?

Granulation tissue is a histopathologic diagnosis based on tissue architecture. The evaluation of architecture is impossible by cytology alone. With cytology, granulation tissue is seen in the face of chronic inflammation. With inflammation, fibroblasts, which are stromal cells, will infiltrate the area. These fibroblasts are reactive and appear anaplastic. Anaplastic changes are difficult to discern from neoplastic changes that are seen with sarcomas.

13. What are the round cell tumors?

Generally, five types of round or discrete cell tumors are recognized: lymphosarcoma, mast cell tumor, plasmacytoma, histiocytoma, and transmissible venereal tumor. The cell population determines the type of round or discrete cell tumor. Occasionally other tumors, like melanoma, can appear as round or discrete cell tumors.

14. How do I determine if this lesion is lymphosarcoma?

Lymphosarcoma is seen in small animals in peripheral lymph nodes, visceral organs, cranial mediastinum, bone marrow, and skin. Both lymphoblastic and lymphocytic lymphosarcoma occur in small animals, with the lymphoblastic form being by far the most common type. As the name implies, lymphoblastic lymphosarcoma is composed primarily of lymphoblasts (more than 50% of the cells present). Lymphoblasts are round, discrete cells, which are larger than a peripheral blood neutrophil. Their nucleus has a stippled chromatin pattern and is round to irregular with the presence of a single or multiple nucleoli (Fig. 2). Lymphoblasts also have a high nuclear-to-cytoplasmic ratio and a medium blue cytoplasm that is usually pushed to one side. A feature consistent with all lymphoid tissue is the presence of lymphoglandular bodies. Lymphoglandular bodies are small cytoplasmic fragments that will be scattered throughout the background of the smear. Seeing these bodies will help differentiate a tumor of lymphoid origin from other round cell tumors. Frequently, lymphocytic lymphosarcoma cannot be differentiated from normal lymphoid proliferation or hyperplasia cytologically. Histopathology is needed to definitively diagnose lymphocytic lymphosarcoma.

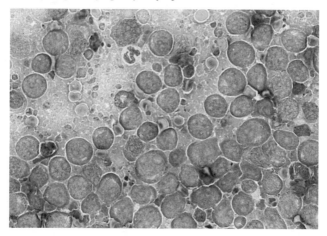

FIGURE 2.   Lymphosarcoma. Numerous lymphoblasts are present and appear as round, medium-sized cells (larger than peripheral blood neutrophils), with irregular shaped nuclei and multiple nucleoli. Lymphoglandular bodies and a few red blood cells are present in the background. (Wright's-Giemsa stain, courtesy Dr. J. Meinkoth, Department of Pathology, Oklahoma State University.)

15. What does a mast cell tumor look like?

Mast cell tumors can be easily diagnosed cytologically. Mast cells are round cells with a round to ovoid nucleus and red-purple intracytoplasmic granules. Because mast cell granules have a high affinity for the stain, the nucleus may have a light basophilic color and be partially obscured from view in the presence of heavy granulation. During slide preparation, some mast cells rupture, spilling their granules into the background of the smear. A diagnosis of mast cell tumor can be challenging with poorly differentiated mast cell tumors and tumors stained with Diff-Quik. With Diff-Quik, mast cell granules stain poorly, and poorly differentiated mast cell tumors have few granules. However, these tumors usually contain cells with sufficient numbers of granules along with the presence of eosinophils to allow for a cytologic diagnosis.

16. What cytologic appearance differentiates plasmacytoma and histiocytoma?

Histiocytoma is a round or discrete cell tumor composed of histiocytes or macrophages. These cells have round to indented large nuclei with finely granular chromatin and a moderate amount of pale blue cytoplasm. Small nucleoli are seen in the nucleus, with multiple nucleoli sometimes being present. The cytoplasm may be difficult to discern when the background is clear. Commonly, histiocytomas appear as button size, raised skin tumors on dogs. Spontaneous regression of these tumors is common. Plasmacytomas are derived from plasma cells. These tumors are characterized by the presence of plasmablasts, which appear as discrete round cells. Their nucleus has a coarse, clumped chromatin pattern, with dark blue cytoplasm generally pushed to one side. A perinuclear clear zone (Golgi area) is sometimes seen. Multinucleated cells are common with plasmacytomas. The lack of lymphoglandular bodies helps differentiate these tumors from lymphoid tumors.

17. What is TVT?

Transmissible venereal tumors (TVT) are round raised tumors that occur in the genitalia of both female and male dogs. They can occur on the face, which is a less common location. TVT is a discrete or round cell tumor. These cells have large round nuclei, with a coarse clumped chromatin pattern and distinctive nucleoli. Multiple nucleoli are sometimes present. A distinguishing feature of TVT is the presence of small vacuoles scattered throughout the cytoplasm. Location of this tumor and cytologic appearance will help diffentiate TVT from other round cell tumor types.

18. What do spindle cell tumors look like cytologically?

Spindle cell tumors are composed of mesenchymal cells (connective tissue cells) and can occur anywhere in the body. Most spindle cell tumors have similar cytologic characteristics, with a few exceptions that will be discussed under specific questions. Mesenchymal cells are medium-sized cells that characteristically have round to ovoid nuclei. Their cytoplasm has indistinct borders, which stream in one or two directions. Criteria of malignancy that are generally present include mild to moderate anisokaryosis, coarse nuclear chromatin, and single to multiple prominent, often bizarre shaped, nucleoli. The cytoplasm may become less fusiform as malignant potential increases, yet it still retains its indistinct borders. Spindle cells can be seen in many samples. In the presence of inflammation, spindle cells will undergo dysplastic change, which is termed fibroplasia. Differentiation between a sarcoma and fibroplasia can be difficult. If the smear is predominantly spindle cells without inflammation, the malignant potential of the sample needs to be determined. It is helpful to remember that most spindle cell tumors with malignant biologic behavior are more common than their benign counterparts.

19. What is the difference cytologically between osteosarcoma and chondrosarcoma?

Cytologically, osteosarcoma (OSA) and chondrosarcoma (CSA) are almost indistinguishable, making histopathology necessary to determine the difference between the two. Often, aspirates from an OSA have good cellularity, with cells that are characteristic of a neoplastic process. Osteoblasts are the primary cell present in OSA. These cells are of medium size, with a flag or flame shape and an eccentrically displaced nucleus that appears almost extracellular. The nucleus also has coarse chromatin, and distinct nucleoli are often present. The cytoplasm is pale blue. Osteoclasts are also seen in aspirates from bony lesions. Osteoclasts are multinucleated cells that contain 6 to 12 separate nuclei in an abundant amount of dark blue cytoplasm (Fig. 3, see top of next page). An intracellular eosinophilic matrix is sometimes present with OSA or CSA. This matrix is considered osteoid or chondroid, respectively, and is an inconsistent finding. Adequate criteria of malignancy need to be present for a diagnosis of neoplasia.

20. Is this lesion a malignant fibrous histiocytoma?

Malignant fibrous histiocytoma, also called giant cell tumor of soft parts, is seen in cats. The tumor is of mesenchymal cell origin and is composed of neoplastic spindle cells, multinucleated

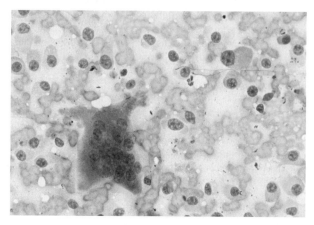

FIGURE 3.   Osteosarcoma. Numerous osteoblasts are present, which are medium-sized cells with eccentrically placed nuclei. Many have multiple nucleoli. A multinucleated osteoclast with abundant basophilic cytoplasm is also visible. Criteria of malignancy are present. (Wright's-Giemsa stain, original magnification 125×, courtesy Dr. J. Meinkoth, Department of Pathology, Oklahoma State University.)

giant cells, and histiocytes. The spindle cells will show consistent criteria of malignancy. The multinucleated giant cells have multiple separate nuclei, with distinct nucleoli, in an abundant amount of basophilic cytoplasm. These cells are similar in appearance to osteoclasts. The histiocytes appear as discrete round cells typical of macrophages and are an inconsistent finding. This admixture of cells is needed for a cytologic diagnosis of malignant fibrous histiocytoma.

21. What are the characteristic findings for a lipoma?

Adipocytes are the predominant cell type in aspirates from lipomas. Several features of the aspirate will help lead to a diagnosis of a lipoma. Adipocytes when expressed onto a slide will appear as an accumulation of fat or grease. After being smeared, the slide will not dry. Often, adipocytes are present in clusters or sheets. They are large cells with small eccentrically displaced pyknotic nuclei, with cytoplasm full of nonstaining fat (Fig. 4). Lipid droplets may be present and appear as circular clear areas in a stained background. Red blood cells and a few white blood cells are generally also observed. Aspirated subcutaneous fat has the same cytologic appearance as a lipoma. Therefore, when making a diagnosis of lipoma, one should be sure the needle is in the lesion and that the lesion was not missed during sampling.

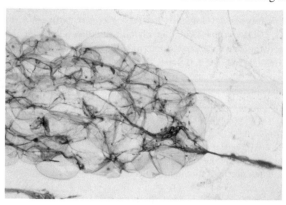

FIGURE 4.   Lipoma. The adipocytes shown have small pyknotic nuclei and cytoplasm full of nonstaining fat. (Wright's-Giemsa stain, original magnification 100×.)

22. Why are so few cells seen on lipoma preparations?

Free fat will not stain with common Wright's stains. Many adipocytes are ruptured during aspiration and smearing. As a result, free fat is left and is dissolved by the alcohol component in the staining process. When this occurs, clear spaces representing dissolved lipid droplets are left and can be identified in the background of the slide.

23. What do carcinomas look like cytologically?

Carcinomas are malignant tumors of epithelial origin. Cytologically, these tumors exfoliate in sheets or groups. Some individual cells are scattered throughout the slide. These are large to very large cells with round to oval nuclei. The nuclear chromatin becomes more coarse and ropey as the malignant potential rises. Most cells will have a prominent round nucleolus that increases in size and changes in shape with the degree of malignancy. Other neoplastic characteristics include anisokaryosis, nuclear molding, perinuclear vacuolization, deep basophilic cytoplasm, and giant cells.

24. What is the cytologic appearance of squamous cell carcinoma?

Squamous cell carcinomas (SCC) are usually ulcerated tumors that can occur on the skin of dogs and cats. Because ulceration is common, imprints and superficial scrapings tend to collect inflammatory cells. This can be avoided by deep aspirations of the lesion. Like other carcinomas, these cells tend to occur in sheets or clumps. Undifferentiated SCC cells are large with easily identifiable criteria of malignancy, unlike well-differentiated SCC, which has less visible criteria of malignancy. Asynchronous maturation of the cytoplasm and nucleus is seen commonly with SCC. This neoplastic change is seen cytologically as a large angular lightly basophilic cytoplasm, which is consistent with mature squamous cells, and a very large nucleus, which is an abnormal finding in mature squamous cells.

25. How do I determine if this lesion is a melanoma?

Melanomas can appear as epithelial, mesenchymal, or discrete or round cell tumors. They have a higher malignant potential when found on the feet or face of domestic animals. Aspirates from these locations tend to have cells that are usually less pigmented. Melanin appears as an intracytoplasmic black-green pigment. In heavily pigmented melanocytes, nuclear detail can be obscured, making an evaluation of malignant criteria difficult. In poorly pigmented melanocytes, melanin granules can appear as a light dusting of the cytoplasm, making cell identification challenging. Malignant criteria include a lightly basophilic cytoplasm with an increase in nuclear-to-cytoplasmic ratio. The nucleus is round to ovoid and contains a large nucleolus (Fig. 5). Normal melanocytes can occur in pigmented skin. These normal melanocytes should not be confused with malignant melanoma, which requires distinct criteria of malignancy to be diagnosed.

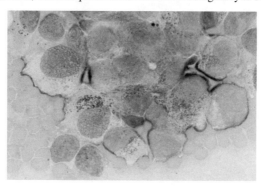

FIGURE 5. Malignant melanoma. Melanocytes have blue-black melanin granules and show marked criteria of malignancy. (Wright's-Giemsa stain, original magnification 330×, courtesy Dr. J. Meinkoth, Department of Pathology, Oklahoma State University.)

BIBLIOGRAPHY

1. Baker R, Lumsden JH: Color Atlas of Cytology of the Dog and Cat. St. Louis, Mosby, 2000.
2. Cowell RL, Tyler RD, Meinkoth JH: Diagnostic Cytology and Hematology of the Dog and Cat, 2nd ed. St. Louis, Mosby, 1999.

7. ROLE OF THE PATHOLOGIST IN VETERINARY ONCOLOGY

Peter H. Rowland, DVM, *Dipl* ACVP

OVERVIEW

1. What information can I expect to gain from submitting tissue for histopathologic examination?

Tissue evaluation is performed in oncology cases to determine if neoplasia is present and, if possible, to identify the histogenesis (cell of origin). A differentiation is made between benign and malignant conditions and, with some types of neoplasms, a histologic grade may be assigned to help with prognosis and therapy. Depending on the type of sample, surgical margins may also be examined, and the extent of infiltration and completeness of excision may be determined.

2. How do I decide whether the removed tissue warrants the extra expense of a biopsy evaluation?

The bottom line is that there really is no decision to make. The safest rule of thumb to follow is that any mass that is worth removing is worth submitting for evaluation. In some cases, the clinical history and gross appearance may be characteristic of a particular condition, but there are always a few cases that have atypical disease that may mimic a more common lesion. An improper gross diagnosis in these cases may have serious consequences for the patient, and it is always safer to confirm the diagnosis histologically.

3. Can I just hold onto some fixed tissue for submission in the event the incision does not heal well or there are other suspicious complications?

In many cases, the delay until a recurrence or other complication is identified may make definitive treatment more difficult than if a diagnosis was established at the time of the initial surgery. Some neoplasms may also warrant adjunct therapy that would be delayed if a biopsy sample was not initially submitted.

4. What can I do to aid the pathologist in the interpretation of my samples?

The quality of the sample is most important. In addition, supplying sufficient clinical history and gross lesion description can be of utmost importance. To avoid potential errors, it is also important to label all submitted containers so they may be identified even if separated from the accession form.

5. What information should be supplied to the pathologist?

This depends on the clinical presentation and the sample submitted. Minimal data to supply include complete signalment, location of lesion, gross description, duration and rate of growth, and any past history of neoplastic disease. With bone lesions, the radiographic appearance is particularly important. Depending on the clinical differential diagnosis and location of the lesion, other clinical or laboratory data may also be useful (such as complete blood count results with suspected lymphoid or hematopoietic neoplasia).

6. What is done with the submitted tissue?

Tissue processing involves a dehydration procedure and infiltration by paraffin wax to allow thin sections to be made using a microtome. These sections are adhered to glass slides and can then be stained with a variety of histochemical stains, and the remaining tissue can be stored indefinitely in the paraffin block. Additional sections can be cut from the block at any time if needed for second opinions, special stains, or other procedures. The processing is usually performed by an automated processor that is run overnight, and prepared slides may be ready to examine in about 24 hours.

SAMPLING

7. What are the sampling options that can be used for the identification of a potential neoplasm?

You first have a basic choice between excisional biopsy (removal of an entire mass, usually with the intent to cure) or removal of a small sample for identification purposes. Small samples can be removed with biopsy instruments or may be taken through a small incision (incisional biopsy). Biopsy instruments include needle biopsy instruments, punch biopsy instruments, trephines, and endoscopic biopsy instruments.

8. When should a small biopsy be taken for tumor identification prior to mass removal?

There are several reasons a biopsy may be indicated prior to an attempt at complete excision. In some cases the type and grade of neoplasm may alter the extent of resection required (wide versus narrow margins). The neoplasm may also be in a location that requires more involved surgery, such as exploratory or amputation, and it may be important to establish the prognosis prior to an attempt at curative resection. There may also be cases where knowledge of type of neoplasia may alter the therapy, such as cases where chemotherapy or radiation are used instead of surgical excision.

9. Are there disadvantages to needle biopsies?

In general, the smaller the sample, the greater the chance that a definitive diagnosis may not be made. More common potential complications include the following:
- Necrosis or hemorrhage within a mass may make a small sample nondiagnostic.
- Small samples often only allow evaluation of cellular features, without an overview of the tissue organization or the architecture of the organ involved, and important criteria, such as peripheral tissue invasion, cannot be evaluated.
- Some neoplasms, such as soft tissue sarcomas, may have extensive variation of morphology within the mass, and small samples may not include the least differentiated areas, possibly causing an incorrect grade to be applied.
- Small samples may also have compression artifact if tissue is fragile, and this may obscure morphology.

Some of the disadvantages can be minimized by taking multiple biopsies.

10. Is an incisional wedge sample preferable?

Small, superficial wedge samples may also be nondiagnostic because many neoplasms, particularly if they are partially necrotic, have a peripheral margin of reactive tissue or inflammation. It is important to sample tissue deep to this peripheral reaction.

11. What are advantages of mucosal biopsies obtained during endoscopy, rhinoscopy, bronchoscopy, or cystoscopy?

These instruments generally sample very superficial tissue. In some cases they provide a definitive diagnosis but, if the mass is deep to the mucosa or if there is associated ulceration and granulation, samples may not contain diagnostic tissue. Compression artifact is also very common, and it may obscure cellular morphology.

12. What size biopsy is too small?

In general, if the largest dimension of a small sample is less than 1 mm, it will be difficult or impossible to process, embed, and section.

13. Is electrocautery OK for sampling tissue?

Electrocautery results in extensive tissue artifact and should generally be avoided. With small samples, this artifact may extend through the entire sample and may make the sample useless. In larger samples, the artifact may be restricted to margins, but this can prevent adequate evaluation of surgical borders and degree of invasion.

14. Bone seems to be particularly problematic. How can I obtain diagnostic biopsies?

Most bone sarcomas are central and have peripheral reactive bone. The reactive bone can plug the biopsy instrument and prevent the deeper, softer tissue from being sampled, even when it is penetrated. To avoid this, the peripheral reaction and areas of lysis may be identified radiographically, and the depth to penetration into the lytic area can be measured. After initial penetration to this approximate depth, any peripheral hard tissue can be emptied from the biopsy instrument and measured, and then the instrument can be reintroduced through the same hole to allow sampling of deeper soft tissue in the area of lysis. With larger lesions, this procedure can be repeated in a few different sites to have the best chance of sampling the primary, underlying lesion.

FIXATION

15. What is fixation?

Fixation performs a few crucial functions, including prevention of postmortem self-digestion (autolysis) of cells, coagulation of cellular components so they will be insoluble for processing and so they will be protected against shrinkage, improved differentiation of cellular components, and improved staining quality.

16. What is the most appropriate fixative?

For routine histopathology, 10% neutral buffered formalin is the most frequently used fixative because it has good penetration, does not dissolve lipids, and allows a variety of post-fixation treatments.

17. Is formalin used for all tissues?

The answer depends on the preference of the pathologist. Some individuals prefer other fixatives, particularly Bouin's fixative, for fixation of the retina or endometrial biopsies, but formalin is a good choice for the fixation of any tissue unless specifically instructed otherwise by your laboratory. Some laboratories have switched to formalin substitutes, but those laboratories will usually supply this.

18. Can formalin be used when immunohistochemistry or immunofluorescence are planned?

Formalin fixation may result in the alteration of some antigens and may decrease or eliminate staining with individual antibodies used in immunostaining. Others work quite well with paraffin-embedded, formalin-fixed tissue samples. Depending on the individual markers and techniques being considered, a different fixative may be required or fresh tissue may need to be submitted for frozen sections. It is best to contact your laboratory to be sure. Even for antibodies that work with formalin-fixed tissue, prolonged fixation should be avoided if immunohistochemical staining is anticipated. Immunofluorescence often works best on frozen sections, and either fresh tissue or tissue immersed in transport solutions are needed (again, the laboratory should be contacted prior to sampling).

19. What volume of fixative should be used?

Classically, a 10:1 ratio of fixative to tissue volume is recommended. Adequate fixation is often achieved with a lower ratio, but stuffing a specimen bottle with a sample that displaces much of the formalin will guarantee poor fixation.

20. How can I fix those huge, hemorrhagic splenic masses?

No matter what volume of formalin is used, penetration is restricted to 1 to 2 cm in most tissues. As a result, masses that are more than 2 to 3 cm in diameter require sectioning prior to immersion in the fixative. Very large splenic masses most often have extensive hemorrhage, and it can be very difficult to identify any underlying neoplasia. In general, with a large, hemorrhagic mass, the following procedure is advised to evaluate for neoplastic tissue:

1. "Bread slice" the large mass perpendicular to the interface with the remaining spleen at 2-cm intervals.

2. Examine the cut margins for areas that appear microcystic or more solid (vs the jelly-like consistency of a blood clot). Sample any suspicious areas.

3. If no suspicious tissue is identified, take two or three 1.5-cm–thick slice sections in different areas perpendicular to the splenic interface, including a small amount of splenic tissue along with the mass. This interface is most likely to have viable neoplastic tissue.

21. How do I handle fixation of other large lesions?

As mentioned above, penetration by the fixative is limited, and these larger masses should be sectioned prior to fixation. The surgeon should note the most worrisome surgical border(s). Slab sections 1.5 cm thick can be taken perpendicular to the border of the mass that includes the narrowest lateral and deep margin(s). This allows examination for invasion as well as determination of completeness of excision. Masses that are small enough to submit whole may still require partial sectioning to allow adequate penetration. Partial-thickness slices can be made at 1.5-cm intervals with retention of an intact deep surgical margin. Larger tissue samples that require a large volume of formalin may be fixed on site in a larger container for 48 hours and then transferred to a smaller container (with a 1:1 ratio of fixative to tissue) for transport.

22. Should the surgical margins be marked, and how is this done?

With smaller masses that can be submitted intact, the surgical margins may be readily apparent, and marking may not be necessary. The same is often true of slab sections from larger masses that have easily recognizable borders. When borders are not easily recognized, there are particularly worrisome borders, or there has been separation of marginal tissue during removal, these borders can be marked with suture material or with india ink. Sets of multiple inks of various colors are also helpful in identifying margins.

23. How long must tissue be immersed in fixative prior to processing?

When using formalin, it should be realized that penetration is relatively rapid, but fixation is progressive and optimal fixation occurs in 24 to 48 hours. The time varies with different tissues, and very small samples may be successfully processed sooner, but 24 hours is generally considered a minimum period for fixation. With today's same-day and next-morning deliveries, some tissues must be held for additional fixation at the laboratory prior to processing.

24. How long can tissues remain in the fixative before processing?

Indefinite fixation in formalin is not a problem unless immunohistochemistry is planned. As previously mentioned, tissue that remains in formalin for weeks or more may lose some staining when using immunohistochemical techniques. When using other fixatives, the maximum time of fixation varies. With Bouin's fixative, for example, months of fixation will result in poor nuclear staining.

25. Does bone require a special fixative?

No, neutral buffered formalin is a good fixative for bone. The processing of bone may be delayed because the tissue must be decalcified prior to sectioning.

26. How should small-needle and mucosal biopsies be fixed?

Needle biopsies may be carefully teased from the instrument directly into the biopsy container. Mucosal biopsies can be adhered to sections of tongue depressor. They may be dislodged during or after immersion, but this is not a problem. It is **not** advised to place these unfixed samples between sponge pads in plastic cassettes because compression artifact results. Tissue and lens papers become very soft in the fixative, and it is not advised to adhere samples to these materials because it may be difficult to separate small, friable samples from the wet paper.

27. What are the most common causes of fixation artifact?

Poor fixation and artifact are commonly related to the following factors:

1. Attempting to fix too large a sample without sectioning
2. Compression of tissue prior to immersion in fixative
3. Delayed fixation, allowing drying or autolysis
4. Cautery artifact, particularly in smaller samples
5. Freezing of tissue when left out for pick-up in cold weather.

TERMINOLOGY AND THE BIOPSY REPORT

28. If hyperplasia can cause a swelling or enlargement, how is hyperplasia differentiated from neoplasia?

Neoplasia involves a loss of control of cellular proliferation and, in neoplastic lesions, there is often disorganization of cells and compression or destruction of adjacent tissue that are not seen with hyperplasia (in which there is proliferation but still under normal control mechanisms). There may also be abnormal cellular morphology in a neoplasm that is more pronounced than seen in cases of hyperplasia. The differentiation between hyperplasia and benign neoplasms that have minimal cellular atypia can be difficult, but common differentiating features are listed below.

Comparison between Morphology of Non-neoplastic Cellular Proliferation, Benign Neoplasia, and Malignant Neoplasia

MORPHOLOGIC FEATURE	HYPERPLASIA	METAPLASIA	DYSPLASIA	BENIGN NEOPLASIA	MALIGNANT NEOPLASIA
Cellular organization	Retained	Retained	Lost	Lost	Lost
Cellular differentiation	Normal	Normal	Mild atypia	Mild atypia	Moderate to marked atypia
Tissue types appropriate for location?	Yes	No	Yes	Yes	Yes, if primary neoplasia
Mitotic index	Low to medium	Low	Low to medium	Low to medium	Medium to high
Atypical mitoses	None	None	None	None	Often present
Pleomorphism (cell, nuclear variation)	None to mild	None to mild	Mild to moderate	Mild to moderate	Moderate to severe
Nuclear and nucleolar enlargement	Mild	Minimal	Mild to moderate	Mild to moderate	Moderate to severe

(Table continued on next page.)

Comparison between Morphology of Non-neoplastic Cellular Proliferation, Benign
Neoplasia, and Malignant Neoplasia (Cont.)

MORPHOLOGIC FEATURE	HYPERPLASIA	METAPLASIA	DYSPLASIA	BENIGN NEOPLASIA	MALIGNANT NEOPLASIA
Bizarre cells	Absent	Absent	Absent	Absent	May be present
Necrosis	None	None	None	None to mild	Mild to severe
Local invasion	None	None	None	Expansile	Invasive
Lymphatic/vascular invasion	None	None	None	None	May be present

29. Is dysplasia a precursor to neoplasia?

Dysplasia indicates an abnormality of organization and growth within mature tissue, often with atypical cell size and shape. This can be a precursor to the development of neoplasia but can also be seen in non-neoplastic conditions, as in a response to chronic irritation (see table at question 28).

30. Is metaplasia associated with neoplasia?

Metaplasia refers to a change to an adult type of tissue that is abnormal for that organ and is a non-neoplastic lesion (see table at question 28).

31. What is the difference between a diagnosis of neoplasia and cancer?

Neoplasia is a more general term that includes both benign as well as malignant proliferation of cells that are no longer under normal control mechanisms. Cancer refers more specifically to malignant neoplasms.

32. What criteria are used to determine if a lesion is malignant?

The amount of nuclear size variation, alteration in cell size and shape, mitotic activity, nuclear morphology, cytoplasmic staining properties, nucleolar appearance, and invasion or destruction of tissue are some common features that can help determine if a lesion is malignant. Some malignant neoplasms are well differentiated and may be difficult to differentiate from a benign lesion. In contrast, there are also benign lesions that have morphologic features suggestive of malignancy, and these also require recognition. Knowledge of these specific neoplasms, sometimes combined with clinical information, may be needed. General morphologic features of benign and malignant lesions are listed in the table at question 28.

33. What does the term "anaplastic" refer to?

Anaplasia is a loss of differentiation and, therefore, the term "anaplastic" is often used interchangeably with "undifferentiated" or "poorly differentiated" in the description of neoplasia. Histologically, the neoplastic cells lack features of the more mature cell of origin, often have prominent cell and nuclear size variation (anisocytosis and anisokaryosis, respectively), and the histogenesis may not be apparent based on histologic examination.

34. "Desmoplasia" is sometimes used in the description of a neoplasm. What does it mean?

Desmoplasia indicates the neoplasm has a prominent, reactive fibrous tissue component and is a feature of some carcinomas. "Scirrhous" or "sclerosing" are other terms sometimes used. The reactive fibroblasts can exhibit pleomorphism, and fine-needle aspirates from these masses may be misleading, being mistaken for fibrosarcomas.

35. How are neoplasms classified by pathologists?

After a lesion has been determined to be neoplastic, an appropriate name is provided based on the histogenesis and the benign or malignant appearance. There are exceptions, but the suffix "-oma" usually indicates a benign neoplasm. The suffix "carcinoma" indicates a malignant neoplasm of epithelial origin. The suffix "sarcoma" is used for malignant neoplasms of mesenchymal origin. In some cases the term "malignant" will be inserted in front of the name of the benign neoplasm to indicate malignancy.

Examples of the Classification of Common Neoplasms in Domestic Animals

HISTOGENESIS (cell of origin)	BENIGN NEOPLASIA	MALIGNANT NEOPLASIA
Epithelial		
Squamous	Squamous papilloma	Squamous cell carcinoma
Glandular/ductular	Adenoma	Adenocarcinoma
Basal cell	Basal cell tumor	Basal cell carcinoma
Transitional cell	Transitional cell papilloma	Transitional cell carcinoma
Mesenchymal		
Fibroblast	Fibroma	Fibrosarcoma
Adipocyte (fat)	Lipoma	Liposarcoma
Osteocyte (bone)	Osteoma	Osteosarcoma
Chondrocyte (cartilage)	Chondroma	Chondrosarcoma
Endothelial cell	Hemangioma	Hemangiosarcoma
Nerve sheath fibroblast	Peripheral nerve sheath tumor (schwannoma, neurofibroma)	Malignant peripheral nerve sheath tumor (neurofibrosarcoma)
Mesothelial cell	None	Mesothelioma
Skeletal muscle	Rhabdomyoma	Rhabdomyosarcoma
Smooth muscle	Leiomyoma	Leiomyosarcoma
Hematopoietic cells and derivatives		
Lymphocytes	None	Lymphoma, malignant lymphoma, lymphosarcoma, lymphocytic leukemia
Myeloid, monocytic	None	Myeloid leukemia, monocytic leukemia
Macrophage	Histiocytoma	Histiocytic sarcoma, malignant histiocytosis
Mast cell	None	Mast cell tumor
Plasma cell	Plasmacytoma	Multiple myeloma
Other		
Melanocyte (neuroectoderm)	Melanoma, melanocytoma	Malignant melanoma, melanosarcoma
Testicular germ cell	Seminoma	Seminoma
Sertoli's cell	Sertoli's cell tumor	Sertoli's cell tumor
Interstitial cell (testis)	Interstitial cell tumor	None

36. What is the difference between a carcinoma and an adenocarcinoma?

The term "adenocarcinoma" is used to describe a malignant epithelial neoplasm that is of glandular origin or that is seen to form glands. The term "carcinoma" is more general, indicating a malignant neoplasm of epithelial origin.

37. Why are lymphoid neoplasms sometimes called lymphoma, other times lymphosarcoma?

As mentioned, "sarcoma" refers to malignant neoplasia of mesenchymal origin. The term "lymphosarcoma" has long been used to refer to lymphoid neoplasms because they are malignant and not epithelial but, more recently, the term has been considered inappropriate because the lymphoid cells are not truly mesenchymal. As in human medicine, the term "lymphoma" is now more commonly used to refer to lymphoid neoplasia, but this is misleading because these neoplasms are not benign. In some cases you may also hear the term "malignant lymphoma" to emphasize the malignant nature. The subclassification of lymphomas is even more problematic because there are several different classification schemes.

38. Are there other classifications of neoplasms that may be confusing?

Unfortunately, yes. As seen in the table below, several neoplasms have somewhat confusing nomenclature. For instance, "seminoma" can refer to benign or malignant neoplasms of germ cell origin. A hemangiopericytoma is a very common canine neoplasm of uncertain histogenesis that metastasizes only very rarely, but it is commonly locally invasive and is considered a low- to intermediate-grade soft tissue sarcoma despite the suffix "-oma." Other terms may not clearly identify the cell of origin, such as "multiple myeloma," a malignant tumor of plasma cell origin. It is important to become familiar with the exceptions to the general rules of nomenclature.

Examples of Confusing Nomenclature of Neoplasia in Domestic Animals

HISTOGENESIS	CLASSIFICATION	POINTS OF CONFUSION
Uncertain (mesenchymal)	Hemangiopericytoma	Behaves as a low- to intermediate-grade soft tissue sarcoma, despite suffix "-oma."
Circumanal gland	Circumanal gland adenoma (carcinoma)	Synonyms are perianal gland adenoma (carcinoma) and hepatoid gland adenoma (carcinoma).
Testicular germ cell	Seminoma	The same name is given whether considered benign or malignant.
Melanocyte	Melanoma	Melanoma has been used for both benign and malignant forms of melanocytic neoplasia. Melanocytoma, compound melanoma, dermal melanoma (benign), malignant melanoma, and melanosarcoma (malignant) are terms that are used to help differentiate.
Mesothelial cell	Mesothelioma	Considered malignant despite suffix "-oma."
Lymphocyte	Lymphoma	Lymphoid neoplasia is a malignancy, and lymphoma, lymphosarcoma, and malignant lymphoma are synonyms.
Nerve sheath fibroblast, Schwann cell	Peripheral nerve sheath tumor	Synonyms include neurofibroma, schwannoma. The more benign form behaves as a low-grade soft tissue sarcoma.
Mast cell	Mast cell tumor	All mast cell tumors are potentially malignant. Grading correlates with behavior.
Plasma cell (malignant form)	Multiple myeloma	The cell of origin is not specifically identified in the name.

(Table continued on next page.)

Examples of Confusing Nomenclature of Neoplasia in Domestic Animals (Cont.)

HISTOGENESIS	CLASSIFICATION	POINTS OF CONFUSION
Sertoli's cell	Sertoli's cell tumor	Most canine Sertoli's cell tumors are benign, but some have features of malignancy. There is no specific term for the malignant variant.
Chemoreceptor	Chemodectoma	These are neuroendocrine carcinomas despite the suffix "-oma." Synonyms (e.g., aortic body tumor, carotid body tumor) may be used depending on the location.
Uncertain (mesenchymal)	Malignant fibrous histiocytoma	The name can be confusing because the histogenesis is uncertain. These are generally intermediate-grade soft tissue sarcomas seen in dogs.
Kulchitsky's cell, entero-chromaffin cell	Carcinoid	The term does not indicate the specific cell of origin or the degree of malignancy. These are generally considered malignant.

39. How did I get two different diagnoses from a single neoplasm cut in half and sent to two different laboratories?

In many cases this is due to differences in terminology used by pathologists that train in different institutions. Commonly there are synonyms that may be used for the same neoplasm. Examples include "neurofibroma" and "peripheral nerve sheath tumor." Another common synonym is "perianal gland adenoma" and "circumanal gland adenoma." In other cases, there may be variation within neoplasms that may result in different classification, particularly grade, depending on the portion of the neoplasm examined. It is also possible that two different pathologists may interpret the same tissue differently and, in those cases, additional studies may be indicated to help differentiate.

40. Assuming adequate tissue is submitted for evaluation, why is a specific diagnosis not always received?

Malignant tumors may be poorly differentiated and, in those cases, may not resemble the cell of origin. Based on morphology alone, the diagnosis may not be specific, and a more generic term may be used, such as "undifferentiated sarcoma" or "undifferentiated malignant neoplasm."

41. Isn't the result obtained from a board-certified veterinary pathologist definitive?

In the ideal world, every histopathology result would be specific and correct, but the interpretation and diagnosis may be affected by many factors. Particularly when a histopathology result does not appear to make sense when taken in context with clinical findings or progression of disease, consultation with the pathologist would be advised. Technical difficulties in accessioning, processing, or labeling are all possible sources of a mistaken diagnosis. Pathologists are human, and the interpretation of histopathologic sections is an art with the potential for error in more difficult cases. Invariably, there will be instances when an interpretation is not correct. In some cases, additional information that can be provided when discussing the case will allow the pathologist to explain any discrepancies by reviewing the submitted sample(s) or may suggest that additional staining techniques should be used. In other cases, a second opinion may be in order, particularly with unusual or poorly differentiated lesions.

42. When and how do I get a second opinion on a histopathology submission?

As discussed above, a second opinion is a good idea when the first interpretation does not correlate with clinical findings, particularly when the therapy of the patient or the prognosis may be affected. In some difficult cases, the pathologist may suggest that additional opinions be elicited, but you should never feel uncomfortable about requesting the second opinion yourself. By contacting the laboratory, additional sections can be cut and stained from the paraffin block, and these slides may be sent for evaluation.

43. What is the purpose of the histologic grade?

With many neoplasms, the grade of the neoplasm has been correlated to some degree with the expected behavior, and the purpose of grading is to aid in determining the prognosis as well as helping to decide on the most appropriate therapy.

44. How are neoplasms graded?

Grading is based on the morphology of the neoplasm and may vary with different types of neoplasms. Common components of grading systems include the following:
- Degree of nuclear and cell size and shape variation (pleomorphism)
- Mitotic index
- Amount of necrosis
- Degree of organization
- Depth of invasiveness
- Degree of cellular differentiation (resemblance between neoplastic cell and cell of origin).

In quantitative systems of grading, a numerical figure may be assigned to each component and the added score determines the grade. In other cases, a more subjective classification of low, intermediate, or high grade is given without the use of a scoring system.

45. Is grading an accurate predictor of behavior?

This depends on the type of neoplasm. For some neoplasms there is good correlation established, such as mast cell tumors, while other neoplasms are incompletely studied or have a less distinct correlation. In some cases the histologic appearance does not correlate with behavior such as cutaneous plasmacytomas.

46. How does grading differ from staging?

There is commonly confusion concerning grade versus stage. Grading is based on the morphology seen in histologic sections, while staging is based on clinical findings and generally includes tumor size and location in addition to the presence or absence of metastatic lesions. There are some features of a neoplasm that may be used both for grading and staging, particularly depth of invasion into the normal tissue. A more detailed description of staging schemes is outlined elsewhere in this text.

47. What is considered complete excision in histologic sections?

This depends on the type of neoplasia. A well-delineated, benign neoplasm such as a basal cell tumor may be cured when there are only narrow margins (0.5 cm or less) of clear tissue, while locally aggressive forms of neoplasia may be difficult to cure even with radical excision. In general, aggressive resection involves removal of 2 to 3 cm of clear tissue along all lateral and deep margins. It should be noted that there is contraction of some tissues, particularly skin, after excision and fixation, and the amount of clear tissue measured in a fixed specimen may be less than that seen prior to removal.

SPECIAL STAINS AND PROCEDURES

48. What stains are commonly used in the diagnosis of neoplasia?

A hematoxylin-eosin stain is routinely used as the initial stain and provides good differential staining of nuclear and cytoplasmic components of cells as well as staining of matrix and interstitial elements. A variety of other stains are available to highlight specific morphologic features, such as mast cell granules.

Histochemical Stains Commonly Used in the Diagnosis of Neoplasia

STAIN	EXAMPLE OF USAGE IN TUMOR DIAGNOSIS
Toluidine blue	Used to identify mast cell granules
Fontana method	Identifies argentaffin granules and melanin granules
Alcian blue	Stains cartilage matrix and mucin in carcinomas
Masson trichrome	A collagen and muscle stain
Congo red	Identifies amyloid, seen in some plasma cell tumors and calcifying epithelial odontogenic tumors
Periodic acid-Schiff	Stains mucin and granules of granular cell tumors
Phosphotungstic acid-hematoxylin	Used to identify granules in globular leukocyte tumors
Reticulin stain	Highlights fine stroma in neuroendocrine tumors
Oil red O	Identifies fat (requires special processing procedure), as seen in liposarcomas and sebaceous carcinomas

49. Immunohistochemistry is being used more commonly, but what is it?

Immunohistochemical staining uses specific antigen-antibody reactions. Antibodies (primary antibodies) are derived that will react with cellular products or components such as intermediate filaments that may provide information concerning the histogenesis. In most techniques, a second antibody (secondary antibody) is combined with an enzyme and will specifically adhere to the primary antibody. The enzyme attached to this secondary antibody can then be exposed to a chromogen that undergoes a color change that can be seen under the microscope. The identified antigens are often referred to as "markers" of histogenesis.

50. What are some immunohistochemical stains that can be helpful in oncology?

Selected, commonly used antigens (markers) in veterinary medicine can be divided into structural proteins, secretory products, cell surface markers, and intracellular proteins such as enzymes (see table, next page).

51. Why is a specific cell of origin not always able to be identified using immunohistochemistry?

Several potential factors might prevent a diagnosis:

1. Specific antibodies are not yet available (particularly in veterinary medicine) to identify all different types of cells.

2. In some cases the detected antigen may be present in more than one type of cell (such as the intermediate filament vimentin, which is a general mesenchymal cell marker), or there may be cross-reactivity with antigens in other types of cells, and a positive result may only help narrow the list of potential differentials.

Selected Immunohistochemical Markers of Histogenesis

CELLULAR COMPONENT STAINED	ASSOCIATED HISTOGENESIS
Intermediate filaments	
Cytokeratins	General epithelial marker
Vimentin	General mesenchymal marker
Desmin	Muscle marker
Smooth muscle actin	Smooth muscle
Glial fibrillary acidic protein	Marker of astrocytes, ependymomas, some Schwann's cell neoplasms
Neurofilament protein	Neurons
Secretory products	
Thyroglobulin	Thyroid follicular cells
Calcitonin	Thyroid C cells
Insulin	Pancreatic islet B cells
Immunoglobulins	Plasma cells
Intracytoplasmic granules and enzymes	
Lysozyme	Histiocytes
Factor VIII-related antigen	Endothelial cells
Chromogranin A	Neuroendocrine cells
Neuron-specific enolase	Neural tissues
Cell surface antigens	
CD1	Langerhans' cells, thymocytes
CD3 (T-cell receptor)	T cells
CD11	Leukocytes
CD68	Macrophages
CD79a	B cells

3. Poorly differentiated, neoplastic cells may no longer produce or express markers of differentiation (as a result, a lack of staining is not particularly helpful in many instances).

4. Fixation may alter antigenic sites and can interfere with the binding of antibodies, causing false negatives (this can be a particular problem with long fixation times).

5. Tissue drying, autolytic change, or other variables can cause excessive background staining that may obscure results.

52. Why isn't electron microscopy used more often?

In many instances the increased magnification provided still does not provide a specific diagnosis in cases that cannot be identified with light microscopy. In addition, formalin fixation does not provide optimal results, although formalin fixed samples can be used. The equipment used and the time involved makes it impractical in most diagnostic settings.

53. How do I handle a case that I suspect may benefit from electron microscopy?

It is best to contact your laboratory and discuss the case ahead of time (prior to the biopsy procedure). If electron microscopy is anticipated, small samples (2-mm cubes) should be harvested and fixed in an appropriate fixative such as a gluteraldehyde solution.

54. Are there other special procedures that may be helpful?

The table summarizes selected laboratory techniques that may be used in oncology cases. Histochemical and immunohistochemical staining have been previously discussed. In some instances, flow cytometry performed on fluid samples can be used to detect surface markers or abnormal DNA content in neoplastic cells. Molecular diagnostics are currently not routinely used as diagnostic tools in veterinary medicine but, if future research identifies specific genetic alterations that are the basis for the development of animal neoplasms and probes become available, polymerase chain reaction, in situ hybridization, and cytogenetic studies may become valuable tools. Cell cultures are used to study neoplastic tissue but are not routinely used in a diagnostic setting.

Special Procedures Used in Tumor Diagnosis

PROCEDURE	USE IN THE DIAGNOSIS OF NEOPLASIA
Histochemical stains	A variety of stains are available that help identify morphologic features associated with specific cells of origin. The uses of selected stains are listed in the table at question 48.
Immunohistochemistry	Allows identification of markers of histogenesis via specific antigen-antibody interactions. Common markers are listed in the table at question 50.
Electron microscopy	Used to visualize subcellular morphologic features, such as cytoplasmic granules or intercellular junctions that may provide clues to histogenesis. Generally limited usage due to cost and technical requirements.
Flow cytometry	Membrane surface antigens and DNA content may be measured in cells from fluid samples.
Molecular diagnostics	Cytogenetic assays, polymerase chain reaction, and in situ hybridization are techniques that may be used to identify gene rearrangements (particularly translocations) that have been associated with neoplasia. The use of these methods is very limited in veterinary oncology because of a lack of appropriate probes and insufficient knowledge of gene alterations that are associated with neoplasia in animals.
Cell cultures	Cultures allow evaluation of cell growth characteristics. They are used in a research setting but are not practical for most clinical, diagnostic cases.

BIBLIOGRAPHY

1. Cotran RS, Kumar V, Collins T: Robbins Pathologic Basis of Disease, 6th ed. Philadelphia, WB Saunders, 1999.
2. Jones TC, Hunt RD, King NW: Veterinary Pathology, 6th ed. Baltimore, Williams & Wilkins, 1997.
3. Patniak AK, Ehler WJ, MacEwen EG: Canine cutaneous mast cell tumor: Morphologic grading and survival time in 83 dogs. Vet Pathol 21:469–471, 1984.
4. Powers BE: The pathology of neoplasia. In Withrow SJ, MacEwen EG (eds): Small Animal Clinical Oncology, 2nd ed. Philadelphia, WB Saunders, 1996, pp 4–15.
5. Presnell JK, Schreibman MP: Humason's Animal Tissue Techniques, 5th ed. Baltimore, The Johns Hopkins University Press, 1997.
6. Stetler-Stevenson M, Medeiros LJ, Jaffe ES: Immunophenotypic methods and findings in the diagnosis of lymphoproliferative diseases. In Jaffe ES (ed): Surgical Pathology of the Lymph Nodes and Related Organs, 2nd ed. Philadelphia, WB Saunders, 1995, pp 22–57.
7. Vail DM, Powers BE, Getzy DM, et al: Evaluation of prognostic factors for dogs with synovial sarcoma: 36 cases (1986–1991). J Am Vet Med Assoc 205:1300–1307, 1994.
8. Withrow SJ: Biopsy principles. In Withrow SJ, MacEwen EG (eds): Small Animal Clinical Oncology, 2nd ed. Philadelphia, WB Saunders, 1996, pp 52–56.

8. IMAGING OF THE ONCOLOGY PATIENT

David S. Biller, DVM, Dipl ACVR, and Laura Armbrust, DVM

1. Why does imaging help in the cancer patient?

Neoplasia almost always alters the normal spatial relationships of tissues and organs. Diagnostic imaging is critical not only for making the diagnosis of cancer, but also for staging the patients and for following response to therapy.

2. Name the imaging modalities available for evaluation of the oncology patient.

At present the most frequently used imaging modalities for the diagnosis of cancer are conventional radiographs and ultrasound, but magnetic resonance imaging (MRI), computed tomography (CT), and nuclear medicine are increasing in availability and usage.

3. Will ultrasound, CT, MRI, and nuclear medicine replace conventional diagnostic radiographs?

No, they will not replace conventional radiography, but rather compliment it. These newer imaging modalities have made assessing tumor margins, evaluating for metastasis, and determining the degree of invasiveness more reliable.

4. Aren't these new imaging modalities quite expensive and unavailable to the practitioner?

Some of these techniques are relatively costly (CT, MRI), but they provide additional information that can decrease cost and patient suffering in the long run. They may also aid in narrowing the differential diagnosis and prevent unnecessary surgery. These modalities, especially ultrasound, can help guide deep-needle aspirations or biopsies as well as assist in the planning of open biopsies and surgical resections. CT and MRI are also very helpful in the planning of radiation treatment.

5. Can these new, expensive, high-tech imaging modalities lend a tissue diagnosis?

No. The clinician is still not able to make a tissue diagnosis based on an image. Cytology or histopathology is necessary to make a definitive diagnosis.

6. What are the advantages and disadvantages of conventional diagnostic radiography for the cancer patient?

Advantages: availability and cost. Radiographs provide good spatial resolution, but have poor contrast discrimination between normal and neoplastic soft tissues. Another advantage is coverage of a large area, such as the abdomen or thorax, in two images (lateral and ventrodorsal/dorsoventral). Radiographs can provide information regarding the size, shape, margination, opacity, position, and organ displacement more easily than other imaging modalities. Therefore, conventional radiographs are a good screening procedure and guide to further diagnostic procedures and imaging modalities.

Disadvantages: invasiveness and inability to assess tissue architecture.

7. What are the advantages of ultrasound in imaging the cancer patient?

The affordability and availability of ultrasound equipment have resulted in a tremendous increase in its use in veterinary practice. Ultrasound excels as an imaging modality to discriminate between cystic and solid masses, to evaluate a body cavity filled with fluid (abdominal or pleural effusion), to determine the internal architecture of an abdominal organ, or to guide fine-needle aspiration or tissue core biopsy.

8. What are the advantages and disadvantages of computed tomography in imaging the cancer patient?

Compared to conventional radiographs, CT has excellent contrast discrimination and the ability to separate deep structures without the superimposition of overlying tissues (Fig. 1). It is possible to visualize the brain without the inconvenience of the surrounding skull. Soft tissues must be significantly altered by disease before changes can be visualized with conventional radiographs, whereas changes can be appreciated earlier and more accurately with CT. However, CT is usually available only in referral and academic institutions, and animals must be anesthetized to be imaged with CT.

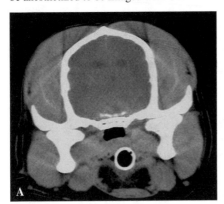 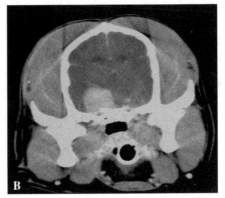

FIGURE 1.   Axial CT of a canine brain with meningioma. *A*, Without contrast. *B*, With contrast.

9. What is the main advantage of magnetic resonance imaging in evaluation of the cancer patient?

The contrast between different soft tissues is superior to all other imaging modalities.

10. Are there disadvantages to using magnetic resonance imaging in evaluation of the cancer patient?

General anesthesia is required, and the procedure usually requires substantially more time than CT. Monitoring of patients can be difficult depending on the type of MRI unit utilized. MRI can be expensive, and availability is not as universal as CT, but nothing is superior for imaging of the central nervous system.

11. Describe the best way to image the lungs for evaluation of the cancer patient.

Conventional radiographs represent the most valuable and cost-effective examination for primary screening of neoplasia of the thorax. Radiographs should be taken of all patients suspected of having cancer and during treatments to monitor response to therapy. Making three views of the thorax (right and left laterals as well as dorsoventral or ventrodorsal) should increase sensitivity for finding lesions.

12. Describe the different appearances of pulmonary neoplastic lesions.
- Solitary or multiple well-defined nodules or masses
- Solitary or multiple ill-defined nodules or masses
- Amorphous ill-defined alveolar opacities
- Diffuse miliary (micronodular) interstitial opacities
- Diffuse interstitial opacities
- Diffuse and lobar alveolar opacities

Solitary nodules with either well- or ill-defined borders are the most characteristic findings of primary pulmonary neoplasia. Cavitation is occasionally present within primary or metastatic pulmonary nodules or masses. Primary lung tumors are most commonly found in the caudal lung lobes.

13. Do you recommend metastasis checks for all oncology patients?

Yes. Demonstrating metastasis plays a large role in therapy recommendations and the prognosis of the patient.

14. Radiographically, how do you tell the difference between pulmonary nodules and mimics such as osseous metaplasia, end-on vessels, and skin nodules?

End-on vessels are typically very circular and very opaque for their size. The size of the vessel should also correspond to the region within the lung (the vessels are larger in the perihilar region and smaller at the periphery). End-on vessels overlie linear vascular markings. *Osseous metaplasia* are nodules less than 3 mm in diameter that are very opaque for their size due to their mineral density. Nipples or *skin nodules* are well circumscribed and dense. These can be ruled out because they will be outside the lung on at least one of the views.

15. Of all the imaging and modalities available for the cancer patient, which would be the best for evaluating the thorax?

Computed tomography, by virtue of its cross-sectional display of anatomy, superior contrast, and anatomic resolution, can differentiate pulmonary lesions from overlying normal superimposed structures. CT is clearly superior to conventional radiography in demonstrating the extent of the primary lesion, invasion of the hilus or mediastinum, body wall or pleural space involvement, and the presence of enlarged lymph nodes. At present, the most sensitive modality in the diagnosis and staging of pulmonary metastatic disease is CT.

16. What imaging modalities are useful in screening the skeletal structures of the cancer patient?

A diagnosis of skeletal neoplasia can often be supported on conventional radiographs. Bone scintigraphy may be used to screen for additional lesions or to evaluate the extent of lesions diagnosed radiographically. MRI and CT are used to supply additional information about the location and extent of the tumor, but not to obtain a diagnosis.

17. What are the radiographic signs of aggressive bone disease? Can you tell the difference radiographically between neoplasia and infectious disease?

When evaluating bone disease radiographically, determine the zone of transition and degree of lysis and bony proliferation. With aggressive bone disease, the periosteal reaction is typically sunburst to amorphous in nature; the zone of transition is long; and osteolysis is present. Primary bone tumors usually begin in the metaphysis. It is unusual for a primary bone tumor to cross the joint. The most common locations for osteosarcoma, which is the most common primary bone tumor, are the proximal humerus, distal radius, ulna, distal femur, and proximal and distal tibia (Fig. 2, see next page). Although the aforementioned are characteristic of neoplasia, cytology or histopathology is required for a definitive diagnosis to differentiate tumor type or infection.

18. Do I really need both right and left lateral radiographs when checking for pulmonary metastatic disease?

Yes! Three views of the thorax include a ventrodorsal or dorsoventral and both the left and right lateral radiographs (Fig. 3). The nondependent (up) lung is best visualized due to the increased air within the pulmonary parenchyma. This results in improved contrast between a pulmonary nodule and aerated lung (Fig. 4). The nondependent lung is partially atelectatic, which results in decreased contrast between a pulmonary nodule and nonaerated lung tissue. The same principle holds true for the dorsoventral or ventrodorsal radiograph. Nodules in the

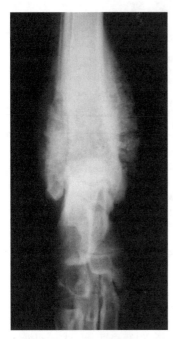

FIGURE 2.   Dorsoplantar radiograph of the distal tibia of a dog with osteosarcoma.

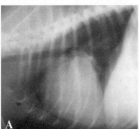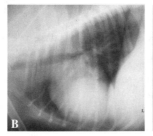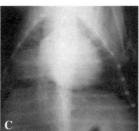

FIGURE 3.   *A*, Right lateral, *B*, left lateral, and *C*, ventrodorsal thoracic radiographs in a dog with a primary pulmonary carcinoma of the right middle lung lobe.

caudodorsal lung field would be best visualized on the dorsoventral radiograph. If a pulmonary lesion is seen in only one view, then it is of questionable significance. The contralateral film should be used to confirm an intrapulmonary lesion.

19. What is the technique of choice for imaging the central nervous system?

Magnetic resonance imaging is the technique of choice for imaging brain and spinal cord neoplasia (Fig. 5). MRI is ideally suited for imaging of intracranial neoplasia because of its inherit property of producing excellent contrast between normal and abnormal tissue. Intravenous gadolinium contrast may also be valuable in helping to demonstrate blood-brain barrier disruption.

20. In animals with suspected brain neoplasia, is conventional radiography of value?

This is one of the few situations where conventional radiography has little value, unless there is adjacent bone involvement.

21. What radiographic changes may be seen with neoplasia of the adrenal glands?

Radiographic changes of the adrenal are detectable if the adrenal tumor is large or mineralized. Large unilateral adrenal masses may displace the kidney or other adjacent abdominal

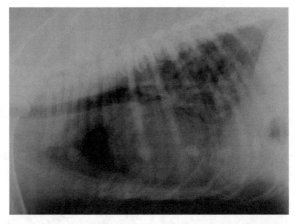

FIGURE 4. Right lateral radiograph of a dog with pulmonary metastatic disease from osteosarcoma.

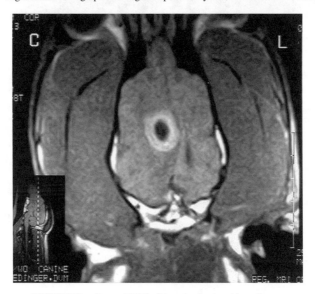

FIGURE 5. Coronal MRI of a canine brain with a glioma.

organs. Other changes that might be radiographically apparent with a functional adrenocortical tumor are large, blunted pulmonary arteries secondary to pulmonary thromboembolism or pulmonary interstitial mineralization; other soft tissue mineralization; and, although nonspecific, a large urinary bladder, pendulous abdomen, and hepatomegaly.

22. Which imaging modality is probably best adapted for diagnosis of adrenal tumors?

Adrenal ultrasound is highly sensitive for the diagnosis of adrenal neoplasia (Fig. 6). The one caveat is that nodular hyperplasia may mimic the appearance of an adrenal adenoma, although adenomas are usually unilateral and may not disrupt the architecture (or disrupt it far less than malignant tumors do). Diagnosis of an abnormal adrenal with ultrasound is not diagnostic for tumor type. The liver, abdominal lymph nodes, and adjacent structures can be evaluated for invasion (caudal vena cava) and metastasis.

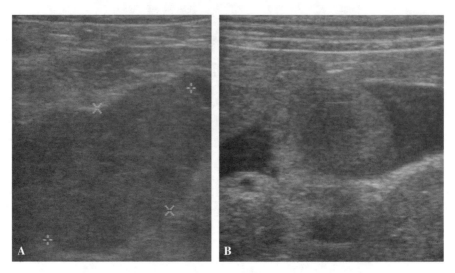

FIGURE 6. *A*, Longitudinal ultrasound of the left adrenal adenocarcinoma, *B*, with invasion of the caudal vena cava through the phrenicoabdominal vein.

23. Describe the proper radiographic series for evaluation and diagnosis of nasal neoplasia.

The skull is a complex structure; therefore, detecting disease within the nasal passages is difficult radiographically. For best results multiple views should be taken, including a ventrodorsal open-mouth view and/or intraoral radiograph. In this manner the mandible is out of the way so that the nasal cavity can be better visualized. A lateral radiograph of the skull and a rostral caudal view to obtain both frontal sinuses should also be obtained. In the case of animals that have small frontal sinuses (brachycephalic dogs or Persian cats), oblique laterals may be helpful.

24. What is the ideal imaging modality for evaluation of nasal tumors?

Computed tomography is superior to conventional radiography for demonstrating changes associated with nasal neoplasia. This superiority is a result of the higher contrast resolution and the ability to minimize superimposition of overlying structures. CT is also more helpful in differentiating fluid versus masses in the frontal sinuses. CT is also recommended when surgery or radiation therapy is a treatment option.

25. List the types of changes that can be visualized by CT scan of a nose with tumor.
- Patchy areas of increased opacity within soft tissue
- Destruction of all or part of the ethmoid bone
- Abnormal soft tissue in the retrobulbar space
- Destruction of the lateral maxilla
- Destruction of the nasal bone or the rostral dorsal maxilla
- Hyperostosis of the lateral maxilla

26. Are there any techniques that can be used to help determine the organ of origin for abdominal masses?

If ultrasound is not readily available, an inexpensive, simple technique that can help determine the origin of a mass is **compression radiography**. This allows for displacement of overlying structures from the mass and provides increased visualization of the margins. This technique is useful in cats and small- to medium-sized dogs and has been used in larger dogs but can be more difficult due to their size. When using compression radiography, decrease your original radiographic technique approximately 10% to allow for the decreased thickness through which you are imaging.

Positional radiography may also be helpful and consists simply of obtaining the opposite lateral view, a dorsoventral view, or an oblique view. Positional radiography may also include horizontal beam projections with erect and decubitus patient positioning.

27. What is the best imaging modality for evaluation of the abdomen for primary tumors or metastatic disease and invasion?

Ultrasound is an excellent follow-up to radiographs, as it can define the organ of origin and internal architecture and evaluate the rest of the abdomen (including other abdominal organs as well as lymph nodes) for metastasis. Abdominal effusion that may be present with cancer (carcinomatosis) usually does not hamper and can even enhance the diagnosis of neoplasia via ultrasound. Ultrasound is also very helpful in guiding fine-needle aspiration or biopsy.

28. Describe the appearance of a tumor of the kidney.

Small mass lesions that do not affect renal opacity, contour, or size are not appreciated on survey radiographs. Neoplasia generally appears radiographically as large irregular or regularly shaped, and smooth or roughly margined. An enlarged neoplastic left kidney displaces the colon ventrally and displaces the small intestine ventrally and to the right. Mass lesions of the right kidney may result in displacement of the small intestine ventrally, caudally, and to the left. As a second-line image, **excretory urography** may be helpful to better define kidney size, shape, contour, and the appearance of the collecting system (Fig. 7).

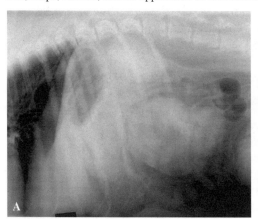 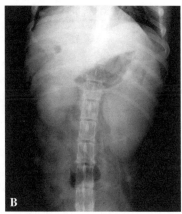

FIGURE 7. *A*, Lateral and *B*, ventrodorsal excretory urogram of a dog with renal carcinoma of the cranial pole of the left kidney.

29. What is the best imaging modality for evaluation of the kidneys for tumors?

Ultrasound allows definition of renal architecture. There are a variety of appearances of renal ultrasound with neoplasia including: hypoechoic or hyperechoic masses, small masses that do not disrupt renal size or contour, masses of mixed echogenicity, multiple mass lesions, and large masses with complete disruption of the normal renal appearance.

30. What type of instrument should be used for ultrasound-guided fine-needle aspirates or biopsies?

For fine-needle aspirate, a 22-gauge needle is generally used. For biopsy, gauges between 14 and 18 are often used. To obtain the best samples for histology, a 14-gauge needle is recommended; however, the organ being biopsied and the patient size must be considered. For example, a 14-gauge needle may work well on the liver or kidney if the dog is large. On a smaller dog or cat, an 18-gauge needle may be more appropriate. A fine-needle aspirate can be obtained first and evaluated cytologically, followed by a biopsy if this is nondiagnostic.

31. Are there any risks associated with biopsies?

Risks that should be considered include neoplastic dissemination, infection, and hemorrhage. With ultrasound guidance, there is a better chance of obtaining diagnostic tissue samples, and risks are decreased. Benefit verses risk dictates that these high-yield, low-risk procedures provide helpful information necessary for the diagnosis and treatment of cancer in veterinary patients.

BIBLIOGRAPHY

1. Brown ML, Collier BD, Fogelman I: Bone scintigraphy: Part 1. Oncology and infection. J Nuc Med 34(12):2236–2251, 1993.
2. Burk RL: Computed tomography of thoracic disease in dogs. J Am Vet Med Assoc 199(5):617–621,1991.
3. Forrest LJ, Thrall DE: Oncologic applications of diagnostic imaging techniques. Vet Clin North Am Small Anim Pract 25(1):185–205, 1995.
4. Park RD, Beck ER, LeCouteur RA: Comparison of computed tomography and radiography, for detecting changes induced by malignant nasal neoplasia in dogs. J Am Vet Med Assoc 201(11)1720–1724, 1992.
5. Shore A: Magnetic resonance imaging. Vet Clin North Am Small Anim Pract 23(2):437–459, 1993.
6. Stickle RL, Hathcock JT: Interpretation of computed tomographic images. Vet North Am Small Anim Pract 23(2):417–435, 1993.
7. Widmer WR, Guptill L: Imaging techniques for facilitating diagnosis of hyperadrenocorticism in dogs and cats. J Am Vet Med Assoc 206(12):1857–1864, 1995.

9. TUMOR MARKERS

Richard Weller, DVM, Dipl ACVIM

1. What are tumor markers?

Tumor markers are molecules occurring in blood or tissue that are associated with cancer and whose measurement or identification is useful in diagnosis or clinical management.

2. Can you give some examples of tumor markers?

Traditionally, tumor markers have included tumor-associated antigens, enzymes, specific proteins, and metabolites. More recently, oncogenes, oncogene products, and tumor suppressor genes have been used as tumor markers. Such markers can be measured in tissue as well as in blood.

3. How are they detected?

They are detected and measured in the laboratory using biochemical or immunochemical means.

4. Are they tumor-specific?

In general, tumor markers are tissue- or organ-specific, not tumor-specific, biologic products. With some tumors, the marker is associated with the normal cell of origin and is produced in excess by the tumor cells. With other tumors, the marker is not associated with the normal cell of origin but is produced normally for a while in fetal life. Tumor markers include many substances that are not readily systematically organized.

Markers resulting from tumor-cell dedifferentiation	Tumor
Carcinoembryonic antigen	Carcinomas of gastrointestinal tract, pancreas, mammary gland, lung
Alpha-fetoprotein	Hepatocellular carcinoma, yolk-sac tumor of testis
Alkaline phosphatase isoenzyme	Various tumors
Ectopic hormones	Various tumors
Markers resulting from over-production by tumor cells	**Tumor**
Prostate-specific antigen	Prostate carcinoma
Calcitonin	Medullary carcinoma of thyroid
Other hormones	Endocrine tumors
Monoclonal gammopathy and Bence Jones protein	Multiple myeloma
Basic fibroblast growth factor	Bladder cancer

5. What would be the characteristics of an ideal tumor marker?

An ideal tumor marker would be a "blood test" for cancer in which a positive result would occur only in patients with cancer, one that would correlate with stage and response to treatment and that was easily and reproducibly measured. It would also be sensitive and specific, with concentrations reflecting size or activity of the tumor, and provide prognostic information. No tumor marker in use today has met this ideal.

6. Why has no molecule met all of the requirements of an ideal tumor marker?

No marker has established itself as a practical cancer-screening tool either in a general healthy population or in most high-risk populations. This is due to the relative lack of sensitivity and specificity of available tests, given the low prevalence of cancers in most population groups. Given the low prevalence of cancer in general, even tests that are highly sensitive and specific may have low predictive values.

7. Why should we bother with the study of tumor markers in veterinary oncology?

Despite their shortcomings, tumor markers can be used for several purposes: (1) screening a healthy population or a high-risk population for the presence of cancer; (2) diagnosing cancer or a specific type of cancer; (3) determining the role of specific oncogenes, oncogene products, or tumor suppressor genes in the pathogenesis of different tumors; (4) determining the prognosis in a patient; (5) monitoring the course of a patient in remission or while receiving surgery, radiation, or chemotherapy; and (6) detecting relapse.

8. Why is it important to determine a specific type of cancer?

The distinction is of great importance from a clinical perspective because germ cell origin will often influence the biologic behavior of a particular neoplasm and choice of treatment.

9. How is this usually accomplished?

Immunohistochemistry and electron microscopy have become important tools for tumor typing through determination of certain internal structures and secretions of individual neoplastic cells. A number of antigenic markers have been shown to be useful in making distinctions among some tumors. Diagnosis can also be facilitated through the use of monoclonal antibodies, cytochemical stains, and flow cytometry. These techniques often allow more precise diagnosis than can be accomplished by assessment of morphologic criteria alone.

10. List some antigenic markers currently used to specifically type tumors in animals.

MARKER	TARGET
CD31 antigen	Endothelial cells
S-100 protein	Cells of neural crest origin or cells with nerve sheath differentiation
Osteosarcoma-associated antigen	Osteosarcoma tumor cells
Vimentin	Mesenchymal cells of nonmuscle origin
Laminin	Basal lamina of smooth muscle and Schwann cells
Keratins	Epithelial and myoepithelial cells
Carboxypeptidase A	Pancreatic acinar cells

11. Have any tumor markers been identified that might lend themselves to screening high-risk populations of animals for the presence of cancer?

While research in this area has been limited, veterinary researchers have obtained some promising results.

MARKER	SOURCE	TARGET
Tumor-associated antigens	Serum	Bovine leukemia cells
Glutathione-S-transferases	Plasma	Malignant lymphoma in dogs
Thymidine kinase activity	Plasma	Malignant lymphoma in dogs
Oncofetal protein 55	Plasma	Various tumors
Tumor-associated antigens	Serum	Canine mammary cancer
Core protein p27	Serum	Ovine pulmonary carcinoma
Alpha-fetoprotein	Serum	Liver tumors in dogs
Carcinoembryonic antigen	Serum	Various tumors
Basic fibroblast growth factor	Urine	Bladder cancer in dogs

12. Can you cite a specific example of how one of these markers has been used to screen a healthy or susceptible population of animals?

Absolutely. Ovine pulmonary carcinoma (OPC) is a contagious pulmonary neoplasm with suspected retroviral etiology. A recombinant enzyme-linked immunosorbent assay was developed using p27 protein. This was used to screen sera obtained from 400 sheep. The results showed that (1) a high prevalence of infection existed with putative OPC retrovirus in sheep with chronic pneumonia; (2) subclinical infection with OPC virus was more common than expected; and (3) an apparent association existed between ovine lentivirus and OPC.

13. Can acid phosphatase and prostate-specific antigen be used as markers for diagnosis of canine prostate disorders in the same way they are used in men?

Serum and seminal plasma concentrations or activities of acid phosphatase (AP), prostate-specific antigen (PSA), and canine prostate-specific esterase (CPSE) were measured in normal dogs, dogs with benign prostate hyperplasia, dogs with bacterial prostatitis, and dogs with prostatic carcinoma. PSA was not detected in serum or seminal plasma obtained from any group of dogs, and AP and CPSE were not significantly increased in dogs with prostatic carcinoma, possibly due to down-regulation of those enzymes by cancer cells. In a different study, however, a novel marker called EphA2 receptor tyrosine kinase was shown to be overexpressed in metastasis-derived canine prostate carcinoma cell lines.

14. How could tumor markers be useful in determining the prognosis in a patient?

Diagnosis and prognosis are mainly based on the somewhat uncertain interpretation of cytologic signs of malignancy in histologic sections. Several studies have been conducted that sought to compare the accuracy of prognosis based on classical morphologic criteria with that provided by several proliferation indices. Indices included potential doubling time (Tpot), argyrophilic nucleolar organizer region (AgNOR) frequency, proliferating cell nuclear antigen (PCNA), and growth fractions as determined by the expression of the Ki-67 antigen.

15. What types of tumors were included in those studies?

Most focused on canine malignant lymphoma, but canine mast cell tumors, canine mammary tumors, and melanocytic tumors in dogs and cats have been studied as well.

16. What are the best predictors of clinical behavior in canine malignant lymphoma?

The AgNOR count, Tpot (based on bromodeoxyuridine-delayed biopsy), Ki-67 antigen expression, and immunophenotype were the best predictors of treatment outcome in dogs with malignant lymphoma. PCNA counts had no prognostic significance in relation to median survival time in treated or untreated dogs.

17. What are the findings with other tumor types?

Histologic grade, AgNOR count, and PCNA counts accurately predicted clinical outcome in dogs with mast cell tumors, while only Ki-67 antigen expression had prognostic value for canine mammary tumors and melanocytic tumors in dogs and cats.

18. Isn't the hypercalcemia often associated with canine malignant lymphoma also considered a tumor marker?

Yes, and it is probably one of the more reliable and cost-effective markers for a veterinary practitioner or oncologist to use for tracking response to therapy, remission, and relapse. It is the most-studied and best-understood paraneoplastic syndrome occurring in veterinary medicine.

19. What are paraneoplastic syndromes?

Paraneoplastic syndromes are disorders associated with cancer that are unrelated to the size, location, metastases, or physiologic activities of the mature tissue of origin. Paraneoplastic disorders (PNDs) occur in approximately 75% of human cancer patients; the true incidence of PNDs in animal cancer patients is unknown. PND, which may present as signs or specific syndromes, may precede tumor diagnosis by weeks, months, or even years. Various types of PNDs, either singly or in multiples, may be associated with either benign or malignant tumors and may involve almost every organ system directly or indirectly. PNDs are significant clinical entities in animals with cancer. They can cause morbidity and mortality in affected individuals, with effects more severe than those caused by the associated tumor.

20. What is on the horizon as far as tumor markers are concerned?

One area of considerable interest involves the measurement of telomerase activity. Studies are underway to look at whether telomerase activity might serve as a marker for canine tumors.

21. What is telomerase, and what is its function?

Telomerase is an enzyme that adds new telomeric sequences to the end of chromosomal DNA. Telomeres are specific structures present at the end of linear chromosomes, and they become progressively shortened by successive cell divisions. By adding telomeric sequences, the enzyme aids in maintaining chromosomal length.

22. How will telomerase be used as a tumor marker?

Telomerase activity is undetectable in normal tissue. The results of two studies using tumor tissues of dogs showed detectable telomerase activity in more than 95% of tumor samples, with an estimated sensitivity of 92% and specificity of 86% tumor detection. One assay system, the telomere repeat amplification protocol assay, can detect telomerase in fluid samples as well as tissues obtained from solid tumors. This suggests that the assay could have significant clinical value in rapid and noninvasive diagnosis of canine tumors.

CONTROVERSY

23. Is total serum sialic acid a specific tumor marker in dogs?

For: Increased total serum sialic acid (TSA) is positively correlated with the presence of both benign and malignant tumors in dogs, but that is strongly influenced by the concentration of the acute-phase protein α1-acid glycoprotein and its influence on TSA.

Against: The nonspecificity of increases makes TSA determinations unsuitable as a tumor marker. TSA levels appear, instead, to be a general disease marker.

BIBLIOGRAPHY

1. Bell FW, Klausner JS, Hayden DW, et al: Evaluation of serum and seminal plasma markers in the diagnosis of canine prostatic disorders. J Vet Intern Med 9:149–153, 1995.
2. Biller BJ, Kitchell BE, Cadile CD: Evaluation of an assay for detecting telomerase activity in neoplastic tissues of dogs. Am J Vet Res 59:1526–1529, 1998.
3. Ferrer L, Fondevila D, Rabanal RM, et al: Immunohistochemical detection of CD31 antigen in normal and neoplastic canine epithelial cells. J Comp Pathol 112:319–326, 1995.
4. Kiupel M, Bostock D, Bergmann V: The prognostic significance of AgNOR counts and PCNA-positive cell counts in canine malignant lymphomas. J Comp Pathol 119:407–418, 1998.
5. Kwang J, Keen J, Rosati S, et al: Development and application of an antibody ELISA for the marker protein of ovine pulmonary carcinoma. Vet Immunol Immunopathol 47:323–331, 1995.
6. Lowseth LA, Gillett NA, Chang IY, et al: Detection of serum alpha-fetoprotein in dogs with hepatic tumors. J Am Vet Med Assoc 199:735–741, 1991.

10. PRINCIPLES OF SURGICAL ONCOLOGY

James A. Flanders, DVM, Dipl ACVS

1. Does surgical manipulation of a malignant tumor cause tumor spread?

This is a common concern of pet owners considering surgery for their pets with cancer. It is true that exision of a tumor may actually spread the tumor at the site of excision and may even promote cancer growth at distant sites. However, the incidence of such spread is very low, and it can be further minimized by adherence to good surgical principals.

2. What is a tumor capsule?

Most noncutaneous neoplasms are surrounded by a zone of fibrous connective tissue known as the tumor capsule. This tissue is intimately associated with the neoplasm and is the result of an inflammatory reaction between the cancerous tissue and the normal tissue around the neoplasm. Depending on the type of neoplasia, the tumor capsule can be only a few cell layers thick or several millimeters thick. Within the inner layers of the tumor capsule are microscopic pockets of neoplastic cells that represent the most recent areas of tumor expansion. Tumor excision should always include the tumor capsule to ensure that these microscopic neoplastic foci are removed along with the tumor.

3. Can contaminated instruments spread cancer in a patient?

This is the most common cause of cancer spread associated with excision of a malignant cancer. If at all possible, a tumor should be excised en bloc without incising into the tumor or into the tumor capsule (fibrous connective tissue surrounding most tumors). If surgical instruments (or a surgeon's gloves) come in contact with a tumor during excision, cancer cells will adhere to the surgical instruments. Viable cancer cells may then be spread to adjacent sites if the contaminated instruments are used to handle or incise adjacent normal tissue.

4. Can hemorrhage from a tumor cause tumor spread?

Malignant cancers usually contain a very primative, leaky vasculature. Tumor cells are often present within the vasculature of a tumor, and this permits the spread of the tumor to distant sites. It is impossible to prevent hemorrhage completely during tumor excision, but efforts should be made to identify and ligate large tumor vessels prior to transection.

5. Should a tumor site be lavaged after excision of a tumor?

Saline lavage of a tumor bed after tumor excision helps remove any residual tissue debris or clotted blood. However, experiments in mice have shown that dispersed tumor cells introduced into a wound bed firmly implant within the walls of the wound within moments. So, while lavage of a tumor bed with sterile, isotonic saline solution is a good idea to reduce inflammation during wound healing, lavage does not make up for sloppy technique during tumor handling.

6. What can be done to reduce the incidence of cancer seeding from a surgery site?

The oncologic surgeon should consider a tumor excision to be like the excision of a contaminated wound.

- Use meticulous surgical technique, delicate tissue handling, careful hemostasis, and sharp dissection whenever possible. Blunt dissection can produce more tissue damage (inflammation) and, more importantly, blunt dissection can obscure tissue planes around a tumor.

- Any instrument that comes in contact with the tumor should be set aside for the remainder of the procedure.
- Gloves should be changed before wound closure is begun.

7. What is the difference between debulking a tumor and en bloc excision of a tumor?

Debulking a tumor consists of removal of part or most of a tumor. Residual tumor remains in the affected animal. Debulking a tumor also necessitates incising within the tumor capsule and potentially contaminating surgical instruments and the surgical field with viable cancer cells. En bloc excision consists of tumor removal by exision through normal tissues surrounding the tumor. A block of normal tissue is removed with the tumor in the center of the block. The tumor capsule is not compromised, and so there is minimal chance of contaminating the wound bed with tumor cells.

8. Should a large malignant tumor be debulked prior to radiation therapy?

If a decision has been made to treat an animal's cancer with radiation therapy, a decision to debulk the neoplasm prior to radiation therapy should be made in consultation with the radiation therapist. In general, it is usually beneficial to debulk a neoplasm prior to radiation therapy if the debulking can be done with minimal morbidity. Debulking a primary tumor prior to radiation therapy is most useful if a poorly vascularized, poorly oxygenated (and therefore radioresistant) portion of the tumor is excised.

9. Should a large tumor be debulked prior to chemotherapy?

It is usually a good idea to debulk malignant tumors prior to chemotherapy. Chemotherapy is most effective against microscopic cancer. The major exception is lymphosarcoma. Tremendously enlarged lymphomatous lymph nodes can shrink rapidly when responsive to chemotherapy and surgical excision (other than biopsy) is not necessary.

10. If no adjuvant therapy (i.e., chemotherapy or radiation therapy) is planned for the management of a dog with cancer, would debulking a primary malignant tumor prolong the life of an animal with cancer?

There are few instances in which debulking a large malignant tumor would actually prolong the life of a pet. At best, debulking a pet's tumor may make the pet owner feel more comfortable that a tumor has been reduced in size, and such an approach should be considered palliative only. This may delay a decision for euthanasia, especially if a necrotic or ulcerated portion of a tumor has been excised. However, regrowth of the tumor is inevitable, and the rate of regrowth will vary with the mitotic rate of the tumor. At all times, quality of life issues are most important. A more malignant tumor (i.e., transitional cell carcinoma of the urinary bladder) will regrow more rapidly than a benign tumor (i.e., lipoma).

11. Should grossly normal local lymph nodes be excised along with a malignant tumor?

Many cancer cells that enter the circulation do so through the blood stream and bypass the lymphatic system. Many of the cancer cells that enter the lymphatics do not lodge in the lymph nodes close to the tumor. The main indication for excision of normal-appearing local lymph nodes is to allow a tumor to be staged: Histologic examination of local lymph nodes determines if microscopic disease is present. Excision of grossly normal lymph nodes does not prolong survival of cancer patients. It should also be remembered that a grossly normal lymph node may still have some useful immunologic function, as opposed to a node effaced by tumor cells, which has clearly lost the battle.

12. Does excision of metastatic nodules prolong survival?

It has recently been shown in both human and veterinary patients that resection of metastatic nodules may indeed prolong the life span of certain cancer patients. Depending on the known biologic behavior of the tumor and the patient's status, metastasectomy may be considered if the metastases are few in number and can be excised without compromising the function of the organ in which they appear. For example, resection of pulmonary metastases prolonged the life span of dogs with appendicular osteosarcoma a median of 6 months in one study. Some of these dogs had two or three separate thoracotomies to remove metastatic lesions. In human patients it has become common practice to resect hepatic metastases from many different primary cancers. Hepatic metastasectomy may be found to be an effective means of prolonging the survival of veterinary patients with certain abdominal cancers as well. However, a large study evaluating the success of this procedure in dogs and cats has not yet been published.

13. Does surgical removal of a primary tumor increase the rate of growth of metastases?

It has been shown in numerous experimental studies that removal of a primary tumor can result in the increased rate of growth of metastases. Some primary tumors produce proteins, such as antiangiogenic factors, that limit the growth of metastatic lesions. If the primary tumor is removed, the regulatory factors are no longer produced in the body of the cancer patient and the metastases can grow rapidly.

The possibility that metastases may grow more rapidly after the excision of a primary tumor is not a reason to avoid primary tumor excision. It is not common to see rapid growth of metastases after primary tumor excision. In most cases, the benefits of excision of a primary tumor far outweigh the small risk of increased rate of metastasis. Research is currently being done to determine which primary tumors are releasing factors that may be controlling metastasis growth; however, dozens of factors that inhibit satellite tumor growth have been discovered, and the interplay of these factors is quite complex.

14. How can a surgeon determine that adequate margins of normal tissue have been included in a tumor excision?

It is obvious that the greater the amount of adjacent normal tissue excised with a neoplasm, the better the chance of preventing local recurrence. However, in many cases, the presence of vital structures near a tumor, or the inability to close the wound if large margins are excised, prevents the surgeon from including large amounts of surrounding normal tissue in a tumor excision. In general, at least 1 cm of normal tissue outside of the tumor capsule (in every direction) should be included with any tumor excision to consider the tumor completely excised. It must be remembered that tumors are three-dimensional, and attention should be paid to obtaining appropriate deep margins during tumor excision. At least one tissue plane deep to the tumor should be included in the excision.

Some neoplasms, such as mast cell tumors, require larger margins because they produce skip metastases. Skip metastases are microscopic foci of cancer cells that appear in local tissue outside of the tumor capsule. Mast cell tumors may produce skip metastases up to 2 cm beyond the primary tumor, so margins of at least 3 cm are recommended as routine for most cell tumors.

15. How is surgery used to assist in clinical staging of a neoplasm?

A biopsy, whether done with a biopsy needle or a scalpel blade, is always included among the procedures necessary to stage neoplasia properly. Histologic analysis of the biopsy provides information about the tumor type and the tumor grade. Biopsy of adjacent or draining lymph nodes provides information about the spread of the neoplasm.

Surgery may also be necessary to stage cancer in animals with deep tumors. In such cases, surgery may be needed to supplement information about local tissue invasion by the neoplasm that could not be completely obtained by noninvasive imaging modalities. Information about the invasiveness and the spread of a cancer is critical for the oncologist to plan therapy and provide as accurate a prognosis as possible. Such findings also allow the owner to make an informed decision about further therapy for an animal with cancer.

16. Why should a biopsy of a tumor be done before a large, deep, or invasive tumor is excised?

Biopsy of an easily accessible tumor is a minor procedure that can be done rapidly and with minimal morbidity. Deeply situated tumors (abdominal or thoracic) can often be safely biopsied without major surgery by using ultrasound guidance. By knowing the biopsy results, the surgeon can give the pet owner a more accurate prognosis prior to major surgery. Furthermore, the surgeon may plan a more aggressive surgery (i.e., mandibulectomy or limb amputation rather than lumpectomy) if the biopsy results indicate that the tumor is malignant.

17. What is the best way to biopsy a small (less than 5 cm), superficial tumor?

If the tumor is easily accessible and easily excisable, remove it completely (with adequate margins) and submit the entire excised sample, properly prepared and fixed, for histologic analysis.

18. What is the best way to biopsy a large tumor?

If a large tumor can be completely excised (i.e., a large, superficial lipoma), remove it completely and submit a portion of the mass for histologic evaluation. Otherwise, a superficial tumor may be biopsied by scalpel excison of a small wedge of tissue. If the tumor is deep to the skin, a needle biopsy device may be used. The best results are obtained if the device removes a core of tissue at least 1 mm in diameter (larger than a hypodermic needle). If at all possible, the center of the tumor should be sampled, and several samples should be submitted for histologic analysis. Avoid the perimeter of a tumor because this area may contain inflammatory cells in the tumor capsule and will not provide an accurate diagnosis.

19. How can ultrasound guidance aid in the safe biopsy of deep abdominal or thoracic tumors?

Needle biopsy devices (and hypodermic needles) passed percutaneously into a body cavity can be visualized with ultrasound. Ultrasound guidance can allow the accurate biopsy of many deep tumors, such as renal masses, hepatic tumors, and mediastinal masses. Some tumors, such as pancreatic or intestinal masses, may not be amenable to ultrasound-guided biopsy because gas in the intestinal tract creates interfering artifact. Gastric, esophageal, and intramural colonic tumors are best visualized and biopsied using endoscopic equipment.

20. Should a biopsy site be included in later tumor excision?

If a needle biopsy device is passed through normal tissue to obtain a biopsy, it is possible that the biopsy tract can become contaminated with tumor cells as the biopsy device is withdrawn. These tumor cells may attach and grow within the biopsy tract. Therefore, it is highly advisable to include the biopsy site in the excision (and to plan your biopsy route so that the tract will be easy to excise!).

21. How should a biopsy or excised tumor be handled prior to submission to a pathologist?

The more tissue that you submit for biopsy, the more likely the pathologist will be able to make an accurate diagnosis. If an excised tumor is submitted, it is very helpful to paint the edges of the excision with an indelible ink such as india ink. A tumor margin marking kit containing several colors of ink is also available. If the histologic analysis shows that tumor cells extend to an inked margin, the surgeon knows that complete tumor excision was not accomplished.

It is very important that the tissue be completely fixed in 10% formalin prior to submission. If india ink was used to mark the margins, make sure that the ink is dry before immersion of the biopsy sample in formalin. If the tissue submitted is greater than 1 cm³, it should be partially sliced into 1-cm segments to enhance formalin penetration.

Provide the pathologist with a careful description of the tumor and a brief clinical history. Time spent enlightening the pathologist about the tumor is usually rewarded with a more complete histologic report.

22. Is laser surgery superior to conventional scalpel surgery or electrosurgery in cancer patients?

A laser should be considered a highly sophisticated means of making an incision. Lasers can be adjusted to make very fine incisions, and they can provide coagulation simultaneous with incising. This can reduce the amount of hemorrhage from small blood vessels during cancer surgery. Certain types of laser energy can be transmitted through fiberoptic cables, making it possible to do endoscopically guided laser surgery. Lasers can be defocused to allow fulguration of a tumor bed, similar to what can done with electrosurgery. Lasers incise tissue without coming in contact with the tissue. This noncontact surgery reduces the possiblity of contaminating adjacent healthy tissue with surgical instruments. However, lasers do not possess any special anticancer properties. A tumor that is incompletely excised using a laser is just as likely to recur as a tumor incompletely excised with a scalpel blade.

23. What are the principles of cryosurgery?

Cryosurgery consists of rapidly freezing a tumor using liquid nitrogen and then allowing the tumor to thaw slowly. Usually, two freeze-thaw cycles are used during each treatment. For the procedure to be effective, the tumor must be frozen solid to a temperature of at least –40°C. This will ensure that ice crystals form within the tumor. During a slow thaw, the ice crystals move and change shape within the tumor cells. This damages cell membranes and causes the release of degradative enzymes from within the tumor cells (and from adjacent frozen normal tissue). Cancerous tissue is more sensitive than normal tissue to damage from freezing because the inefficient vascular supply of tumors allows more complete freezing and prevents rapid thawing.

After two complete freeze-thaw cycles, the tumor slowly necroses over 5 to 14 days. Liquid nitrogen can be applied as a liquid or by using cotton-tipped applicators, but specialized devices that make use of metal probes and thermocouples to measure the temperature in the frozen area are much more effective.

24. What are the benefits of cryosurgery?

No incisions are made when cryosurgery is used to treat cancer, and therefore no wound bed is created immediately and no sutures are needed. Cryosurgery may be used to treat some tumors that are not surgically excisable, especially broad-based, superficial oral tumors. Cryosurgery should be avoided in areas where unrecognized freezing beyond the scope of accurate measurement could lead to fistula formation. It can also be used to treat multiple small tumors, such as papillomas, without requiring local anesthesia, incisions, or sutures.

25. What are the drawbacks to cryosurgical treatment of cancer?

Cryosurgery is usually not faster than traditional surgery. Freezing a tumor larger than 2 cm into a solid ball of ice requires 3 to 10 minutes. The tumor must then be allowed to slowly thaw (10 to 20 minutes), and then the freeze-thaw cycle must be repeated. Anesthesia is required for cryosurgical treatment of tumors bigger than a few millimeters to provide analgesia and to prevent motion during the procedure.

The greatest detriment to cryosurgical treatment of cancer is the postoperative necrosis of the tumor 5 to 14 days following treatment. During this time the necrotic tumor may have a bad odor, an unpleasant appearance, and bleed. The pet owner must be carefully prepared for this phase of therapy.

The surgeon should anticipate potential complications associated with healing of the necrotic area induced by cryotherapy. For example, an oronasal fistula may form if the hard palate or maxilla is involved in the freezing of oral tumor. Excessive wound contraction may ensue after treatment of a large cutaneous tumor.

In general, cryosurgery is no more effective than traditional surgery for cancer treatment. Complete necrosis of a malignant tumor treated with cryotherapy may provide effective local control, but metastatic spread is not curtailed.

26. What surgical options are available if a tumor regrows at the primary site?

Tumor regrowth at the site of the original excision indicates that gross or microscopic amounts of cancer tissue remained within or adjacent to the wound bed of the original surgery. If a tumor regrows at the primary site and a careful evaluation of the patient reveals no evidence of metastasis, further therapy can be recommended. If the pet owner will consent to further cancer surgery, it is certainly better to initiate the surgery as soon as a recurrence is noticed and the recurrent tumor is small than to wait until the regrowth has attained a large size.

Usually, surgical excision of a recurrent tumor is more difficult than the initial surgery. Because the initial tumor excision usually includes incision into tissue planes beyond the tumor, cancer regrowth can advance through compromised tissue layers and grow deeper in the patient's body. Furthermore, it is often difficult to differentiate scar tissue from recurrent tumor tissue; therefore, a greater amount of tissue must be excised during the second surgery to ensure that no cancerous tissue is left behind.

Chemotherapy, radiation therapy, or a combination of both therapies should be strongly considered if a tumor has recurred at a primary surgical site. Nonsurgical therapy could be used as an adjunct or an alternative to repeated surgical therapy of recurrent cancer.

BIBLIOGRAPHY

1. Baker DG, Masterson TM, Pace R, et al: The influence of the surgical wound on local tumor recurrence. Surgery 106:525–532, 1989.
2. Crane SW: Surgical lasers. In Statter D (ed): Textbook of Small Animal Surgery, 2nd ed. Philadelphia, WB Saunders, 1993, pp 197–203.
3. Fisher B, Gunduz N, Coyle J, et al: Presence of a growth-stimulation factor in serum following primary tumor removal in mice. Cancer Res 49:1996–2001, 1989.
4. Gilson SD: Clinical management of the regional lymph node. Vet Clin North Am Small Anim Pract 25:149–167, 1995.
5. Gilson SD, Stone EA: Surgically induced tumor seeding in eight dogs and two cats. J Am Vet Med Assoc 196:1811–1815, 1990.
6. McEntee MC: Principles of adjunct radiotherapy and chemotherapy. Vet Clin North Am Small Anim Pract 25:133–148, 1995.
7. O'Brien MG, Straw RC, Withrow SJ, et al: Resection of pulmonary metastases in canine osteosarcoma: 36 cases (1983–1992). Vet Surg 22:105–109, 1993.
8. Rochat MC, Mann FA, Pace LW, et al: Identification of surgical biopsy borders by use of india ink. J Am Vet Med Assoc 201:873–878, 1992.
9. Salisbury, SK: Principles of oncologic surgery. In Morrison WB (ed): Cancer in Dogs and Cats. Baltimore, Williams & Wilkins, 1998, pp 223–240.
10. Soderstrom MJ, Gilson SD: Principles of surgical oncology. Vet Clin North Am Small Anim Pract 25:97–110, 1995.
11. Withrow SJ, Grenier TR, Liska WD: Cryosurgery: Veterinary considerations. Cryosurgery 11:271–282, 1975.

11. RADIATION ONCOLOGY

G. Neal Mauldin, DVM, Dipl ACVIM, Dipl ACVR

1. How does radiation therapy work?

Therapeutic radiation is radiation that is of high enough energy to result in ionizations when it interacts with matter. These ionizing "packets" of energy, called photons, may either arise from radioactive decay (cobalt 60) or through the production of x-rays (orthovoltage, linear accelerator). The term *ionization* refers to the fact that an atom has had an electron ejected from one of its outer shells, leading to a highly unstable state. These ionizations result in the formation of reactive free radical species and in the direct damage of DNA. Free radical generation is the most important component of cellular cytotoxicity due to radiation therapy. The formation of reactive oxygen species and hydroxyl radicals, among others, results in the formation of DNA cross-linkages, which interfere with DNA replication and cellular division. If the damage is severe enough, the tumor cell should die when it attempts to divide into daughter cells. However, much of the free radical damage caused by radiation therapy can be repaired if enough time elapses between treatments.

2. Do cancer cells always have to attempt division before they manifest the effects of radiation?

No, some cells undergo apoptosis when exposed to even small doses of radiation. This means that irradiation will trigger cellular mechanisms of programmed cell death. The most important clinical example of a cell type that responds to radiation via apoptosis is the lymphocyte. Tumors arising from lymphoid cells (lymphoma, multiple myeloma, plasmacytoma) tend to have a very dramatic and rapid response to even a single dose of radiation.

3. What kinds of radiation generators are available to veterinarians?

Most radiation therapy in veterinary oncology is delivered as external beam therapy. This means that a machine is used to generate a radiation beam that is then directed toward the patient.

Orthovoltage units are older, lower-energy radiation therapy units that are still used in veterinary oncology. Orthovoltage machines are not suitable for treating deeply seated tumors and typically cause more severe cutaneous reactions in patients because of their poor penetrating ability.

Megavoltage radiation therapy units are high-energy machines (by definition more than 1 million electron volts) that have much better penetrating ability than orthovoltage units. Additionally, megavoltage machines cause fewer cutaneous reactions because they actually pass through the superficial layers of the skin before depositing their maximum energy. Examples of megavoltage machines used in veterinary oncology include cobalt 60 units and linear accelerators.

Electrons can also be used as a therapeutic form of radiation and are available from some forms of linear accelerators. Electrons are characterized by extremely limited penetration depths because they are charged particles. Electrons are especially useful for treating superficial tumors that lie over deeper critical structures that should be protected from radiation.

4. What is brachytherapy?

Brachytherapy is the placement of radioactive sources within the tumor volume to provide a high dose of radiation to the tumor while sparing normal surrounding tissue. Brachytherapy requires appropriate equipment for manipulation of the radioactive sources and proper isolation facilities for the patients after implantation. Animals treated with radioactive implants do pose an exposure risk to their handlers.

5. What is a radionucleide?

A radionucleide is a radioactive compound that may be administered by injection. Radionucleides may be useful for both diagnostic and therapeutic purposes. For example, technetium 99m is used to perform bone, lung, and renal scans, and iodine 131 is used to treat hyperthyroidism.

6. What is fractionation?

The total dose of radiation to be delivered to a patient is broken down into multiple small doses called fractions. These doses of radiation are expressed in units called Grays (gy), although an older unit known as the rad (radiation absorbed dose) is still sometimes used.

Fractionation permits the radiation oncologist to deliver a large total dose of radiation to the tumor while allowing time between fractions for the normal tissue within the field to repair some of the radiation damage. It is important to remember that neoplastic cells can also repair some of the radiation damage, so there should not be too much time between fractions. In veterinary oncology, most fractionation schemes are based on 5-day (Monday through Friday) or 3-day (Monday, Wednesday, Friday) per week treatment protocols.

7. What are the four R's of radiotherapy?

Repopulation: refers to cellular proliferation following the repair of sublethal radiation damage. In theory, neoplastic cells are less efficient at repair than normal tissues.

Redistribution: refers to the fact that cells will redistribute themselves to different parts of the cell cycle, some of which are more responsive to radiation damage than others. For instance, cells in the M phase of mitosis are the most sensitive to radiation, while those in S phase (synthesis) are the most resistant.

Reoxygenation: refers to the fact that normally hypoxic cells will gain access to the vasculature as the more radiosensitive well-oxygenated cells die following radiation exposure. Because oxygen is a potent radiation sensitizer, reoxygenation is an important component of the radiocuability of any tumor that contains hypoxic regions.

Repair: refers to the ability of cells to repair sublethal radiation damage between fractions.

8. What cellular characteristics make a tumor most responsive to radiation therapy?

Damage to DNA is the primary cause of cell death following exposure to ionizing radiation, and cell division is necessary for radiation damage to be expressed in most instances. Additionally, certain phases of the cell cycle are more sensitive than others to the effects of radiation. This means that tumors that are rapidly growing (short T1/2) and that have a high growth fraction (low numbers of cells in the resting phase of the cell cycle, G_0) will be the most sensitive to radiation therapy. Large, bulky tumors tend to have many cells in G_0 as well as having significant areas of hypoxia due to an inadequate blood supply. These factors combine to make radiation therapy a poor choice as the primary therapy for large, slow-growing tumors.

9. What are the goals of radiation therapy?

Radiation therapy can be used as curative or palliative therapy. Curative therapy is usually reserved for patients that have locally aggressive, nonmetastatic tumors. Cutaneous mast cell tumors and soft tissue sarcomas are good examples of tumors that can be cured with radiation therapy. Palliative therapy is appropriate for patients that have systemic tumor spread and also have some local complications of their tumor that may be alleviated by radiation. Alleviation of pain secondary to bone metastases, or treatment of an osteosarcoma in a patient that is not a candidate for amputation, are examples of the palliative applications of radiotherapy.

10. What is the most important step in treating a patient with external beam radiation therapy?

The most important part of treating a patient with radiation therapy is an accurate staging and assessment of tumor volume. Most tumors will respond to radiation therapy, but a geographic miss will lead to local tumor recurrence. The increasing availability of cross-sectional imaging, such as computed tomography and magnetic resonance imaging scans, has greatly improved our ability to define tumor volumes in our patients. After the tumor volume is accurately determined, the next major hurdle is appropriate radiation dose delivery. As with imaging, veterinary access to radiation therapy treatment-planning computers is improving, resulting in better dose delivery to our patients.

11. Can radiation therapy be used as a single-treatment modality?

Radiation therapy is rarely used as primary therapy. For reasons discussed above, the combination of radiation and surgery is just about ideal for treating locally aggressive tumors. Radiation therapy is not an appropriate primary therapy for pets with systemic tumors.

12. If I have resected a tumor with inadequate margins, should I refer that patient for radiation therapy immediately or wait until I see signs of recurrence?

The best time to treat an animal with residual microscopic disease is as soon as the surgical incision has healed. In this situation, the residual tumor burden should be very low, and the remaining tumor cells would be expected to be well oxygenated. If you do wait until recurrence has occurred, a second surgery should be performed, if possible, before radiation therapy is initiated.

13. What tumor types are most appropriately treated with radiation therapy?

Radiation therapy is most appropriate for tumors that are locally aggressive but have a low incidence of metastasis. Examples of such tumors include cutaneous grade II mast cell tumors, the soft tissue sarcomas, and nasal tumors. Metastatic tumors are usually only treated with radiation in a palliative setting.

14. What is the dose-limiting toxicity of radiation?

The dose-limiting toxicity of radiation is always the normal tissue within the radiation field. The total dose of radiation that can be safely delivered to a tumor is determined by the radiation tolerance of the most sensitive tissue within the field. The tissues most sensitive to radiation therapy include gastrointestinal mucosa, bone marrow, lung, kidney, and the lens of the eye. Resistant tissues include muscle, bone, connective tissue, and peripheral nerve.

15. What does *acute radiation toxicity* mean?

This term is used to describe radiation effects that occur during or shortly after a course of radiation therapy. Examples include radiodermatitis, mucositis, or acute keratoconjunctivitis sicca. These acute reactions are generally self-limiting and are treated symptomatically. Acute toxicities occur because of the clonogens present in the normal tissue, which typically have growth characteristics similar to cancer cells. This suggests that acute toxicities due to radiation damage of normal tissue clonogens mimic the damage being done to tumor cells.

16. What does *delayed radiation toxicity* mean?

This term is used to describe radiation effects that occur several months after a course of radiation therapy is complete. Such delayed toxicities may present in an acute or peracute manner months to years after the completion of a course of radiotherapy. Examples include bone necrosis, second tumor formation, muscle fibrosis, radiation pneumonitis, and central nervous system infarct. The delayed toxicities of radiation therapy are the ones most likely to result in life-threatening complications.

17. What toxicities are commonly associated with radiation therapy?

Fortunately, most of the toxicities seen with radiation therapy are of the acute and self-limiting variety. Radiodermatitis is the most common toxicity seen. This is due to damage of epithelial clonogens in the skin and results in a moist dermatitis and desquamation. Topical drying agents and antibacterial or steroid creams in a nonocclusive base work well. Similar reactions may be seen if the oral mucosa is irradiated, resulting in anorexia. The acute skin and mucosal reactions usually resolve within 10 to 14 days following the completion of the radiotherapy protocol. Acute keratoconjunctivitis sicca may be seen if the lacrimal gland is in the radiation field and may be a permanent change. Patients receiving ocular or periocular radiation need to have their tear production monitored. Fortunately, nausea, vomiting, and diarrhea are uncommon toxicities in veterinary patients, but they may be seen if a significant portion of the abdomen is irradiated.

18. Should a patient showing signs of discomfort due to acute radiation toxicity be rested until some of the clinical signs resolve?

Radiation damage to acutely responding tissue clonogens closely mimics the damage being done to tumor cells. Resting a patient to allow the signs of acute toxicity to resolve will also allow the tumor cells to repair some of the radiation damage they have suffered and may negatively affect the outcome of therapy. As a general rule, acute radiation toxicity is not a reason to discontinue or delay therapy—unless the patient is severely affected or systemically ill.

19. Can a patient with recurrence of their cancer in a previously irradiated field be retreated?

This depends on the amount of time that has passed between the first radiation treatment and recurrence.

If a tumor recurs within the radiation field a few weeks to months after completing a course of radiation therapy, one should suspect that the tumor is resistant to radiation therapy or that an inadequate dose was delivered. The benefit of reirradiation in these patients is questionable, and reirradiation should be undertaken with extreme caution to prevent undesirable radiation toxicity.

Tumors that recur outside of the radiation field are due to a geographic miss and poor tumor staging or treatment planning. These types of marginal recurrence can be treated, but great care must be taken to avoid excessive doses in the overlapping treatment fields.

If the tumor recurs many months to years after the initial course of radiation therapy, retreatment is a feasible consideration. The dose delivered will need to be modified somewhat, but it is possible to effectively reirradiate a recurrent tumor and regain some measure of local control.

20. Other than surgery, what treatment modalities can be used as an adjunct to radiation therapy?

Other treatment modalities that can be used with radiation therapy include chemotherapy, hyperthermia, and radiation sensitizers. Some chemotherapeutic agents have potent antitumor activity as well as improve the effects of radiation therapy. This setting provides a dual benefit from the chemotherapeutic agent: primary antitumor activity and radiation sensitization. Hyperthermia is a modality that holds theoretical promise as an adjunct to radiation therapy. However, there are still many technical issues surrounding the consistent and uniform delivery of heat to neoplastic tissues. Radiation sensitizers are agents that, while having no inherent antitumor activity, potentiate the cytotoxicity of radiation.

CONTROVERSIES

21. When combining radiation therapy with surgery, should the radiation be done before or after the surgical resection?

This is an area of active investigation in the veterinary radiation oncology community. The advantages to preoperative radiation include a smaller radiation field, better definition of the tumor volume, and lack of postoperative vascular compromise, or hypoxia. The primary disadvantage to preoperative therapy is that the surgery must be performed in an acutely irradiated field, and wound complications are possible.

Because postoperative radiation is performed after the tumor is resected and the sutures are removed, wound complications are uncommon. However, postoperative radiation requires that you deliver radiation to a poorly defined target volume based on surgical scar, comparative cross-section images, or radiopaque markers placed by the surgeons at the time of the resection.

It is currently unknown if one technique is better than the other. At the present time, most radiation therapy in veterinary oncology is performed postoperatively, primarily because veterinary patients are usually referred after the initial resection has been performed.

22. Which fractionation protocol is best—3 days or 5 days per week?

Traditionally, most veterinary radiation therapy protocols follow a 3-day per week fractionation scheme. However, this is based on convenience and the fact that veterinary patients must be anesthetized for each treatment rather than on any sound radiobiologic principles. Five-day per week protocols are becoming more common and may have the benefit of decreasing the amount of time available for repopulation of tumor cells and repair of radiation damage between fractions. However, there are no controlled studies to suggest that 5-day per week protocols are, in fact, superior to 3-day per week protocols. As these data become available, it may become obvious which fractionation scheme is superior.

BIBLIOGRAPHY

1. Burk RL, Giel T: A selected review of the physics of radiation therapy. Vet Clin North Am Small Anim Pract 1997;27(1):7–20.
2. Harris D, King GK, Bergman PJ: Radiation therapy toxicities. Vet Clin North Am Small Anim Pract 1997;27(1):37–46.
3. Mauldin GN: Radiation therapy: A radiation oncologist's point of view. Vet Clin North Am Small Anim Pract 1996;26(1):17–27.
4. McEntee MC: Principles of adjunct radiotherapy and chemotherapy. Vet Clin North Am Small Anim Pract 1995;25(1):133–48.
5. McNiel EA, LaRue SM: Principles of adjunctive therapy. Clin Tech Small Anim Pract 1998;13(1): 33–7.
6. Siegel S, Cronin KI: Palliative radiotherapy. Vet Clin North Am Small Anim Pract 1997;27(1):149–55.
7. Thrall DE: Biologic basis of radiation therapy. Vet Clin North Am Small Anim Pract 1997;27(1): 21–35.
8. Thrall DE, Ibbott GS: Physics and treatment planning. Semin Vet Med Surg (Small Anim) 1995;10(3): 135–47.

12. THEORY OF CHEMOTHERAPY

Ruthanne Chun, DVM, *Dipl* ACVIM

1. Why should I use chemotherapy for my cancer patients?

Cancer is a common problem that has been reported to be the main medical reason for euthanasia in dogs. Many clients actively seek therapies for their companion animals with cancer. As people become more knowledgeable about the available treatment modalities to treat humans, they will demand more sophisticated treatment options for their pets. Provided they have an understanding of the treatment goals, numbers of visits required, and costs, most owners are appreciative of honest attempts to control disease and prolong the lives of their pets.

2. How can I justify using toxic drugs to treat dogs and cats with cancer?

Although we use many of the same chemotherapeutics as we use to treat humans with cancer, we see much less toxicity in our patients than is traditionally associated with chemotherapy in people. Veterinary protocols tend to use lower doses and less aggressive combinations of drugs than most human chemotherapy protocols. Quality of life is as much of a goal as disease control; most dogs and cats undergoing chemotherapy have a normal quality of life.

3. How does chemotherapy work?

In general, chemotherapeutic agents damage DNA and result in cellular death or inability to undergo mitosis. Specific drugs have different mechanisms of action. Drugs are grouped based on their mechanism of action. Categories of commonly used chemotherapeutics include alkylating agents (cyclophosphamide, chlorambucil, melphalan, lomustine); antitumor antibiotics (doxorubicin, mitoxantrone, actinomycin D); plant alkaloids (vincristine, vinblastine); hormones (prednisone); antimetabolites (methotrexate, cytosine arabinoside); and miscellaneous drugs (asparaginase, cisplatin, carboplatin).

4. Do I really need to know the mechanism of action of each chemotherapy agent I am using?

Ideally, yes. To maximize antitumor effect, drugs with the same mechanism of action should not be used in combination against a tumor.

5. Do I also need to know how each drug is eliminated?

Again, the answer is ideally, yes. Some animals with cancer will have preexisting organ failure or will have organ failure secondary to their tumor. Most chemotherapy drugs are activated or eliminated through the kidneys or liver. Doses of drugs may need to be decreased in the face of organ failure.

6. How do you know what drugs work against a certain tumor type?

The drug development process includes screening potential anticancer drugs against a wide range of neoplasms, both in tissue culture and in laboratory animals. When a drug is being evaluated for clinical potential, there are three basic phases of testing. Phase I is a dose escalation study, where groups of patients are treated with progressively higher doses of the drug until unacceptable toxicity occurs. Phase II uses the drug at the maximally tolerated dose and evaluates tumor response either against a specific tumor type or against a wide range of malignancies. Phase III is when the drug is known to have activity against a specific tumor type, and the new treatment is actively compared to previously existing treatment protocols. After Phase II, we know whether a drug can induce a remission against a certain tumor type. After Phase III, we know how the new treatment compares with other treatment options.

7. When is chemotherapy indicated?

Chemotherapy is indicated when an animal has systemic (i.e., lymphoma) or metastatic (i.e., osteosarcoma, hemangiosarcoma, some mast cell tumors) disease. It may also be indicated for localized disease if surgery or radiation therapy are not feasible options.

8. Why do some protocols use multiple drugs when others rely on only one?

Drugs need to undergo much testing before we know if they work against a certain type of cancer. Drugs should only be combined when we know that each individual drug has activity against the tumor in question. Many chemotherapy drugs are known to be effective against lymphoma, and therefore these patients are often placed on multiple-drug protocols. In theory, using multiple drugs with different mechanisms of action is more likely to control disease than using only one drug.

9. Why does chemotherapy not work in some patients?

Chemotherapy drugs may not be able to penetrate all sites of the body equally, resulting in inadequate exposure; sites such as the brain or skin may be sequestered regions where metastatic tumor cells can be successful in forming a clinically significant lesion. At the cellular level, drug resistance can be classified as intrinsic or acquired. Although there are many different ways in which drug resistance arises, one of the most common forms is due to the presence of P-glycoprotein. P-glycoprotein is a pump that sits on the cellular membrane. In normal individuals, P-glycoprotein is important in keeping toxins outside of cells. In malignant neoplasms, P-glycoprotein is overexpressed and, even though the drugs are able to enter the cell, they are recognized and pumped back out again. Unfortunately, P-glycoprotein is not drug specific; its activity confers cellular resistance to multiple structurally unrelated chemotherapy drugs.

10. Why is variation in any tumor cells important?

Chemotherapy resistance is the bane of the medical oncologist. By the time most cancers are detected, there are more than 1 billion cells within the mass. Due to the unstable nature of cancer cells, genetic differences (also known as tumor heterogeneity) will exist in this new mass. Tumor heterogeneity means that not all cancer cells are equal in their abilities. Some cells will have natural resistance to chemotherapy. Other cells will have the special abilities to break down extracellular matrix, escape notice by the immune system, or produce growth factors that will promote metastases and tumor growth.

11. What are the adverse effects of chemotherapy, and why do they occur?

The general adverse effects of chemotherapy are myelosuppression (primarily neutrophils and platelets), gastrointestinal (GI) upset (manifested as inappetence, diarrhea, or vomiting) and alopecia.

Myelosuppression occurs because chemotherapy damages cells that are growing and dividing rapidly. Neutrophils and platelets have short circulating half-lives and must be continuously replaced by new cells from the bone marrow. It is in the bone marrow that rapidly dividing cells are killed. Red blood cells have a life span of 70 to 120 days (cats and dogs, respectively), and therefore a mild anemia may occur with chronic chemotherapy administration.

GI upset occurs for a variety of reasons. GI epithelial cells replace themselves every 3 to 5 days. Therefore, onset of diarrhea secondary to decreased absorptive capacity is usually delayed by 3 to 5 days after treatment. Inappetence, nausea, and vomiting arise because of stimulation of the central chemoreceptor trigger zone (CRTZ), either directly or via distention and ileus of the GI tract, which activates vagal efferents that connect to the CRTZ.

Alopecia is associated with chemotherapy administration because hair follicles are constantly growing and causing active hair growth. The only breeds in which alopecia is of concern are those with continuously growing hair, such as Maltese and some terriers. However, both dogs and cats continuously replace their whiskers. Animals that are on extended chemotherapy protocols may lose their whiskers.

12. How do I manage chemotherapy-induced neutropenia?

All animals treated with chemotherapy should have a complete blood count evaluated 1 week after therapy. If the neutrophil count is low (less than 2500 cells/µl), no chemotherapy should be administered that week. If the neutrophil count is less than 1000 cells/µl and the patient is not febrile, broad-spectrum oral antibiotic therapy (i.e., a cephalosporin or a trimethoprim-sulfa combination) is indicated. If the neutrophil count is less than 1000 cells/µl and the patient is febrile, broad-spectrum intravenous antibiotic therapy (i.e., ampicillin and enrofloxacin) is indicated, as are urine and blood cultures.

13. How do I manage chemotherapy-induced GI upset?

Most cases of GI upset following chemotherapy are mild and self-limiting. If necessary, animals may be fasted for 24 hours or may be fed a bland diet of boiled rice mixed with boiled chicken or beef. Rarely, animals will have intractable vomiting or diarrhea. In these cases, hospitalization for intravenous fluid therapy and antiemetics is necessary.

14. Based on the answer to question 11, are there specific adverse effects of concern for each individual drug?

There are several specific adverse effects that are important to keep in mind when using these agents.

Perivascular irritation or sloughing may occur following extravasation of vincristine, vinblastine, and doxorubicin (or other antitumor antibiotic-type agents). There are no specific antidotes for these drugs. After extravasation, be sure that these drugs are given through a perfectly placed intravenous catheter.

Cardiac toxicity is a cumulative problem with doxorubicin, typically arising after six doses. Dogs with preexisiting cardiomyopathy should not be given doxorubicin.

Sterile hemorrhagic cystitis arises secondary to cyclophosphamide therapy. It may occur after chronic therapy or after a single bolus dose. Like perivascular irritation, there is no antidote for this problem. Owners must be advised to let their dog outside to urinate frequently for 2 days after cyclophosphamide therapy. Some protocols use cyclophosphamide concurrently with prednisone, which helps minimize the chances of sterile hemorrhagic cystitis by keeping the patient polyuric.

Allergic reactions have been reported during doxorubicin administration and within 30 minutes of asparaginase therapy. Dogs should be monitored for urticaria, hyperemia, or vomiting. Cats may develop respiratory distress or vomiting. Should these signs arise during doxorubicin administration, stop giving the drug and treat the patient with diphenhydramine and dexamethasone (as you would a vaccine reaction). Chemotherapy may be initiated as a slower intravenous bolus following dissipation of the allergic reaction. Animals having allergic reactions should be premedicated with diphenhydramine and dexamethasone before subsequent treatments with that drug.

Finally, cisplatin and 5-fluorouracil are **fatal to cats** and should not be used in this species.

15. Is it safe to start chemotherapy if my patient is still healing from the biopsy site or the site of surgical excision?

In most situations it is appropriate to initiate chemotherapy after surgery so long as there is not a lot of tension at the surgical site. Although chemotherapy may delay wound healing, it is rarely a clinically significant effect. One clinical example is appendicular osteosarcoma, for which chemotherapy is initiated within 24 hours of limb amputation. There are no reports of delayed wound healing or increased infection rates in this patient population.

16. What safety precautions do I need to take when I am working with chemotherapy?

When in doubt, common sense is a good guide. At a minimum, wear a clean buttoned-up laboratory coat and chemotherapy administration gloves. These gloves are thicker than regular latex examination gloves, and they are also impermeable to chemotherapeutic agents. Chemotherapy drugs should be stored well away from other medications, and they should never be in the same refrigerator as food items. When reconstituting and drawing up these drugs into a syringe, a laminar flow hood is ideal. However, chemotherapy safety valves are available to help diminish the risk of aerosolization. These valves have a sharp pin that is inserted into the drug vial, a filter that catches aerosolized drug, and an attachment for the syringe.

17. Do I need a special license to purchase and administer chemotherapy drugs?

No.

18. Do owners need to worry about chemotherapy drug in the urine or feces of their pet?

No studies have ever shown problems with owners of dogs or cats treated with chemotherapy. However, chemotherapy drugs are eliminated in urine and feces for up to 48 hours after the drugs are given. We advise our clients to wear gloves when cleaning up after their pet for the first 48 hours, just to err on the side of caution.

BIBLIOGRAPHY

1. Ban T: Pleiotropic, multidrug-resistant phenotype and P-glycoprotein: A review. Chemotherapy 38:191–196, 1992.
2. Bergman PJ, MacEwen EG, Kurzman ID, et al: Amputation and carboplatin for treatment of dogs with osteosarcoma: 48 cases (1991 to 1993). J Vet Intern Med 10:76–81, 1996.
3. Cornell K, Waters DJ: Impaired wound healing in the cancer patient: Effects of cytotoxic therapy and pharmacologic modulation by growth factors. Vet Clin North Am Small Anim Pract 25:111–131, 1995.
4. Henry CJ, Marks SL, Tyler JW: Comparison of chemotherapy safety procedures used in veterinary teaching hospitals and human oncology centers. J Am Vet Med Assoc 209:974–976, 1996.
5. Jain RK: Barriers to drug delivery in solid tumors. Sci Am 271:58–65, 1994.
6. Marks SL, Cook AK, Griffey S, et al: Dietary modulation of methotrexate-induced enteritis in cats. Am J Vet Res 58:989–996, 1997.
7. Moore A: Recent advances in chemotherapy for nonlymphoid malignant neoplasms. Compend Cont Educ 15:1039–1052, 1993.
8. Slater MR, Barton CL, Rogers KS, et al: Factors affecting treatment decisions and satisfaction of owners of cats with cancer. J Am Vet Med Assoc 208:1248–1252, 1996.
9. Stewart J, Gorman NT: Multi-drug resistance genes in the management of neoplastic disease. J Vet Intern Med 5:239–247, 1991.

13. CHEMOTHERAPEUTIC AGENTS

Carolyn Henry, DVM, MS, Dipl ACVIM

1. What chemotherapy drug dosages should be adjusted for patients with hepatic disease?

Doxorubicin, vincristine, and vinblastine dosages should be reduced in patients with hepatic disease. In general, a dosage reduction of 50% is recommended for the first dose when bilirubin is above 1.5 mg/100 ml. Subsequent dose escalation can be performed if the initial treatment is well tolerated.

2. What chemotherapy drug dosages should be adjusted for patients with renal disease?

Carboplatin, etoposide, cyclophosphamide, cisplatin, streptozocin, methotrexate, and bleomycin should be used with care in patients with renal disease. Doxorubicin has been associated with nephrotoxicity in cats and should also be used cautiously in those with preexisting renal disease. For most of the drugs listed, dosage reduction is recommended in proportion to changes in creatinine clearance. However, cisplatin and streptozocin, drugs requiring intense diuresis, even in patients with a normal renal function, should generally not be used at all in patients with preexisting renal disease.

3. Which antineoplastic agents are unsafe for use in cats?

Cisplatin causes a fatal pulmonary edema in cats when given intravenously. Intralesional administration appears to be safe. Cats can be treated with carboplatin as an alternative drug with similar antineoplastic properties. Fluorouracil (5-FU) causes fatal neurotoxicity in cats. Doxorubicin can be safely used in cats but has different dose-limiting toxicity in cats than dogs. Cardiotoxicity is unlikely in cats, but nephrotoxicity is more likely. A different prescription method is used for cats. The dose of doxorubicin is 20 to 25 mg/kg every 21 days in cats and 30 mg/kg in dogs.

4. What are cell-cycle specific drugs?

They are agents that affect cells in specific portions of the cell cycle only. For example, antimetabolites (e.g., cytosine arabinoside, 5-FU) work in the S-phase of the cell cycle, L-asparaginase is specific for the G_1 phase, and plant alkaloids (e.g., vincristine, vinblastine) arrest cells in the M-phase.

5. Do any antibiotics have adverse interactions with chemotherapy drugs?

Yes. Competitive protein binding by antibiotics such as tetracyclines, chloramphenicol, and sulfonamides affects the plasma concentrations of protein-bound drugs such as methotrexate and enhances their toxicity. Likewise, cephalothin and penicillins have been shown to decrease cellular uptake of methotrexate. In some cases, antibiotics may interfere with metabolism of antineoplastic agents. An example is the decreased efficacy of cyclophosphamide when given in conjunction with chloramphenicol, owing to decreased cyclophosphamide activation. Nephrotoxicity of cisplatin is reportedly enhanced when it is used in conjunction with a cephalothin-gentamicin combination antibiotic therapy, and aminoglycosides generally enhance the risk of ototoxicity and nephrotoxicity associated with platinum compounds. Cytosine arabinoside reportedly decreases the efficacy of gentamicin against *Klebsiella pneumoniae* and is physically incompatible with the antibiotic as well as with cephalothin and penicillins. Other physical incompatibilities include bleomycin and cephalothin, cefazolin, and penicillins; doxorubicin and cephalothin; and 5-fluorouracil with penicillins and tetracyclines.

6. What is the fluid of choice for diluting chemotherapy drugs?

Most drugs are diluted in 0.9% saline or sterile water. Some advise using 5% dextrose water to dilute carboplatin, however, because the presence of chloride ions favors the conversion of carboplatin to cisplatin.

7. What is the best route for administering L-asparaginase?

Because L-asparaginase is associated with type I hypersensitivity reactions, intravenous and intraperitoneal routes are generally avoided. One study comparing intramuscular with subcutaneous administration of L-asparaginase in dogs with lymphoma suggested a response and survival advantage using the intramuscular route.

8. What chemotherapy drugs are most often associated with neurotoxicity in animals?

Vinca alkaloids (vincristine and vinblastine), cisplatin, and fluorouracil. Vincristine and vinblastine can cause a peripheral neuropathy. Cisplatin may induce ototoxicity, especially in combination with other ototoxic drugs. Fluorouracil causes fatal neurotoxicity in cats, possibly due to metabolism of the drug to flurocitrate, a neurotoxicant. Neurotoxicity may also occur in dogs but is less severe. Signs may include hyperesthesia, hyperexcitability and nervousness, muscle tremors, cerebellar ataxia and, in severe cases, seizures.

9. What causes the allergic reactions seen following intravenous etoposide or paclitaxel (Taxol) administration in dogs?

Hypersensitivity reactions to both drugs are primarily due to vehicles or carriers used in the drug formulations. The incriminated component in Taxol is Cremophor EL and in etoposide is polysorbate 80.

10. Should I expect to see hair loss in veterinary patients receiving chemotherapy?

Alopecia and delayed hair growth is most commonly an adverse effect in dog breeds with continuous hair growth (e.g., poodles, terriers, Old English sheepdogs) due to the sensitivity of the anagen phase of the hair cycle to the effects of chemotherapy. In other breeds, hair and coat changes are generally limited to thinning of the coat and loss of tactile hairs around the muzzle. Cats may lose whiskers. Hair loss may be more apparent in areas of friction (under collars or harnesses). Where hair is clipped, regrowth may be slow.

11. How often does sterile hemorrhagic cystitis occur with cyclophosphamide administration?

In one study of cyclophosphamide-induced cystitis in dogs and cats, the incidence rate was 7% in dogs and 3% in cats treated with oral cyclophosphamide. Although cystitis is a well-known toxicity, myelosuppression is actually the most common adverse effect of cyclophosphamide administration.

12. What causes the cystitis induced by cyclophosphamide?

A metabolite of cyclophosphamide called acrolein causes direct mucosal and arteriolar damage to the bladder wall. This effect is enhanced by prolonged exposure time to the mucosal surface. Although generally associated with prolonged use of oral cyclophosphamide, peracute hemorrhagic cystitis has been reported after intravenous cyclophosphamide doses in dogs (100 to 250 mg/m^2).

13. Which commonly used chemotherapy drugs are excreted in the urine?

Actinomycin D, chlorambucil, cisplatin, carboplatin, cyclophosphamide, cytosine arabinoside, DTIC, lomustine, and methotrexate.

14. Which commonly used chemotherapy drugs are excreted in the feces?

Doxorubicin, mitoxantrone, vincristine, and vinblastine.

15. How can I avoid inducing cardiotoxicity with doxorubicin?

Avoid using doxorubicin in breeds at risk for cardiomyopathy, and keep cumulative doses below 150 to 180 mg/m^2. Patients should be screened for underlying cardiac disease and monitored regularly with echocardiography. Avoiding high peak serum concentrations by slowly infusing the diluted drug over 20 to 30 minutes is advised. Pretreatment with diphenhydramine or corticosteroids to reduce mast cell degranulation may be useful, because histamine has been implicated as a mediator of cardiotoxicity. Dexrazoxane is an iron chelator that has been shown to reduce doxorubicin cardiotoxicity, but it is not widely used in veterinary oncology.

16. Which veterinary chemotherapy drugs cross the blood-brain barrier?

Cytosine arabinoside and the nitrosoureas such as CCNU (lomustine) and BCNU (carmustine) are able to cross the blood-brain barrier and achieve potentially beneficial drug concentrations in the cerebrospinal fluid.

17. Are some chemotherapy agents inactive until they are metabolized?

Yes. The classic example is cyclophosphamide, which is inactive until metabolized by the liver.

18. How are combination chemotherapy protocols devised?

Although there are several theories about the best way to combine or schedule drugs, the choice of drugs for combination protocols generally should adhere to three guidelines:
- The drugs should be active when used alone against the tumor.
- The drugs should have different mechanisms of action.
- The drugs should have different dose-limiting toxicities.

19. Do some antineoplastic agents have a delayed onset of myelosuppression?

Yes. BCNU, CCNU, and mitomycin C typically produce myelosuppression 3 to 4 weeks after administration. Of these drugs, only CCNU is in common use in veterinary medicine, and the dose/schedule issues have not been fully evaluated.

20. Of the chemotherapy drugs used in veterinary oncology, which exhibit cross-resistance in multidrug resistance (MDR) due to P-glycoprotein?

Alkylating agents and antimetabolites are usually not affected by MDR cross-resistance. Doxorubicin, vincristine, mitoxantrone, daunorubicin, vinblastine, mitomycin C, actinomycin D, taxol, and etoposide are known to be affected by MDR. Imagine two veterinarians discussing MDR over lunch and the mnemonic DVM DVM ATE may help with remembering this list.

21. What is the difference between adjuvant and neoadjuvant chemotherapy?

Adjuvant chemotherapy refers to the use of chemotherapy in conjunction with localized therapy (such as surgery or radiation) to prevent or delay recurrence and metastasis. Neoadjuvant chemotherapy refers to the use of chemotherapy to reduce tumor burden prior to surgery or radiation of the primary tumor.

22. For which antineoplastic agents used in veterinary medicine is extravasation a concern?

Doxorubicin, mechlorethamine, actinomycin D, vincristine, and vinblastine are vesicants.

BIBLIOGRAPHY

1. Bergman PJ: Multidrug resistance. In Bongura JD (ed): Kirk's Current Veterinary Therapy XIII. Philadelphia, WB Saunders, 2000, pp 479–482.
2. Carter SK: Principles of cancer chemotherapy. In Theilen GH, Madewell BR (eds): Veterinary Cancer Medicine, 2nd ed. Philadelphia, Lea & Febiger, 1987, pp 167–182.

3. Chabner BA, Collins JM: Cancer Chemotherapy Principles and Practice. Philadelphia, JB Lippincott, 1990.
4. Frimberger AE: Anticancer drugs: New drugs or applications for veterinary medicine. In Bongura JD (ed): Kirk's Current Veterinary Therapy XIII. Philadelphia, WB Saunders, 2000, pp 474–478.
5. Hammer AS: Prevention and treatment of chemotherapy complications. In Kirk RW, Bonagura JD (eds): Kirk's Current Veterinary Therapy XI. Philadelphia, WB Saunders Company, 1992, pp 409–414.
6. Henry CJ, Brewer WG: Drug interactions with antineoplastic agents. In Bongura JD (ed): Kirk's Current Veterinary Therapy XII. Philadelphia, WB Saunders, 1995, pp 482–487.
7. Kisseberth WC, MacEwen EG: Complications of cancer and its treatment. In Withrow SJ, MacEwen EG (eds): Small Animal Oncology, 2nd ed. Philadelphia, WB Saunders, 1996, pp 129–146.
8. Kitchell BE, Dhaliwal RS: CVT Update: Anticancer drugs and protocols using traditional drugs. In Bongura JD (ed): Kirk's Current Veterinary Therapy XIII. Philadelphia, WB Saunders, 2000, pp 465–473.
9. Ogilvie GK: Chemotherapy. In Withrow SJ, MacEwen EG (eds): Small Animal Clinical Oncology, 2nd ed. Philadelphia, WB Saunders, 1996, pp 70–86.

14. SAFE HANDLING OF CYTOTOXIC AGENTS

Mary Lynn Higginbotham, DVM

1. How can exposure to cytotoxic agents occur?

Inhalation secondary to aerosolization, drug absorption through the skin, and ingestion of contaminated food or cigarettes are three common modes of exposure to cytotoxic agents. The risk of exposure is greatest during drug preparation and administration.

2. What are common situations in which exposure to cytotoxic agents occurs?

- Aerosolization of a drug by removing a needle from a pressurized drug vial
- Opening glass ampules
- Expelling air from syringes
- Breaking tablets
- Exposure to excreta from recently treated animals

3. How can employees be educated about the handling of cytotoxic agents?

A videotape series called "Cytotoxic Drug Safety," available from the American Animal Hospital Association, is specifically designed for the veterinary community. The Occupational Safety and Health Administration (OSHA) has published guidelines for controlling occupational exposure to hazardous drugs. A series of published guidelines for cancer chemotherapy also has been published by the Oncology Nursing Society.

4. What information should be available in each practice where cytotoxic agents are used?

Each antineoplastic agent that is available in the hospital pharmacy should have a material safety data sheet and drug insert that are kept in a notebook with all written hospital policies.

5. Who should handle cytotoxic agents?

Only employees who have been trained to handle cytotoxic agents should be involved with these drugs. Pregnant women should avoid handling these agents, and women of childbearing age should be especially careful.

6. During which trimester of pregnancy is there the highest potential for fetal malformations in the people handling these agents?

The first trimester.

7. How and where should cytotoxic agents be stored?

Cytotoxic agents should be stored according to the manufacturer's recommendations. If refrigeration is necessary, these drugs should be stored away from other medications or foodstuffs. If a reconstituted drug is to be stored, it should be in a Ziploc-style bag that is clearly labeled.

8. Where should cytotoxic agents be prepared?

Ideally, these agents are prepared in a biological safety cabinet (BSC) or class II vertical-flow fume hood with the exhaust or fan on at all times.

9. Where should cytotoxic agents be prepared if a biological safety cabinet is not available?

In the setting where no BSC is available, the drugs should be prepared in a low-traffic, well-ventilated area that is not near food preparation areas. All drafts should be eliminated, and drinking, eating, smoking, and cosmetic application should be prohibited in these areas. These areas should be dedicated—with no other activities occurring while cytotoxic agents are being prepared.

10. What equipment should be available in the hood?
- A plastic-backed absorbent pad, which can be replaced if contaminated
- Gauze squares
- Alcohol pads

11. What kinds of protective wear are recommended when preparing or administering cytotoxic agents?

Chemo-safety gloves are the ideal gloves to be worn while preparing, administering, or disposing of cytotoxic agents. If these are not available, disposable, nonpowdered, latex gloves should be worn. Double gloving is recommended because thickness is more important than material. Vinyl is more permeable than latex. A nonpermeable gown with long sleeves, closed front, and closed cuffs is recommended. Protective eyewear and a respiratory mask with a filter are recommended as well.

12. How can aerosolization of a drug be avoided?

Chemo-dispensing pins, or chemo-pins, are ideal to help prevent aerosolization of cytotoxic agents. These are venting devices that attach directly to the vial and release pressure through a 0.2-μm hydrophobic filter. One must be familiar with these devices because improper use may actually increase the risk of aerosolization. If chemo-pins are not available, pressure buildup can be minimized by the removal of air before adding diluent to the drug vials. For added protection, an alcohol-moistened gauze pad should surround the needle to prevent aerosolization of droplets as the needle is removed. Placing the bottle and syringe within a Ziploc-style bag prior to removing the needle will also help prevent aerosolization.

13. What steps should be taken to prepare injectable drugs?

Cytotoxic agents should be prepared using aseptic technique. First, the top of the vial from which the agent is to be drawn should be wiped with an alcohol swab. Ideally a chemo-pin is inserted into the vial. A Luer-lok syringe is used and attached to the chemo-pin while keeping the vial upright. If diluent needs to be added, it is slowly pushed into the vial and the bottle shaken gently. The vial is then inverted and drug slowly drawn into the syringe to help avoid excess air bubbles. Any excess drug should be pushed back into the vial. The vial should be turned upright before removing the syringe. A gauze square should be placed around the syringe and the top of the pin to absorb any drug that may have leaked or become aerosolized. A covered needle should be placed on the syringe.

14. How should cytotoxic agents be transported after being prepared for use?

Transportation should be done by placing the previously prepared agents into Ziploc-style bags. All bags, syringes, and bottles should be carefully labeled with agent and patient information.

15. How should equipment used for drug preparation and administration be discarded?

All equipment used for drug preparation and administration should immediately be discarded into a chemotherapy waste container. This container should be puncture-proof and specifically designated for chemotherapy waste. Thick, leak-proof bags that are of a differing color from other hospital trash bags should be used to dispose of used gloves, gowns, and other materials that have been used for preparation, administration, or transportation of cytotoxic agents. These bags should then be placed in puncture-proof containers designed for chemotherapy waste. Needles should not be clipped or recapped after use. Any needles, syringes, or breakable items should be placed in a sharps container before being placed in the chemotherapy waste container. The waste container should always be covered, and a separate waste container should be located in each designated area for preparation and administration. Chemotherapy waste can be incinerated at temperatures of 1000°C or buried in a landfill.

16. How should oral cytotoxic drugs be prepared for use?

Oral cytotoxic agents ideally should be counted within a BSC class II hood with the preparer wearing gloves. If this is not available, tablets may be counted within a Ziploc-style bag to minimize aerosolization.

17. Should cyclophosphamide tablets be divided?

Cyclophosphamide tablets should not be broken. The active drug within the tablets is within the core of the tablet and not evenly distributed throughout the tablet. Therefore, when tablets are divided, the active drug concentration will not be the same in both halves. Cyclophosphamide can also be aerosolized when the tablets are broken. To prevent overdosing the patient and to avoid breaking tablets, the calculated dose should be rounded down to use whole tablets.

18. What should be included in a chemotherapy spill kit?

A spill kit should be located near each area designated for preparation and administration of chemotherapy agents. According to OSHA recommendations, these should contain goggles, two separate pairs of gloves, utility gloves, a gown, two 1' × 1' sheets of absorbent material, 250-ml and 1-L spill control pillows, a sharps container, a small scoop to collect glass fragments, and two large hazardous drug waste disposal bags.

19. How should chemotherapy spills be managed?

One individual should be designated to clean up spills. Personal protective equipment should be worn. Absorbent pads should be used to absorb all liquid, or cat litter may be used to absorb liquid cytotoxic agents. Glass materials should be handled with a scoop and placed in a sharps container. All material used to clean a spill should be disposed of in chemotherapy waste containers.

20. Which drugs commonly used in veterinary oncology are excreted as active drug?

Actinomycin D, bleomycin, cisplatin, and doxorubicin (ABCD).

21. Which drugs commonly used in veterinary oncology are excreted as metabolites?

Busulfan, chlorambucil, cyclophosphamide, cytosine arabinoside, DTIC, lomustine, and vincristine.

22. For which drugs commonly used in veterinary oncology is the primary route of elimination urinary excretion?

Actinomycin D, chlorambucil, cisplatin, carboplatin, cyclophosphamide, cytosine arabinoside, DTIC, lomustine, and methotrexate.

23. For which drugs commonly used in veterinary oncology is the primary route of elimination fecal excretion?

Doxorubicin, mitoxantrone, vincristine, and vinblastine.

24. What are the clearance times for handling excreta from animals treated with common cytotoxic agents?

DRUG	CLEARANCE TIMES
Cyclophosphamide	Urine for 72 hours
Doxorubicin	Feces for 7 days
Vincristine	Urine for 4 days and feces for 7 days
Cisplatin	Urine for 72 hours
Mitoxantrone	Urine for 5 days and feces for 7 days

25. How can owners decrease exposure to excreta?

Dogs should be walked with a leash in restricted areas only for 1 to 3 days following treatment. Cats litter boxes should be cleaned frequently and litter disposed of in closed plastic containers or bags.

26. How should owners dispose of excreta if necessary?

Owners should wear latex gloves when handling vomitus, urine, or feces. Feces should be flushed down the toilet, and household areas that have been contaminated with any excreta should be cleaned with a bleach solution. Spray bottles should not be used, because this will aerosolize active drug that may be excreted. Paper towels used to clean messes should be disposed of in closed plastic containers. Any rugs, towels, or other items that become soiled with excreta should be laundered separately from other items.

BIBLIOGRAPHY

1. Dickinson K, Ogilvie GK: Safe handling and administration of chemotherapeutic agents in veterinary medicine. In Kirk RW, Bonagura JD (eds): Current Veterinary Therapy XII. Small Animal Practice. Philadelphia, WB Saunders, 1995, pp 475–478.
2. Henry CJ: Safe handling of chemotherapy drugs. In August JR (ed): Consultations in Feline Internal Medicine 3. Philadelphia, WB Saunders, 1997, pp 534–540.
3. Ogilvie GK: Chemotherapy. In Withrow SJ, MacEwen EG (eds): Small Animal Clinical Oncology, 2nd ed. Philadelphia, WB Saunders, 1996, pp 82–83.
4. Ogilvie GK, Moore AS: Clinical briefing: Safe handling of chemotherapeutic agents. In Ogilvie GK, Moore AS (eds): Managing the Veterinary Cancer Patient. Trenton, NJ, Veterinary Learning Systems, 1995, p 53.
5. OSHA Directives: Guidelines for Cytotoxic (Antineoplastic) Drugs. OSHA Instructional Publication 8-1.1. Washington DC, Office of Occupational Medicine, 1986.

15. BIOLOGIC RESPONSE MODIFICATION

Philip J. Bergman, DVM, MS, PhD, Dipl ACVIM

1. What is biologic response modification (BRM)?

BRM is the use of natural or synthetic substances/methods to alter the host/tumor relationship, which may result in an anti-tumor effect.

2. What observations support the idea that BRM may be useful in the treatment of cancer?
- The presence of monocytic, lymphocytic and plasmacytic cellular infiltrates in tumors
- The presence of extremely specific cytotoxic T cells from local lymph nodes
- An increased incidence of cancer in immunocompromised humans
- Documentation of cancer remission with the use of immunomodulators
- Rare demonstration of remission without any form of treatment

3. BRM is not a member of the classic cancer therapy triad (surgery, radiation, and chemotherapy). Does this mean I don't have to understand it?

Absolutely not! An increased understanding of the immune system over the last 10–15 years has translated into a number of human and veterinary, BRM-based, anti-cancer clinical trials. Many clinical oncologists and cancer researchers (this author included) believe that BRM-based therapies will translate into cancer cures, thereby making a greater understanding of BRM necessary.

4. Define Coley's toxins.

One of the pioneering pieces of work in the BRM field was described in 1909 by Coley. Coley's toxins are mixtures of various components of bacteria that were used as vaccines to stimulate an anti-tumor response. This work was based on the anecdotal observations of longer survival times and remarkable remissions in cancer patients treated with coincident bacterial infections.

5. What are the two major categories of the immune system, and what are the components of each?

In an effort to achieve a better understanding of BRM, it's important to have a basic level of knowledge of the immune system. The two major categories are:

Innate immune system (nonspecific or natural)
- Phagocytic cells (natural killer [NK] cells or macrophages)
- Complement system
- Physicochemical barriers

Acquired immune system (specific)
- Humoral system (antibody dependent cellular cytotoxicity)
- Cellular system

6. Divide the categories of immunotherapy, subdividing where appropriate, and provide examples for each.

Active immunotherapy (i.e., immunization)
- Specific active immunotherapy (e.g. tumor cell vaccine)
- Nonspecific active immunotherapy (e.g. IL-2, interferons, levamisole, etc.)

Passive immunotherapy (i.e., transfer of immunologic reagents)

• Cellular passive immunotherapy (i.e., "adoptive immunotherapy")
• Antibody passive immunotherapy (e.g. rituxan monoclonal antibody)
Indirect immunotherapy (e.g., removal of inhibitory or blocking immunologic factors)

7. What is the greatest difficulty that BRM-based therapeutics face?
The immune system is innately designed for tolerance to "self." Unfortunately, tumors are comprised of "self" and therefore the generation of an immune response against a tumor can be difficult.

8. Describe ways that tumors undergo immune avoidance.
Major histocompatibility complex (MHC) I loss
• MHC gene structural defects
• Changes in B2-microglobulin synthesis
• Defects in transporter-associated antigen processing
• MHC gene loss (e.g., allelic or locus loss)
MHC I antigen presentation gene loss
B7-1 loss (B7-1 is co-stimulatory molecule of CD28)
• Prevents T-cell receptor and MHC engagement
• Very common when MHC system remains intact

9. How can antibodies (endogenous or exogenous) be used to fight cancer?
Antibody-directed targeting via coupling the Ab with:
• Immunotoxins (e.g., ricin)
• Chemotherapy (e.g., doxorubicin)
• Radioisotopes (e.g., radioactive iodine)
• Cytokines (e.g., IL-2, G-CSF)
Antibody binding to tumor cell with Fc receptor engagement (e.g., neutrophils, macrophages, NK cells)

10. List the advantages and disadvantages for the immune system using tumor-associated antigens (TAAs) for the generation of an anti-tumor response.
Advantages:
• Virally induced tumors (e.g., FeLV, Epstein-Barr) express unique TAAs.
• Malignant progression may induce overexpression of fetal antigens, growth factors, or growth factor receptors.
• Mutated peptides related to carcinogenesis or malignant progression (e.g., p53 tumor suppressor gene) may be unique TAAs.
• Changes in differentiation antigen (e.g., tyrosinase and other melanoma antigens) expression levels may reach detection threshold and promote response.
Disadvantages:
• Most TAAs are present in low levels of normal tissues; therefore, cytotoxic T lymphocytes (CTLs) against these TAAs may be removed by self-tolerance mechanisms.
• TAA presentation by MHC may lead to development of highly specific CTLs; however, such an "immunodominant" CTL response may be too focused for an anti-tumor effect.

11. Are there a variety of methods for anti-cancer BRM?
Yes, methods include:
  Cytokines
  Antibodies (monoclonal and polyclonal)
  Nonspecific immunomodulators
  Gene therapy
  Tumor vaccines
  Superantigens

Bone marrow transplantation
Others (e.g., bacterial vectors, anti-angiogenic treatments)

12. Describe the ideal BRM agent.

The ideal BRM agent can discriminate between cancer and normal cells (**specificity**); is potent enough to kill small or large numbers of tumor cells (**sensitivity**); and can prevent recurrence of the cancer (**durability**).

13. Which BRM agent has been found to be active against canine osteosarcoma (OSA) and hemangiosarcoma (HSA)?

L-MTP-PE (liposome-encapsulated muramyl tripeptide phosphotidylethanolamine) has been shown by MacEwen et al. to have activity against canine OSA and HSA. Its mechanism of action of L-MTP-PE is by potent nonspecific activation of macrophages and monocytes. The origin of L-MTP-PE is muramyl dipeptide, which is from mycobacterium cell walls and has immunostimulatory properties.

14. Is cimetidine a useful BRM agent?

Yes, cimetidine is a useful BRM agent. It is a histamine-2 (H_2) receptor antagonist with immunomodulatory activities. Mechanisms of action include: direct lymphocyte activation through H_2 receptors on T-suppressor cells; blockade of growth promotion of histamine; blockade of inhibition of cell-mediated cytotoxicity of histamine; and direct inhibition of tumor cell proliferation. Cimetidine can be employed in equine melanoma, papillomatosis, myelodysplastic syndromes, and some leukemias.

15. What cytokine has been found to be useful in vitro or in vivo against canine tumors?

Interleukin 2 (IL-2) has extraordinary LAK-associated anti-tumor effects in rodent models of cancer. Human recombinant IL-2 binds canine peripheral blood lymphocytes and induces them to proliferate. Nebulized liposomal IL-2 has been found to be useful in early clinical canine studies of metastatic OSA and primary lung tumor.

16. Name two FDA-approved monoclonal antibodies for the treatment of human cancer. Which cancers do they target?

These two monoclonal antibodies (MABs) recently were approved for the treatment of human cancer:
- Herceptin (Trastuzumab), an anti-HER2/neu MAB for human breast cancer
- Rituxan (Rituximab), an anti-CD20 MAB for human non-Hodgkin's lymphoma

17. Briefly describe how monoclonal antibodies are produced.

MABs are produced by fusion of malignant plasma cells with normal Ig-producing splenic cells grown in selective media. Immortalized cells with MAB of choice are used.

18. How may classic MABs be problematic in the treatment of cancer?

MABs are made from mice, and therefore an immune response can take place against the MAB if administered in a different species.

19. Describe two types of MABs that can reduce the above-mentioned problem.

Chimeric MABs (murine Fab and species of interest Fc) and bispecific MABs (one Fab against TAA and other Fab against CTL antigen receptor).

20. Which MAB has been used against canine lymphoma?

MAB 231 recognizes canine lymphosarcoma cells. It has been reported to prolong median survival times of dogs treated with chemotherapy and MAB 231 when compared to historical control chemotherapy-only dogs. Properly controlled randomized trials are necessary to address the potential usefulness of MAB 231 in canine lymphoma.

21. Compare and contrast the mechanism of action, sensitivity, specificity, response time, and durability of response between chemotherapy and BRM-based tumor vaccines.

TREATMENT TYPE	MECHANISM OF ACTION	SENSITIVITY	SPECIFICITY	RESPONSE TIME	DURABILITY OF RESPONSE
Chemotherapy agent	Cytotoxicity	Variable	Poor	Hours to days	Variable
Anti-tumor vaccine	Immune response	Good	Good	Weeks to months	Long

22. List three or more methodologies presently used as BRM agents in the treatment of advanced canine malignant melanoma.
- Surgery and liposomal MTP-PE
- Autologous melanoma vaccine transfected with hGM-CSF
- Local tumor transfection with superantigen (staphylococcal enterotoxin B) and cytokine genes
- Intramuscular human tyrosinase DNA vaccination

BIBLIOGRAPHY

1. Curti B:. Adoptive immunotherapy. Cancer Chemother Biol Response Modif 1999;18:239–249.
2. Dow SW, Elmslie RE, Willson AP, et al: In vivo tumor transfection with superantigen plus cytokine genes induces tumor regression and prolongs survival in dogs with malignant melanoma. J Clin Invest 1998;101:2406–2414.
3. Hogge GS, Burkholder JK, Culp J, et al: Preclinical development of human granulocyte-macrophage colony-stimulating factor-transfected melanoma cell vaccine using established canine cell lines and normal dogs. Cancer Gene Ther 1999;6:26–36.
4. Jeglum KA: Chemoimmunotherapy of canine lymphoma with adjuvant canine monoclonal antibody 231. Vet Clin North Am Small Anim Pract 1996;26:73–85.
5. MacEwen EG, Kurzman ID: Canine osteosarcoma: amputation and chemoimmunotherapy. Vet Clin North Am Small Anim Pract 1996;26:123–133.
6. MacEwen EG, Kurzman ID, Vail DM, et al: Adjuvant therapy for melanoma in dogs: Results of randomized clinical trials using surgery, liposome-encapsulated muramyl-tripeptide, and granulocyte macrophage colony-stimulating factor. Clin Cancer Res 1999;5:4249–4258.
7. Mihich E: Historical overview of biologic response modifiers. Cancer Invest 2000;18:456–466.
8. Pettit SJ, Seymour K, O'Flaherty E, Kirby JA: Immune selection in neoplasia: Towards a microevolutionary model of cancer development. Br J Cancer 2000;82:1900–1906.
9. Schilder R: Rituximab immunotherapy. Cancer Biother Radiopharm 1999;14:237–240.
10. Vail DM, MacEwen EG, Kurzman ID, et al: Liposome-encapsulated muramyl tripeptide phosphatidylethanolamine adjuvant immunotherapy for splenic hemangiosarcoma in the dog: A randomized multi-institutional clinical trial. Clin Cancer Res 1995;1:1165–1170.
11. Wolchok JD, Livingston PO, Houghton AN: Vaccines and other adjuvant therapies for melanoma. Hem/Onc Clinics North Am 1998;12:835–848.

16. HYPERTHERMIA

J. Paul Woods, DVM, Dipl ACVIM

"Those diseases that medicines do not cure are cured by the knife. Those that the knife does not cure are cured by fire. Those that fire does not cure, must be considered incurable."

—Hippocrates

1. What is hyperthermia?
Hyperthermia indicates any elevation in body temperature above the normal range designated for any species of animal. Hyperthermia, also called thermotherapy, is currently an investigational therapeutic modality that may join surgery, chemotherapy, and radiotherapy as an established treatment modality in the management of cancer.

2. Who first used hyperthermia?
The anticancer effects of elevated (noncauterizing) temperature (i.e., hyperthermia) were observed thousands of years ago in ancient Egypt. In the late 19th century, the serendipitous observation of tumor regression following acute febrile episodes of bacterial infections, principally erysipelas, led to the treatment of malignant tumors with injections of bacterial toxins ("Coley toxins"). In the last two decades, with the availability of improved heat delivery equipment from new technology, there has been renewed interest in hyperthermia as an adjuvant treatment for cancer.

3. What causes hyperthermia?
Hyperthermia is produced by an uncompensated disequilibrium in the body's heat balance equation whereby heat gain or production exceeds heat loss. Energy, as heat, is stored within the body, with a resultant rise in body core temperature. A net heat gain may occur due to changes in metabolic heat production, radiation, convection, conduction, or evaporation caused by physical, pathologic, or pharmacologic interventions.

4. What is therapeutic hyperthermia?
In this context, hyperthermia specifically refers to the therapeutically induced elevation of body temperature. Therapeutic hyperthermia, for most mammals, is usually in the range of $42° ± 3°C$. Therapeutic hyperthermia is induced by manipulating and overwhelming the body's thermoregulatory system, causing net heat gain, which is opposed by the body's thermoregulatory mechanisms.

5. What is the difference between hyperthermia and fever?
In contrast to fever (pyrexia), current methods of hyperthermia induction do not involve the production of endogenous pyrogen (EP) and its action on the thermoregulatory center in the preoptic anterior hypothalamus. In fever, the action of EP on the thermoregulatory center results in an increase of the body's set point, and the elevated body temperature is actively defended by thermoregulatory behavioral and physiologic mechanisms.

6. What is malignant hyperthermia?
Malignant hyperthermia, unlike therapeutic hyperthermia, is a pharmacogenetic myopathy reported in human beings, swine, dogs, cats, and horses. Affected animals are susceptible to drugs (e.g., inhalant and local amide anesthetics, skeletal muscle relaxants) or stress, triggering an acute uncontrolled malignant hyperthermic reaction, circulatory failure, and death. Malignant hyperthermia results from increased heat production due to a number of factors,

including catabolism of muscle glycogen and liver lactate, accelerated hydrolysis of adeno-sine triphosphate by myosin adenosine triphosphatase, and uncoupling of oxidative phospho-rylation by calcium. There may also be decreased heat loss due to peripheral vasoconstriction.

7. What is the rationale for hyperthermic treatments?

The use of hyperthermia in cancer treatment is based on the increased sensitivity of tumors to heat compared with normal tissue, which may be due to variations in intrinsic cellu-lar heat sensitivity or to variations in the cellular microenvironment milieu (i.e., hypoxia, aci-dosis, and nutritional deficiencies). Hyperthermia (greater than 41°C) can be directly cytotoxic, or heat can sensitize cells to the effects of radiation or chemotherapy. Hyperthermia has had minimal clinical response when heat is used alone; however, hyperthermia combined with radiation or chemotherapy has demonstrated an enhanced anticancer effect. In contrast to ionizing radiation and some chemotherapeutic agents, hyperthermia is not carcinogenic, al-though it is weakly mutagenic.

8. What is the mechanism of heat killing?

Heat is an entropic disordering agent that disrupts highly ordered structures and processes in cells. Temperatures above 45°C destroy cells by nonselective coagulation and denaturation of proteins; however, the mechanism leading to tumor cell death by 41° to 45°C hyperthermia is not fully understood. Hyperthermia affects many cellular components and functions (e.g., cell metabolism, lysosomes, nucleic acid synthesis, and cell membranes), but it is not known which of these effects, if any, represents the lethal hyperthermic event. Heat may act at several cellular sites, and the net effect may be influenced by environmental fac-tors. The reduction in DNA repair from hyperthermia may explain the synergistic activity of heat when associated with radiation and cytotoxic drugs.

9. What is the effect of hyperthermia on tumor vasculature?

The microcirculatory physiology of normal and neoplastic tissues differs strikingly in their response to heating. Blood flow plays a major role in heat dissipation. In response to heat, normal tissue blood vessels vasodilate and can increase blood flow to increase blood cooling and prevent excessive temperature rise. Tumor tissues, in contrast, lack smooth muscle capable of causing vasodilation and therefore are limited in their ability to increase heat dissipation by augmenting blood. Hyperthermia takes advantage of the abnormal tumor circulatory physiology because (*a*) hyperthermia is preferentially cytotoxic to hypoxic-aci-dotic cells; (*b*) tumor microvasculature is more sensitive than normal microvasculature to direct destruction by heat (42° to 46°C), which leads to further reduced pH, anoxia, and is-chemic necrosis; and (*c*) the relative absence of smooth muscle vasodilating response in tumors leads to preferential tumor heating because blood flow is the major conduit for heat exchange.

10. Why is hyperthermia used with radiation (heat radiosensitization)?

Hypoxic cells, such as are present in most solid tumors because of their poor vascular supply, are resistant to ionizing radiation, but hypoxic cells are very sensitive to heat treat-ment. Hence, the synergistic effect is based on different activities of the treatments, with the radiotherapy more active on the oxygenated regions of the tumor and the hyperthermia more active on the anoxic, hypovascular cells of the hypoxic regions of the tumor. In addition, hy-perthermia and radiation have complementary effects because they act on different phases of the cell cycle. Hyperthermia primarily affects cells in the DNA synthesis (S) phase, which are usually resistant to radiotherapy, whereas radiation is most damaging to cells in the mitosis (M) phase. Together, the combined modalities will attack different cell populations in the tumor. Depending on the time interval between treatments and the temperatures achieved, the interaction between hyperthermia and radiation can be independent, additive, synergistic, or antagonistic. An advantageous thermal enhancement ratio (TER) has been achieved by delivering radiation and heat in sequence at 2- to 4-hour intervals. TER is the ratio between the minimal dose of radiation inducing an effect and the dose of radiation required when radiotherapy is administered in combination with hyperthermia to induce the same effect.

11. Why is hyperthermia used with chemotherapy (thermochemotherapy)?

Mild to moderate hyperthermia (40° to 43°C) can enhance the cytotoxicity of some chemotherapeutic agents. An increased therapeutic index has been observed for hyperthermia with melphalan, cyclophosphamide, bleomycin, doxorubicin, cisplatin, mitomycin C, and the nitrosoureas (CCNU). The effect of hyperthermia may be due to enhanced or inhibited drug transport, increased permeability of the cell membrane, increased rate of reaction between the drug and its target molecules, accelerated alkylation, increased inhibition of DNA repair mechanism of drug-induced lesions, or a combination of these effects. Similar to heat radiosensitization, the interaction of hyperthermia and chemotherapy depends on the time interval between the treatments and the temperatures achieved (e.g., doxorubicin administered after hyperthermia is less cytotoxic).

12. What is thermal dose?

The degree of cell killing is dependent on both time and temperature. Many combinations of these two factors can result in the same degree of cell killing. A physical quantity (e.g., the gray for ionizing radiation absorbed dose) is difficult to define for hyperthermia because power absorbed per unit mass of tissue has little biologic significance. Thermal isoeffect based on the Arrhenius relationship is a possible means of predicting biologic effects resulting from various time-temperature combinations (i.e., expressing time-temperature combinations in equivalent minutes at a standard temperature of 43°C). Although minimum monitored tumor temperature is strongly correlated with treatment efficacy, it is difficult to measure because temperature in tissues is a function of the power deposited and the heat transfer due to conductivity and blood perfusion, which is variable and difficult to characterize.

13. What is the Arrhenius relationship?

The time-temperature relationship is described by the Arrhenius equation, $k = 1/D_0 = Ae^{-d/RT}$ where k is the reaction rate constant, D_0 is the time required to reduce cell survival to 37% (e^{-1}), A is the Arrhenius constant, d is the activation energy, R is the universal gas constant (2 cal/degree/mol), and T is the absolute temperature (K). There is a "break" in the Arrhenius plot at about 42.5°C such that above the break point, for every 1°C temperature increase, the duration of heating required to produce a given level of reaction (thermal effect) is halved. Whereas, below the break point, for every 1°C temperature decrease, the duration of heating must be four to six times greater to produce the same level of reaction. The break point may be due to a different mechanism of cell killing or to the induction of thermotolerance.

14. What is thermotolerance?

Thermotolerance is a dramatic heat-induced resistance in normal and neoplastic cells or tissues to further heat killing that occurs at temperatures below 43°C. Thermotolerance can be induced in a number of ways: by continuous heating at low temperatures (41.5° to 42.5°C), heating to temperatures greater than 43°C followed by cooling to normal body temperature, heating cells or tissue to sublethal temperatures (40° to 41°C), or by using some solvents (ethanol). The magnitude and kinetics of thermotolerance are dependent on a variety of factors, including the initial heat dose, tissue pH, cell kinetics, and the pathophysiologic changes during or after hyperthermia.

15. What causes thermotolerance?

Although the mechanism of thermotolerance is unknown, the development of thermotolerance is associated with the enhanced synthesis of heat shock proteins (HSP; particularly an

HSP of molecular weight 70 kda [HSP70]). HSPs are families of similar proteins of various molecular weights that are synthesized in increased amounts by a wide variety of cells in response to heat and other environmental stresses (chemical or mechanical). It has recently been found that most HSPs have a molecular chaperone activity that provides a cellular defense mechanism by inhibiting the aggregation of partially denatured proteins and refolding them using the energy of adenosine triphosphate.

16. What is the significance of thermotolerance?

Regardless of the degree of induction, thermotolerance is transient—decaying in 72 to 168 hours. Thermotolerance is clinically significant because hyperthermia fractions must be timed to avoid heating thermotolerant tissues (i.e., fractional intervals to allow for the reversing of thermotolerance). In addition, differential thermotolerance induction between tumor and normal tissue may be possible by manipulating tissue pH, cell cycle kinetics, and temperature distribution homogeneity, depending on tumor type and location. The interactions between thermotolerance and radiation or chemotherapy are complicated, contradictory, and not well worked out.

17. What is step-down heating?

Minimally lethal or nonlethal temperatures become toxic when they are preceded by acute heat treatments at higher temperatures (e.g., 45°C). The mechanism is unknown, but after acute hyperthermia, lesions induced by minimally lethal temperatures (e.g., 39° to 43°C) may not be repaired, thus resulting in a lethal outcome.

18. How is hyperthermia induced?

Historically, the nonphysical method of inducing hyperthermia involved the injection of pyrogenic agents (e.g., mixed bacterial toxins, or Coley toxins) into the subject. Current methods of producing hyperthermia use physical methods including surface heating or volume heating. Surface heating involves hyperthermia induced by infrared or visible radiation, or hot air/water/wax bath, where heat is added to the skin surface area interacting with the heat source. Heat transfer subsequently occurs from the skin to the underlying tissue by conduction and convection. In volume heating, the temperature of the underlying tissue is elevated by perfusion with preheated blood or by exposure to ultrasound, microwave, radiofrequency currents, or laser. Hyperthermia induced by ultrasound, microwaves, or radiofrequency currents adds heat to the section of the body being heated. During hyperthermia with blood perfusion, the afferent blood temperature is set at a desired value, and the efferent blood is circulated to the central blood pool or to the extracorporeal device used for heating the blood.

19. What are the forms of hyperthermia?

Depending on the surface area or volume heated, hyperthermia can be divided into local, regional, and whole-body hyperthermia (WBH). Local (or interstitial) hyperthermia involves the heating of the tumor and minimal surrounding tissue; regional hyperthermia involves the heating of the tumor and surrounding tissue (e.g., limb, pelvis); and WBH elevates the temperature in the entire body.

20. What are the indications for local hyperthermia?

Local hyperthermia is suitable for tumors that are not widespread or situations in which only a portion of the body needs to be treated. The more heat-sensitive organs (i.e., liver or brain) are usually outside the heated field; therefore, higher temperatures may be used in local hyperthermia than with WBH. The higher temperature has the clinically significant advantage of killing more tumor cells. Disadvantages include inability to treat disseminated tumors, uneven temperature distributions, and inadequate tissue coupling and penetration with external local hyperthermia devices.

21. What are the indications for regional hyperthermia?

Regional perfusion of limbs requiring invasive surgery is suitable for those few situations in which a patient's tumor is confined to a distal portion of an extremity. Regional heating of large regions of the body (e.g., pelvis, abdomen, thorax) poses problems of nonuniform power deposition when attempting to heat a large volume of tissue with minimal toxicity. Problems are also associated with determining dosimetry.

22. What are the indications for whole-body (systemic) hyperthermia?

WBH has the significant advantage with widely disseminated cancer of treating all foci of disease. WBH also has a more homogeneous temperature distribution. A disadvantage of WBH is the maximum temperature limitation in the 41.8° to 42°C range due to systemic toxicity. Another disadvantage is the requirement for general anesthetic or sedation during the procedure.

CONTROVERSY

23. What is the future for hyperthermia in cancer therapy?

In the past 25 years, renewed interest and intense research into hyperthermia as an emerging cancer therapy has resulted in a substantial increase in the understanding and knowledge of the biologic effects of hyperthermia on normal and malignant tissues and advances in the technical capability to induce hyperthermia. There is much evidence suggesting that the combination of hyperthermia with other antitumor therapies (radiation and chemotherapy) may result in synergistic tumor response effects, especially when therapies with different cell-killing mechanisms are combined. However, despite the advances, clinically hyperthermia has been hindered by the unrefined technology of current equipment, which cannot consistently deposit heat within tumors or provide highly accurate thermal dose administration. Future endeavors to make therapeutic hyperthermia an adjuvant modality for cancer therapy will require the cooperation of oncologists, biologists, and physicists to determine the most important biologic parameters affecting hyperthermia, to manufacture devices that can heat deeply and homogeneously, and to determine temperature reliably, consistently, and noninvasively. Hyperthermia offers potential benefit to pets with recurrent, progressive, resistant cancer not amenable to standard therapies.

BIBLIOGRAPHY

1. Bisht KS, Devi PU: Hyperthermia in cancer research: Current status. Ind J Exp Biol 34:113–118, 1996.
2. Dewhirst MW, Connor WG, Sim DA: Preliminary results of a phase III trial of spontaneous animal tumors to heat and/or radiation: Early normal tissue response and tumor volume influence on initial response. Int J Radiat Oncol Biol Phys 8:1951–1961, 1982.
3. Dewhirst MW, Sim DA, Sapareto S, et al: Importance of minimum tumor temperature in determining early and long-term responses of spontaneous canine and feline tumors to heat and radiation. Cancer Res 44:43–50, 1984.
4. Kurzman ID, Keller ET, MacEwen EG: New developments in cancer therapy. In Withrow SJ, MacEwen EG (eds): Small Animal Clinical Oncology, 2nd ed. Philadelphia, WB Saunders, 1996, pp 157–160.
5. Page RL: Recent advances in hyperthermia. Comp Cont Educ 15:781–792, 1993.
6. Page RL, Thrall DE: Clinical indications and applications of radiotherapy and hyperthermia in veterinary oncology. Vet Clin North Am 20:1075–1092, 1990.
7. Page RL, Thrall DE, Dewhirst MW, et al: Whole-body hyperthermia rationale and potential use for cancer research. J Vet Intern Med 1:110–120, 1987.
8. Robins HI, Woods JP, Schmitt CL, Cohen JD: A new technological approach to radiant heat whole body hyperthermia. Cancer Lett 79:137–145, 1994.
9. Thompson JM: Advances in the use of hyperthermia. In Gorman NT (ed): Oncology, Contemporary Issues in Small Animal Practice, Vol 6. New York, Churchill Livingstone, 1986, pp 89–119.
10. Woods JP, Robins HI, Rosenthal RC: Hematological effects of radiant heat-induced whole body hyperthermia in the dog. Can J Vet Res 60:75–78, 1996.

17. PHOTODYNAMIC THERAPY

Dudley McCaw, DVM, Dipl ACVIM

1. What is photodynamic therapy?

Photodynamic therapy (PDT) is the effect of light and a photosensitizing drug to produce biologic damage of therapeutic value. The light or drug alone has little or no effect.

2. Is the process of PDT new?

The first report of successful treatment of tumors in animals was in 1975. PDT was slow to gain acceptance because good light sources were not available. The light sources for the early treatments were slide projectors with filters to obtain the proper wavelengths. Lasers have provided light of the needed wavelength and the ability to deliver the light through fiberoptic cables.

3. How do agents localize in tumor tissue?

Concentration around tumor blood vessels and decreased clearance by immature tumor blood vessels and lymphatics enhance the ability of the agent to enter cells.

4. How is tissue killed?

The interaction of photosensitizing agent and light causes the formation of toxic singlet oxygen. The oxygen radicals cause destruction of cells. Secondary reactions that contribute to tumor cell destruction are alteration of the tumor vasculature, inflammation, and tumor immunity.

5. How many agents are available?

One agent is approved for use by the Food and Drug Administration (FDA): hematoporphyrin derivative (porfimer sodium, Photofrin). Other agents being used in experimental trials include 5-aminolevulinic acid (ALA), tin etiopurpurin ($SnET_2$), meta-tetra (hydroxyphenyl) chlorin (mTHPc), benzoporphyrin derivative-monoacid ring A (BPD), and pyropheophorbide alpha-hexyl ether (HPPH).

6. What light sources are used?

Argon-pumped dye lasers and Nd:YAG lasers are the only light sources approved by the FDA. Less expensive and portable diode lasers are used in Europe and can be used for investigational purposes in the United States.

7. How is the light delivered to the tissues?

The advantage of lasers is that light can be directed through fiberoptic cables. This allows the light to be directed to the tumor tissue without unwanted exposure of normal tissue. A lens at the end of the fiberoptic cable allows for even distribution of the light. The most commonly used lenses diffuse the light in a circular pattern used for surface treatment and in a lateral pattern used for implanting the fibers into the tissue.

8. How long is the patient exposed to light?

The light dose is measured in joules per square centimeter of tissue. This is the product of light intensity (mW) and time. The typical dose is 100 J/cm^2. Although high output and short times can produce this dose, evidence suggests that longer exposure times are better. The typical treatment time for each "spot" is 16 to 20 minutes.

9. What tumors are most sensitive?

Carcinomas appear to be more sensitive than mesenchymal tumors. In humans, PDT has been approved for lung, esophageal, bladder, and gastric cancers in various countries. Published veterinary uses include transitional cell carcinoma, canine oral squamous cell carcinomas, and feline facial squamous cell carcinomas. We have also had success with some canine mast cell tumors.

10. What are the adverse effects?

The primary reaction is extensive tissue swelling, which begins during treatment and resolves within approximately 3 days. Treatment of lesions near the pharynx requires the placement of a tracheotomy tube. Pulmonary edema has been observed in some cats. Sensitivity to light until the agent has been cleared from the skin is also a problem. Using Photofrin, this is a concern for 4 to 6 weeks, but the newer agents are cleared more quickly. Unwanted reactions can be prevented by short exposures to sunlight and covering exposed skin. Commercially available sunscreens are of no value because the photosensitizing agents are activated by light wavelengths not filtered by these agents. The agents can also be activated by sunlight through window glass and strong artificial lighting. Short exposures to sunlight appear not to be a problem in animals. Wound infection during the period of tissue sloughing is common but can be resolved with appropriate antibiotic therapy.

11. Does PDT kill only tumors?

No. Normal tissue contains the photosensitizer and, if exposed to light, will be killed. During treatment of canine oral squamous cell carcinomas, teeth that were included in the treatment field were lost, and in some cases bone sequestrum developed, probably from destruction of the blood supply. Because the toxic oxygen radicals have a very short half-life, the cell killing away from the treated area is small. Therefore, normal tissue can be protected by shielding it from light.

12. How well do PDT lesions heal?

One of the outstanding things about PDT is the complete and usually cosmetic healing that occurs, possibly due to preservation of the collagen architecture. The healing is prolonged with up to 6 weeks in some cases, but most heal within 4 weeks.

13. What are the most apparent limitations?

Delivering light to the targeted tissue is the biggest challenge. Treatments use light in the red spectrum (wavelength between 630 and 690 nm), and the tissue penetration varies between 0.5 to 1.0 cm. Larger tumors can be treated by insertion of fibers into the tissue, but they need to be positioned no more than 0.8 cm apart. This leads to long treatment periods in large tumors. If photosensitizers that are activated at wavelengths above 700 nm are developed, larger tumors could be treated because tissue penetration is much better at longer wavelengths. The problem with deeper penetration of light is that normal structures could be more easily damaged.

14. Are there interactions with PDT and other forms of cancer therapy?

No significant interactions—either synergistic or antagonistic—have been noted with surgery, radiation therapy, chemotherapy, or hyperthermia.

15. Can PDT be used more than once?

Yes. There appear to be no lasting effects on normal tissue. Retreatment has been performed as early as 2 weeks with Photofrin. In that instance, no additional drug was administered because an adequate amount was still present in the tissue. Repeated palliative treatment with PDT is of considerable benefit, especially when removal of the trachea or esophagus would be necessary. There appears to be no acquired resistance of tumors to PDT.

16. How are the photosensitizing agents administered?

Most are administered intravenously. ALA is unique because it can be administered intravenously, orally, or topically.

17. What precautions are needed when handling these drugs?

Most of the agents need to be protected from light. The agents are nontoxic and therefore do not require precautions. ALA is absorbed through the skin, and therefore skin contact should be avoided.

18. What properties would an ideal photosensitizing agent possess?

The desirable qualities of a photosensitizing agent are to: (1) be obtainable in pure form, (2) localize strongly to tumor tissue and spare normal tissue, (3) be nontoxic, (4) be lipophilic and able to cross cell membranes, (5) have a short half-life, and (6) be activated by light wavelength between 700 to 800 nm.

BIBLIOGRAPHY

1. Beck ER: Lasers in veterinary oncology. In Bonagura JD (ed): Current Veterinary Therapy XI, Philadelphia, WB Saunders, 1992, pp 414–418.
2. Liu FF, Wilson BC: Hyperthermia and photodynamic therapy. In Tannock IF, Hill RP (eds): The Basic Science of Oncology, 3rd ed. New York, McGraw-Hill, 1998, pp 453–465.
3. Magne ML, Rodriquez CO, Autry SA, et al: Photodynamic therapy of facial squamous cell carcinoma in cats using a new photosensitizer. Lasers Surg Med 20:202–209, 1997.
4. McCaw DL, Pope ER, Payne JT: Treatment of canine oral squamous cell carcinomas with photodynamic therapy. Br J Cancer 82:1297–1299, 2000.
5. Peaston AE, Leach MW, Higgins RJ: Photodynamic therapy for nasal and aural squamous cell carcinomas in cats. J Am Vet Med Assoc 202:1261–1265, 1993.

18. COMPLEMENTARY AND ALTERNATIVE CANCER THERAPY: CURE OR QUACKERY?

Greg Ogilvie, DVM, Dipl ACVIM

1. What is complementary or alternative veterinary medicine?

Complementary or alternative veterinary medicine (CAVM) is the use of nontraditional therapies that can include acupuncture, massage, chiropractic, herbal, botanic, nutritional, biofield, and homeopathic methods to treat or support patients.

2. Has CAVM ever been shown to cure cancer patients of any species?

No.

3. How common is CAVM?

More clients are using complementary therapies for their pets and for themselves despite the limited data on efficacy and toxicity. Approximately 4 billion people, or 80% of the world's population, use herbal and botanic medicine, and many of these people seek this type of care for their pets. Conservative estimates indicate that one-third of all Americans routinely use alternative and complementary therapies, especially as a supplement to conventional health care methods. In fact, Americans visit alternative practitioners more often than physicians, at a cost of more than $14 billion per year. In addition, Americans spend an additional $4 billion annually on alternative products such as vitamins and herbs.

This same trend is occurring in veterinary health care. Anyone who has practiced during the past 5 years can appreciate clients' growing demand for complementary medicine. This is true especially in the treatment of cancer patients for whom traditional treatment options are limited and often toxic. Because these treatment modalities have been entrenched in traditional veterinary medicine as the standard of care, until recently there have been few western-style studies to document the efficacy of complementary medicine. However, this has changed in the past several years as scientists have undertaken and published studies using traditional research methods to discover the efficacy of such treatments. With the results of each new study, our comfort level in using these treatments grows. Despite the increased use of complementary or alternative medical treatments, none has ever been documented of ever curing a cancer patient. Their potential place in veterinary oncology and medicine is to support the patient. The practitioner should first be aware of the definition of these modalities to be at least conversant with their clients. Second, clinicians should know that while almost nothing is known about the efficacy and toxicity of complementary therapies in veterinary medicine, there are some documented efficacies and toxicities in other species.

4. What is acupuncture?

Acupuncture involves the stimulation of specific anatomic points on the body for therapeutic purposes with needles, heat, pressure, friction, suction, or impulses of electromagnetic energy. This ancient healing art is generally well accepted and widely used by human and veterinary health care professionals to treat a wide variety of ailments.

5. What is the mechanism of action of acupuncture?

Acupuncture is used to normalize or correct the flow of qi (pronounced *chee*, which refers to the body's vivifying force) to restore health. Sound scientific data have shown that the stimulation of specific points in the body alters the chemical neurotransmitters in the body. Acupuncture is one of the most commonly used complementary therapies in veterinary medicine.

6. What are the indications for the use of acupuncture?

Well-designed studies show efficacy for the treatment of osteoarthritis, chemotherapy-in-duced nausea, asthma, back pain, headaches, and others. The most dramatic reports on the efficacy of acupuncture have been its use in surgical analgesia. In 1973, up to 25% of all surgeries in mainland China were performed using acupuncture analgesia, with efficacy reported in up to 90% of the cases. Acupuncture surgical anesthesia is not widely used in the United States in human or veterinary medicine. This modality obviously has the potential for benefiting veterinary cancer patients where surgery is the mainstay of therapy.

7. What is chiropractic science?

Chiropractic science uses a healing method that concerns itself with the relationship between structure and function. The structure of the spine and function of the nervous system are the primary areas of interest of many practitioners.

8. What is the mechanism of action of chiropractic science?

Healing occurs by manual procedures and interventions, not surgical or chemotherapeutic treatments. Chiropractic care involves integration of the disciplines of radiology, sports-medicine, neurology, osteopathy, and orthopedics.

9. What are the indications for the use for chiropractic science?

Research in this area has been performed since the early days. However, research within the profession is still very much in its infancy. Little data exist concerning the efficacy of this treatment discipline in veterinary medicine. Areas of efficacy include back and other orthopedic pain and somatovisceral disorders such as hypertension. Chiropractic care for the veterinary cancer patient revolves primarily around improving function and reducing pain, especially in areas of orthopedic or neurologic disorders.

10. What is massage therapy?

Massage therapy is the manipulation of soft body parts to a state of normalcy.

11. What is the mechanism of action of massage therapy?

This modality incorporates the use of fixed or movable pressure and holding or causing the body to move. This ancient healing art affects the musculoskeletal, circulatory-lymphatic, and nervous systems. Healing by touch in massage therapy involves *vis medicatrix naurae* (helping the body heal itself). Techniques include Swedish massage, deep-tissue massage, neuromuscular massage, and manual lymphatic massage and involve reflexology, zone therapy, tuina, acupressure, the Rolfing, Trager, Feldenkrais method, and Alexander technique. Various adaptations of these techniques in human medicine are being used in veterinary medicine, although few data exist documenting efficacy in cats.

12. What are the indications for the use of massage therapy?

Trials have shown efficacy in acute and chronic pain, acute and chronic inflammation, chronic lymphedema, nausea, muscle spasm, various soft tissue dysfunction, grand mal epileptic seizures, anxiety, and depression. Massage has also been shown to stimulate the body's ability to control pain naturally by producing endorphins. Some suggest that massage therapy is contraindicated in the cancer patient because of increased blood flow that may result in increased metastases. Applications of massage therapy for the veterinary cancer patient may revolve around relieving pain and discomfort and maintaining function.

13. What is biofield therapy?

Biofield therapeutics is the ancient art of laying on of hands. The earliest record of this healing method dates between 2500 and 5000 years ago.

14. What are the mechanisms of action of biofield therapy?

Healing appears to come from two sources. The first is from a source other than the practitioner, such as God, the cosmos, or another supernatural entity. A second source is from the practitioner, who modifies or amplifies the patient's biofield. During this type of healing, the practitioner places his or her hands on or near the patient's body to improve general health or to improve a disease condition. Practitioners note that a biofield emanates for a distance beyond the physical body and that the strength, distance, and color of the field depends on the health and emotional state of the individual.

Three forms of biofield therapeutics are used: healing touch (Reiki), therapeutic touch, and SHEN therapy. Reiki originated from Japan in the 1800s and has a theoretical basis in providing spiritual energy with innate intelligence, channeled through the practitioner. In Reiki, the spiritual body is healed and is then expected to heal the physical body. In SHEN therapy, healing is reported to occur through a biofield, conforming to the natural laws of physics with a discernible flux pattern throughout the body. Therapeutic touch involves a practitioner who restores correct vibrational component to the patient's universal, unitary field. Few, if any, published data document efficacy of these modalites in the pet.

15. What are the indications for the use for biofield therapy?

In an overall report, Benor and colleagues reported an analysis of 151 healing studies. Sixty-one were controlled. Fifty-six percent showed significant results, leading to decreased anxiety of hospitalized patients (four studies), improved hemoglobin levels in hospitalized human patients (four studies), increased speed and completeness of healing of full-thickness wounds (one study), and improved tension headaches (one study). A number of rodent or tissue culture studies were completed, including one showing the efficacy of treating cancer cells. There are no good studies documenting the efficacy of biofield therapy in veterinary medicine.

16. What is homeopathy?

Homeopathic medicine is practiced worldwide, especially in Europe, Latin America, and Asia. These homeopathic remedies are made of naturally occuring substances from plants, animals, and minerals. These substances are recognized and regulated by the Food and Drug Administration. The remedies are diluted to as low as 10^{-30} to $10^{-20,000}$.

17. What is the mechanism of action of homeopathy?

Diseases or disorders are treated with extreme dilutions of like substances. For example, radiation illness could be treated with extreme dilutions of radium. Critics of homeopathy suggest that such extreme dilutions of compounds preclude any probability for efficacy. Scientists who have not rejected the potential benefits of homeopathy suggest that the efficacy can be explained by quantum physics, where the electromagnetic energy of these remedies may interact with the body for beneficial purposes. A phenomenon known as the memory of water is used to explain how extreme dilutions can result in retained efficacy. In this theory, the structure of water and alcohol solution is altered during the procedure of making the remedies so that the structure of the molecule is retained even after none of the actual substance remains.

18. What are the indications for the use of homeopathy?

The *British Medical Journal* published a meta-analysis on 96 published reports of 107 controlled trials. Trials were scored using a predefined system, and 22 were designated as well-designed clinical trials involving homeopathy; 15 of the 22 showed positive results but rarely in any cancer patients. The types of human patients that were improved included those with conditions such as allergic diseases and arthritis. Therefore, homeopathy may be of benefit for supporting a cancer patient, but little data exist to suggest that it can be used to directly treat or prevent a malignant process. The issue of vaccine-associated sarcomas in cats has led many homeopathic practitioners to suggest that homeopathic remedies should be used instead of traditional vaccines. This may have great appeal; however, efficacy data are very limited to nonexistent in veterinary patients.

19. What are pharmacologic and biologic treatments, and what are their indications?

Pharmacological and biological treatments use a wide variety of drugs and vaccines that are not yet accepted by mainstream medicine and surgery. There are no data published documenting the efficacy of these agents in veterinary medicine. Some of the more common agents being used include the following:

- *Antineoplastons* are peptide fractions originally derived from blood and urine and are being used to treat a wide variety of malignancies in people. This controversial treatment is being evaluated in a National Institutes of Health–funded study. Early studies showed efficacy in a number of tumors.
- *Cartilage products*, especially those from sharks and cattle. Cartilage has been shown to have antiangiogenic properties. In addition, they have tissue inhibitors of metalloproteinases that inhibit tumor metastasis. Shark cartilage has become very popular because reports from Mexico and Cuba suggest that this product resulted in the effective treatment of cancer in people. These original studies were soundly criticized because of faulty study design, lack of controls, and failure to confirm that patients had a malignancy. Current studies are being performed in several human cancer centers; however, final reports are not published. One investigator reported rapid reductions in prostate cancer in men. Despite the fact that 50,000 Americans use cartilage products and spend $7000 per year per person on this product, little data exists to document its efficacy. One report published in the *Proceedings of the Veterinary Cancer Society* in 1995 failed to confirm the efficacy of shark cartilage for the treatment of cancer in veterinary patients. Recently closed clinical studies in human cancer patients have failed to document the efficacy of shark cartilage.
- *Ethylenediaminetetraacetic acid (EDTA) chelation therapy* has been used to treat a number of conditions; however, the mechanism for treating cancer has not been clearly stated. It is interesting that metalloproteinases, especially those of gelatinase capability, are indeed inhibited by EDTA. Metalloproteinases 2 and 9 are critical for tumor growth and invasion. Therefore, there may be a reasonable explanation for the potential value of this type of therapy.
- *Immunoaugmentive therapy* is an experimental form of cancer therapy consisting of daily injections of blood products. Work done in dogs with osteosarcoma suggests that specific immunoaugmentive therapy improves disease-free intervals and survival. Similarly, dogs that have limb-sparing surgery for osteosarcoma and get an infected allograft have a significantly longer disease-free interval than those that do not have infected allografts. This may be due to enhancement of factors that augment the immune system. Other studies suggest efficacy by administering derivatives of aloe vera. Therefore, there may be some basis in logic for this type of therapy.
- *714-X* is a nitrogen-producing compound that is injected into the lymphatic system to treat a number of malignancies.
- *Coley's toxins* are derived from *Streptococcus pyogenes* and *Serratia marcescens* and have been touted as a treatment for cancer.
- *MTH-68* is a vaccine from the Newcastle disease virus of chickens that may interfere with oncornoviruses.
- *Iscador* is a lipid extract of mistletoe plants that has been used to treat many tumors.

HERBAL AND BOTANIC MEDICINE

20. What are herbal and botanic treatments?

Approximately 4 billion people use herbal and botanic medicine. Almost every native medicine around the world uses herbal treatments. Despite this widespread use, acceptance differs throughout the world. In the United States, herbal remedies are considered to be without efficacy by many members of regulatory bodies although many drugs routinely used today are derived from plants. European governments, especially German and French government bodies, have formally approved herbs for therapeutic purposes. Indeed, some of the best data on the efficacy of these herbs have been compiled in Europe.

21. What are the mechanisms of action of herbal and botantic treatments?
The mechanism of action depends on the active ingredient of the individual herb or botanic agent. In many cases, the mechanism is unknown. Agents used in China include sesquiterpenes, diterpenes, triterpenes, quinones, podophyllotoxins, Taxol, alkaloids, and others. Many of these have been adapted for western-style cancer therapy.

22. What are the indications for the use of herbal and botanic treatments?
In China and elsewhere in the world, herbs and other plant derivatives have been used to treat a number of disorders, including cancer, chemotherapy-induced nausea, and depression associated with the diagnosis of cancer. The number of herbs and other plant-based materials used therapeutically is staggering and beyond the scope of this chapter. As an example of the potential benefit of these agents, in 1981 the United States Department of Agriculture, in conjunction with the National Cancer Institute, concluded a 25-year study of plants with anticancer properties. The work includes 365 folk medicinal species and identifies more than 1000 pharmacologically active phytochemicals.

23. What is nutrition therapy?
Nutrition therapy revolves around the notion that nutrients can be used to prevent, support, and treat people and animals with cancer and a wide variety of other diseases. Indeed, nutrients have been used as a therapeutic tool for as long as records have been kept. Orthomolecular medicine is a discipline that promotes improving health and treating disease by using the optimum amount of substances normally present in the body. Advocates of orthomolecular medicine insist that, to be effective in preventing overt deficiencies and diseases, the intake of such nutrients needs to be increased drastically. This has been linked to positive responses for the treatment of AIDS, bronchial asthma, cardiovascular disease, strokes, and cancer.

24. What is the mechanism of action of nutritional therapy?
A large quantity of data exists documenting the beneficial and adverse effects of nutrients. Animals and humans have evolved considerably from our original paleolithic diets. The increased use of energy-dense foods rich in animal fats; partially hydrogenated vegetable oils; refined carbohydrates; but lacking whole grains, fruits, and vegetables has resulted in significant health problems. It seems reasonable, therefore, that improving the diet of all animals has many beneficial consequences. Similarly, the use of specific nutrients as a therapeutic tool is taking greater prominence. A great deal of information has been gained by the study of lifestyle diets. For example, Asian and Mediterranean diets have been shown for different reasons to reduce cardiovascular disease and cancer. This has led to research in veterinary medicine where eicosanoids of the n-3 series (eicosapentaenoic acid and docosahexaenoic acid) are being used to treat dogs with lymphoma and hemangiosarcoma. There is logic for this approach. Omega-3 (n-3) fatty acids have also been shown to inhibit tumorigenesis and cancer spread in animal models, and they form the basis for exciting work in prevention and treatment of cancer in humans. As a general rule, n-3 fatty acids (eicosapentaenoic acid, docosahexaenoic acid) have an inhibiting effect on tumor growth. Metastases are enhanced by the n-6 fatty acids (linoleic acid, gamma-linolenic acid). In vivo studies have shown that eicosapentaenoic acid has selective tumoricidal action without harming normal cells.

25. What are the indications for the use of nutritional therapies?

Veterinary food companies have pioneered the use of diets to treat a wide variety of diseases, including obesity, renal disease, heart disease, and urinary disease. Recent research suggests that specific diets can benefit veterinary and human cancer patients. Dietary therapy has taken several approaches. Some advocate increasing supplementation of specific nutrients to prevent or treat diseases such as cancer and the metabolic consequences of cancer. For example, some advise supplementing the diet with n-3 fatty acids, betacarotene, or vitamin C for the cancer patient. Others suggest a massive supplementation of certain nutrients, and still others suggest revision of the entire dietary profile for optimization of health. An example of the latter is a vegan vegetarian diet.

26. Should CAVM therapies be used in veterinary medicine?

Caution needs to be employed when assessing the efficacy of complementary therapies; however, existing data suggest that some of these modalities may be helpful to treat the veterinary cancer patient. Well-controlled studies are essential to document efficacy and toxicity. The biggest concern may be that unproven therapies may be used instead of known treatments. Therefore, the client should be informed of all the benefits and risks of traditional and nontraditional therapies.

BIBLIOGRAPHY

1. Eisenberg DM, Kessier RC, Foster C, et al: Unconventional medicine in the United States. Prevalence costs and patterns of use. N Engl J Med 328:246–252,1993.
2. Helms JM: Acupuncture Energetics: A Clinical Approach for Physicians. Berkeley, CA, Medical Acupuncture Publishers, 1995, pp 42–57.
3. Diamond EG: Acupuncture analgesia: Western medicine and Chinese traditional medicine. J Am Med Assoc 218:1558–1561, 1971.
4. Report of the Medical Delegation to the People's Republic of China, June 15–July 6, 1973. Washington DC, National Academy of Sciences, Institute of Medicine, 1973.
5. Lee MHM: Acupuncture analgesia in dentistry. A clinical investigation. NY State Dent J 39:288–301, 1973.
6. Filshie J, Redman D: Acupuncture and malignant pain problems. Eur J Surg Oncol 11:389–394, 1985.
7. Filshie J: Acupuncture for malignant pain. Acupuncture in medicine. BMJ 8:38–39, 1990.
8. Dundee JW: Reduction in the emetic effects of opioid preanesthetic medication by acupuncture. BMJ 22:583–584, 1986.
9. Dundee JW: Traditional Chinese acupuncture: A potentially useful antiemetic. BMJ 293:583–584, 1986.
10. Ghally RG: Antiemetic studies with traditional Chinese acupuncture: A comparison of manual needling with electrical stimulation and commonly used antiemetics. Anesth 42:1108–1113, 1987.
11. Ghaly RG: Acupuncture also reduces the emetic effects of pfethidine. Br J Anesth 59:135–137, 1987.
12. Yang LC: Comparison of P6 acupoint injection with 50% glucose in water and intravenous droperidol for the prevention of vomiting after gynecological laparoscopy. Acta Anaesthesiol Scand 37:192–194, 1993.
13. Dundee JW: Acupuncture prophylaxis of chemotherapy-induced sickness. J R Soc Med 82:268–271, 1989.
14. Sato T, Yu Y, Guo SY, et al: Acupuncture stimulation enhances splenic natural killer cell cytotoxicity in rats. Jpn J Physiol 46:131–136, 1996.
15. Jianguo Y, Rongxing Z, Mingsheng Z, Qimei G: Effect of acupuncture on peripheral T lymphocytes and their subgroups in patients with malignant tumors. Int J Clin Acupunct 4:53–58, 1993.
16. Xunshi W, Zhaolin Z, Chenrang S, et al: Clinical study on the use of second metacarpal holographic acupoints for re-establishing gastrointestinal motility in patients following abdominal surgery. Am J Acupunct 22:353–356, 1994.
17. Aglietti L: A pilot study of metoclopramide, dexamethasone, diphenhydramine and acupuncture in women treated with cisplatin. Cancer Chemother Pharmacol 26:239–240, 1990.
18. Lewis GBH: An alternative approach to premedication: Comparing diazepam with auriculotherapy and a relaxation method. Am J Acupunct 15:205–214, 1987.
19. Muxeneder R: Die konservative Behandlung chronischer Hautveränderungen des Pferdes durch Laserpunktur. Der praktische Tierarzt 69:12–21, 1988.

20. Liaw M, Wong AM, Cheng P: Therapeutic trial of acupuncture in phantom limb pain of amputees. Am J Acupunct 22:205–213, 1994.
21. Blom M, Dawidson I, Fernberg J-O, et al: Acupuncture treatment of patients with radiation-induced xerostomia. Oral Oncol, Eur J Cancer 32B:182–190, 1996.
22. Filshie J, Penn K, Ashley S, Davis CL: Acupuncture for the relief of cancer-related breathlessness. Pal Med 10:145–150, 1996.
23. Alternative Medicine: Expanding Medical Horizons: A Report to the National Institutes of Health on Alternative Medical Systems and Practices in the United States. 1994.
24. Bennor DJ: Healing research. Helix Verlab 1:1–29, 1992.
25. Kaarda B, Tosteinbo O: Increase of plasma beta endorphins in connective tissue message. Gen Pharmacol 20:487–489, 1989.
26. Sharma HM, Dwvedi C, Satter HA, et al: Antineoplastic properties of Maharishi 4 against DMBA-induced mammary tumors in rats. J Pharm Biochem Behav 35:767–773, 1990.
27. Arnold JT, Korytynski EA, Wilkinson BP, et al: Chemopreventative activity of Maharishi Amrit Kalash and related agents in rat tracheal epithelial and human tumor cells. J Proc Am Assoc Cancer Res 32:128–151, 1991.
28. Kleijnen J, Knipschild P, Reir GT: Clinical trials of homeopathy. BMJ 302:316–323, 1991.
29. Bertelli A, Mathe G: Antineoplastons (1). Drugs Exp Clin Res 12(Suppl 1), 1985.
30. Bartelli A, Mathe G: Antineoplastons (2). Drugs Exp Clin Res 13(Suppl 1), 1987.
31. Simone C: Presentation at a hearing on alternative medicine before a subcommittee of the Committee on Appropriations, US Senate, 103rd Congress, June 24, 1993.
32. Meyer JA, Dueland RT, et al: Canine osteogenic sarcoma treated by amputation and MER. Cancer 49:1613–1616, 1982.
33. MacEwen EG, Kurzman ID, Rosenthal RC, et al: Therapy for osteosarcoma in dogs with intravenous injection of liposome-encapsulated muramyl tripeptide. J Natl Cancer Inst 81:935–938, 1989.
34. Harris C, Pierce K, King G, et al: Efficacy of acemannan in treatment of canine and feline spontaneous neoplasms. Mol Biother 3:207–213, 1991.
35. Lin J-H, Rogers PAM, Yamada H: Chinese herbal medicine: Pharmacological basis. In Schoen AM, Wynn SG (eds): Complementary and Alternative Veterinary Medicine. St. Louis, Mosby, 1998, pp 379–404.
36. Lien EJ, Li WY: Structure Activity Relationship Analysis of Chinese Anticancer Drugs and Related Plants. Taiwan, Oriental Healing Arts Instutute, 1985, pp 1–140.
37. Duke JA, Ayensu ES: Handbook of Medicinal Herbs. Boca Raton, FL, CRC Press, 1985.
38. Begin ME, Ellis G, Das UN, et al: Differential killing of human carcinoma cells supplemented with N-3 and N-6 polyunsaturated fatty acids. J Natl Cancer Inst 77:2053–2057, 1986.
39. Begin ME, Das UN, Ellis G, et al: Selective killing of human cancer cells by polyunsaturated fatty acids. Prost Leuk Med 19:177–182, 1985.
40. Mengeaud V, Nano JL, Fournel S, Rampal P: Effects of eicosapentaenoic acid, Gamma-linolenic acid and prostaglandin E_1 on three human colon carcinoma cell lines. Prostaglandins Leukot Essent Fatty Acids 47:313–319, 1992.

19. NUTRITIONAL CONSIDERATIONS

Glenna E. Mauldin, DVM, MS, Dipl ACVIM

1. What is cancer cachexia?

Cancer cachexia is the term applied to protein-energy malnutrition when it is specifically associated with malignant disease. Protein-energy malnutrition results when the intake of both protein and calories is inadequate to meet the patient's needs. The detrimental clinical effects of protein-energy malnutrition are numerous and well described and include anemia; hypoproteinemia; delayed wound healing; decreased immune function; compromise of gastrointestinal, pulmonary, and cardiovascular function; and death. Cancer cachexia is the single most common cause of death in human patients with malignant disease.

2. Why is weight loss important in the cancer patient?

In addition to being the most common cause of death in human cancer patients, the presence of weight loss is of great clinical importance because it is an independent predictor of prognosis. Human cancer patients with documented weight loss are less likely to respond favorably to therapy and have statistically significantly shortened survival times. They are also more likely to experience treatment-related complications.

3. What tumors are most commonly associated with cancer cachexia?

The prevalence of weight loss in human cancer patients varies with tumor type. It is most common among patients with gastric or pancreatic cancers: 80% to 90% of these patients are reported to have weight loss at the time of diagnosis. Weight loss is relatively less common in patients with treatment-responsive lymphoma, breast cancer, or sarcomas, occurring in approximately 30% to 40% of affected individuals. Weight loss will be present in 50% to 60% of patients with nontreatment-responsive lymphomas or colon, prostate, or lung cancer. The prevalence of weight loss by tumor type in veterinary cancer patients has not been systematically investigated and is not known.

4. How prevalent is cancer cachexia in veterinary cancer patients?

The prevalence of actual weight loss (i.e., cancer cachexia) in veterinary cancer patients has not been thoroughly studied. However, preliminary work suggests that weight loss may be less common in dogs and cats with malignant disease than it is in human patients: In one study, 25% of dogs and 40% of cats had weight loss at the time of their cancer diagnosis; weight loss occurred in approximately 15% of dogs during the course of cancer therapy (radiation therapy, chemotherapy, or a combination of both). Differences in the prevalence of weight loss between species may be related to differences in the frequency of occurrence of various types of malignancies. The tumors least likely to cause weight loss in human patients, such as lymphoma, breast cancer, and soft tissue sarcomas, are commonly diagnosed and treated in dogs and cats. The human tumors most likely to be associated with weight loss—for instance, gastric, pancreatic or colon cancers—are rarer.

5. What causes weight loss in the cancer patient?

Three primary etiologies are responsible for the weight loss associated with neoplastic disease in both human and veterinary cancer patients.

First, the tumor or its metastases may have physical consequences that result in decreased nutrient intake: Tumors affecting the oral cavity, pharynx, or esophagus prevent normal food prehension, mastication, and swallowing; mass lesions of the abdominal viscera cause nausea and vomiting; and tumors diffusely infiltrating the wall of the small bowel impair nutrient digestion and absorption.

Secondly, the complications of anticancer therapy can result in significant compromise of nutrient intake: Drug-induced alterations in smell or taste perception and learned food aversions cause treatment-related anorexia; some chemotherapeutic agents interact directly with neuroreceptors in the gastrointestinal tract or the hypothalamic chemoreceptor trigger zone to cause nausea, anorexia, and vomiting; radiation- or chemotherapy-induced damage to the rapidly proliferating cells lining the intestinal tract results in ulcerative stomatitis, diarrhea, and abnormal nutrient digestion and absorption; and treatment-related myelosuppression predisposes the patient to infectious complications that may affect food intake, such as mycotic stomatitis or even sepsis.

Finally, an intriguing group of human and veterinary patients develop cancer cachexia despite an apparently adequate food intake. Weight loss in these individuals is hypothesized to occur secondary to unique, tumor-related changes in host metabolism that result in the inefficient use of consumed calories. Losses in both lean body mass and adipose stores are typical. Specific abnormalities involving the intermediary metabolism of carbohydrate, protein, and lipid have been demonstrated in human and canine cancer patients as well as in rodents bearing implanted tumors.

The clinician must recognize that cancer cachexia is likely to be the result of a complicated interaction between all three of these potential etiologies. This interaction is likely to change significantly through the course of an individual patient's disease and therapy, necessitating the combined or sequential use of various management strategies.

6. Name the metabolic abnormalities typically associated with the tumor-bearing state.

The most common biochemical alterations reported in association with the tumor-bearing state are related to carbohydrate metabolism. Malignant cells are incapable of significant aerobic glycolysis, or fat oxidation, and derive their energy from anaerobic glycolysis. Thus, they may consume large quantities of host glucose; host hepatocytes also expend additional energy to resynthesize glucose from the lactate produced. Increased serum lactate concentrations are frequently reported. Increased rates of whole-body glucose turnover and disposal, with markedly increased rates of gluconeogenesis from lactate and amino acids, have been documented in human beings as well as rodents. Hyperinsulinism, insulin resistance, and abnormal glucose tolerance have also been observed.

Concurrent derangement of protein metabolism is frequently present. Altered serum amino acid profiles have been reported in both human and canine cancer patients and are believed to reflect tumor-induced changes in amino acid synthesis and use. In addition to increased rates of gluconeogenesis from amino acids, as noted above, increased whole-body protein turnover, decreased protein fractional synthetic rates in skeletal muscle, and increased protein fractional synthetic rates in liver have been demonstrated.

Finally, while older reports frequently suggest that lipid metabolism is normal in tumor-bearing subjects, recent work has repeatedly demonstrated that this is not the case. Cancer patients with tumor-associated weight loss suffer profound depletion of body adipose stores—the result of markedly accelerated lipolysis. Hypertriglyceridemia may be present and is associated with decreased lipoprotein lipase activity in some rodent models. Increased rates of hepatic triacylglycerol and very low-density lipoprotein (VLDL) synthesis, as well as elevated serum concentrations of nonesterified fatty acids, acetoacetate, beta-hydroxybutyrate, and VLDL, are reported.

It is important to distinguish between the presence of these metabolic abnormalities and actual "cancer cachexia." Demonstration of some or even all of these changes does not invariably mean that the subject currently suffers from cancer cachexia or will do so in the future. Cancer cachexia by definition refers to weight loss in a tumor-bearing host: If weight loss is not present, the subject does not have cancer cachexia—regardless of the biochemical perturbations that may exist.

7. What are the primary pathophysiologic mechanisms that are hypothesized to result in the metabolic abnormalities typical of the tumor-bearing state?

The causes of decreased nutrient intake and weight loss secondary to direct tumor effects or complications of cancer therapy are readily apparent and easily understood. However, the pathophysiology underlying the metabolic changes characteristic of the tumor-bearing state is less clear.

There are two primary possibilities: first, that substances elaborated by the tumor itself interfere with the host's intermediary metabolism or, second, that the host's own neural, endocrine, and cytokine response to the presence of neoplastic disease is responsible for the observed changes. The latter seems most likely and is supported by studies documenting alterations in plasma and urine catecholamine concentrations as well as changes in both the absolute and relative concentrations of insulin and glucagon. Increased host production of various cytokines has also been implicated as a contributing cause of these biochemical alterations. The roles of tumor necrosis factor-α (TNF-α) and interleukin-6 (IL-6), for example, have been studied extensively in specific implanted rodent tumor models, where increased production of one or the other appears to be largely responsible for host weight loss.

However, study in human patients with naturally occurring disease indicates that the situation is much more complex: While TNF-α and IL-6 may have roles to play, many other factors are also involved. The underlying causes of the tumor-associated alterations in intermediary metabolism that may lead to weight loss in a specific patient are likely to be numerous, unique to that individual, and variable over the course of disease.

8. What role does the patient's metabolic rate play in the development of cancer cachexia?

It is apparent that futile cycling and increased flux through certain metabolic pathways are characteristic of many of the biochemical abnormalities associated with the tumor-bearing state, including increased serum lactate concentrations, increased whole-body glucose and protein turnover, and increased rates of gluconeogenesis. The transfer of energy through these pathways is not perfectly efficient, and it is tempting to hypothesize that this type of cycling increases the cancer patient's energy expenditure, thereby resulting in hypermetabolism and weight loss. Unfortunately, studies using indirect calorimetry to measure energy expenditure in human and canine patients with naturally occurring tumors as well as in rodents with implanted tumors have yielded widely variable results, and the role of the patient's metabolic rate in the development of cancer cachexia is poorly defined. Energy expenditure is increased in some studies, unchanged in others, and actually decreased in still others.

Again, it is clear that variations in the individual manifestations of cancer cachexia exist: Metabolic rate changes with tumor type, stage of disease, and the patient's preexisting nutritional status. However, the difficulties inherent in the use of indirect calorimetry must also be considered as a potential explanation for some of the observed variation. The technique involves the use of equipment so sensitive that results are difficult to consistently reproduce, and they may certainly vary between investigators. Furthermore, careful analysis of indirect calorimetry work carried out in tumor-bearing subjects reveals potentially significant differences in the types of individuals studied. The relevance of isolated energy expenditure measurements in tumor-bearing subjects prior to the development of weight loss is debatable. In addition, some authors compare weight-losing cancer patients to healthy, weight-stable controls, while others use weight-losing patients with nonmalignant disease. The unavoidable conclusion is that many questions regarding energy expenditure in the cancer patient remain unanswered, and work in this area continues.

9. How is cancer cachexia diagnosed?

Identification of patients suffering from cancer cachexia is accomplished through nutritional assessment, which involves the systematic collection and integration of clinical information to evaluate protein and energy status. In most veterinary patients, it consists of a complete diet history, a thorough physical examination, morphometric assessment in the form of body condition scoring, and evaluation of a few widely available hematologic and biochemical parameters.

10. What physical examination findings are characteristic of cancer cachexia?

With the exception of the tumor itself, the physical examination abnormalities associated with cancer cachexia are the same as those present in protein-energy malnutrition of any etiology. The difficulty is that clinical signs are nonspecific and often subtle, and an increased index of suspicion must be preserved to identify affected individuals. One or more abnormalities may be present, including muscle wasting, pallor, weakness, poor hair coat, hepatomegaly, splenomegaly, evidence of chronic infections, lymphadenopathy, and peripheral edema.

Body condition scoring is a useful technique that is easily performed as part of the physical examination in veterinary cancer patients. In human patients, protein or lean body mass and adipose stores are evaluated through the use of standardized morphometric measurements such as triceps skinfold thickness or midarm circumference. While the large variation in body size and conformation between breeds and individuals makes adaptation of these specific techniques very difficult in dogs and cats, body condition scoring systems developed for use in canine and feline patients provide a practical alternative. When used carefully and consistently, these systems provide much of the same information as morphometric measurements. A five- or nine-point scale is used, in which each point corresponds to a particular body condition as defined by specific, standardized criteria: for instance, "cachectic" (no detectable body fat); "optimal" (good muscle mass and tone, some body fat present but ribs still easily palpable); or "obese" (large quantities of subcutaneous and abdominal fat completely obscure underlying anatomic structures). Published studies confirm that there is good correlation between body condition score and between the proportion of lean body mass to adipose tissue (i.e., body composition) in canine and feline patients.

11. Describe the routine hematologic and biochemical parameters likely to be affected in veterinary patients with cancer cachexia.

Abnormalities in several widely available hematologic and biochemical parameters may be used as supporting evidence of the presence of cancer cachexia, although none are particularly sensitive or specific. Normochromic, normocytic, nonregenerative anemia (anemia of chronic disease), and lymphopenia are considered typical of protein-energy malnutrition. Biochemical abnormalities may include decreased blood urea nitrogen concentrations secondary to decreased protein intake, decreased serum creatinine concentrations due to attrition of lean body mass, and hypoalbuminemia due to catabolism and decreased protein synthesis. The unusually high protein requirement of the cat likely predisposes this species to protein-energy malnutrition and may lead to additional serum biochemical abnormalities: Increased serum concentrations of hepatocellular leakage enzymes and alkaline phosphatase reflect fatty infiltration of the liver and cholestasis, and increased serum concentrations of creatine kinase may occur as skeletal muscle is catabolized for its constituent amino acids.

12. Why is serum albumin concentration an insensitive indicator of nutritional status in veterinary patients with cancer cachexia?

The serum half-life of albumin is relatively long in mammalian species, reaching approximately 8 days in the dog. Thus, dietary protein deficiency, catabolism exceeding the rate of albumin synthesis, or both must be present for a prolonged period before hypoalbuminemia will result. Not surprisingly, serum proteins with shorter half-lives have been shown to be more sensitive for assessing protein status in human patients. Potentially useful proteins investigated for this purpose have included transferrin, fibrinogen, retinol-binding protein, and insulin-like growth factor-1. The utility of short–half-life proteins for the assessment of nutritional status in canine and feline patients is largely unknown.

13. What primary methods are available for the nutritional support of the veterinary patient with cancer cachexia?

Three primary methods are available for the nutritional support of the veterinary patient with cancer cachexia: **voluntary intake, assisted enteral feeding,** and **assisted parenteral feeding**. The optimal route for any individual patient will be determined primarily by the underlying disease process, although cost must often be considered as well. Voluntary intake is preferred if it will meet the patient's needs: It is the simplest, cheapest, and most convenient method. It is essential that any patient's voluntary food intake be carefully monitored over time and compared with the patient's estimated requirement. If a deficit is present, some form of nutritional support is necessary. Several techniques may be used to maximize voluntary intake: hand feeding of small, frequent meals; use of highly palatable and aromatic foods; warming of canned products to body temperature before offering; and use of calorie- and nutrient-dense commercial rations to maximize nutrient intake in the volume of food consumed. However, assisted feeding should be instituted without delay if none of these measures are successful. Nasoesophageal, pharyngostomy, esophagostomy, gastrostomy, or jejunostomy tubes may be used to facilitate assisted enteral feeding, and intravenous catheters are necessary to permit assisted parenteral feeding.

14. Describe the advantages and disadvantages of enteral nutritional support in the veterinary patient with cancer cachexia.

Assisted enteral feeding is the optimal method of nutritional support for most veterinary patients with cancer cachexia who are unable to support themselves through voluntary intake. Placement of nutrients directly into the intestinal tract takes advantage of existing pathways and physiologic adaptations that are more efficient and helps to promote normal organ function. Specifically, the presence of food within the intestinal tract supports enterocyte health, preventing villous atrophy; it also maintains gut immune function, preventing the bacterial translocation that may lead to systemic bacterial infection and sepsis. In general, assisted enteral feeding is less complicated than assisted parenteral feeding, has fewer potential complications, and is less expensive.

There are few disadvantages associated with assisted enteral feeding. However, it is obviously contraindicated if the gastrointestinal tract is nonfunctional. In addition, long periods of transition may occasionally be required to reach the full volume of intake necessary to meet calculated requirements, particularly in patients with long preceding periods of complete or near-complete anorexia.

15. Describe the advantages and disadvantages of parenteral nutritional support in the veterinary patient with cancer cachexia.

Assisted parenteral feeding is the only option for nutritional support in a selected group of veterinary patients in whom the gastrointestinal tract is nonfunctional because of decreased digestive or absorptive capacity or anatomic or physiologic obstruction. Parenteral feeding may benefit patients with inflammatory gastrointestinal conditions such as inflammatory bowel disease or pancreatitis because it permits bypass of the entire gastrointestinal tract and allows complete bowel rest. The lack of ingesta within the upper gastrointestinal tract during parenteral feeding may be advantageous in comatose patients who are at high risk for aspiration. Finally, assisted parenteral feeding may be considered for animals not sufficiently stable to withstand the general anesthesia that may be required for feeding tube placement or for patients with severe coagulopathies.

Despite these advantages, parenteral feeding has numerous potential disadvantages that must be recognized. Mechanical, infectious, and biochemical complications (i.e., hyperglycemia, hypertriglyceridemia, and refeeding syndrome) are all possible, and patients must be carefully monitored to avoid them. The lack of ingesta within the intestinal tract during parenteral nutrition promotes clinically significant villous atrophy and predisposes critically ill patients to bacterial translocation from the gut. An increased level of nursing care and specialized equipment and products are required. Finally, assisted parenteral feeding is often considerably more costly than assisted enteral feeding. The use of parenteral nutrition should be restricted to those patients in whom it is clearly indicated.

16. What primary features characterize the commercial rations typically recommended for veterinary cancer patients?

The commercial rations typically recommended for use in veterinary cancer patients are highly palatable, highly digestible, and nutrient-dense. It is not unreasonable to expect that such diets might minimize or reverse some of the deleterious nutritional effects of neoplastic disease as well as the modalities used to treat it. Potential benefits to the patient could include improved ability to tolerate aggressive antineoplastic therapy, enhanced quality of life, and even increased survival times. Rations may also be chosen in a specific attempt to take advantage of the metabolic differences between normal host tissues and tumor cells: A diet high in fat and low in readily available carbohydrate should theoretically supply energy to the host at the expense of the tumor. Beneficial effects have been documented in both human and canine cancer patients fed such diets, including improved preservation of lean body mass and adipose stores, decreased glucose intolerance, and prolonged survival times.

Not all veterinary cancer patients, however, are likely to benefit equally from highly palatable, high fat rations. It appears that a minority of canine and feline patients suffer from cancer cachexia: Preliminary work suggests that more than 60% of dogs with cancer are actually overweight. Careless use of high-fat diets in such patients will simply promote additional weight gain and all of the health problems associated with obesity. As with any commercial pet food, high-fat diets should initially be fed to meet the estimated caloric requirement of the cancer patient and the intake adjusted up or down as necessary to maintain optimal body condition over time.

17. What types of commercial rations are most likely to meet this profile?

The types of commercial rations most likely to fit the profile described above—highly digestible, very palatable, nutrient-dense, high in fat, low in carbohydrates—are prescription products designed for use during performance or stress, "premium" dog and cat foods, and puppy or kitten foods. A prescription product specifically designed for use in dogs with neoplastic disease is also available. Complete and balanced commercial products made by a reputable manufacturer, which have been tested using animal feeding tests using Association of American Feed Control Officials procedures, are preferred over home-cooked diets for long-term use. Either dry or canned foods may be appropriate, although dry foods are often more energy-dense than canned products and may provide additional benefit in veterinary cancer patients with ongoing weight loss.

18. How do the nutrient requirements of dogs and cats with neoplastic disease differ from those of healthy dogs and cats?

Commercial rations intended for use in weight-losing dogs and cats with cancer are frequently enriched with a variety of nutrients. However, these additions have been made based largely on studies carried out in human cancer patients: Very little is known regarding the specific nutrient requirements of dogs and cats with neoplastic disease. Furthermore, most products have numerous potentially beneficial nutrients added, making it virtually impossible to elucidate the effects of any one with certainty.

Regardless, in addition to being high in fat and low in carbohydrates, the rations commonly recommended for use in dogs and cats with cancer contain ample protein so that the increased protein needs characteristic of critical illness can be met. Most are enriched with n-3 (omega-3) fatty acids; these nutrients are known to modulate the immune response in dogs and may also have specific anticancer and anticachectic effects. However, neither the optimal intake of n-3 fatty acids nor the most appropriate ratio of n-3 to n-6 fatty acids for the veterinary cancer patient is known. (Both are currently subjects of great debate among pet food manufacturers). Other nutrients playing potential roles in the immune response (i.e., zinc) or protecting against oxidative stress (i.e., vitamin E) also are commonly added. Finally, the amino acids arginine and glutamine are often present in increased quantities, although specifically increased dietary requirements in canine or feline cancer patients have yet to be demonstrated. Arginine supplementation in critically ill human patients has been shown to improve nitrogen balance, stimulate immune function, improve wound healing, and decrease morbidity and mortality. Glutamine is a "conditionally" essential nutrient during illness, and supplementation supports protein synthesis, improves gastrointestinal repair and regeneration, and augments both the systemic and gastrointestinal immune response in human patients.

19. What is the best diet to feed a dog or cat with cancer?
The best diet for an individual dog or cat with malignant disease is determined by careful assessment of that animal's current body condition, consideration of the underlying disease processes present, and evaluation of the previous dietary history. Based on these criteria, it is obvious that no single ration will be optimal for all animals. However, high-fat, low-carbohydrate, nutrient-dense diets may be beneficial for patients with cancer-associated weight loss. High-fat diets should probably be avoided in significantly obese patients or in patients that are likely to tolerate fat poorly (i.e., dogs with a history of pancreatitis). Additional nutritional therapies may be indicated in some patients to address concurrent underlying diseases or conditions, such highly digestible diets for gastrointestinal disease, or protein restriction for significant renal or hepatic dysfunction. Finally, consideration should be given to individual flavor and formulation (dry vs canned vs semi-moist) preferences as well as to historical episodes of food intolerance: A diet must be readily consumed, digested, and absorbed to provide benefit to the patient. Regardless of the specific product recommended, a complete and balanced commercial ration made by a reputable manufacturer is always preferred.

20. What equation should be used to calculate the target caloric intake for a dog or cat with cancer?
The best equation for calculation of the target caloric intake in a dog or cat with cancer depends on the patient's clinical situation. The resting energy requirement (RER) in kilocalories per day is given by

$$RER = 70(BW_{kg})^{3/4}$$

for both dogs and cats of all weights and is most appropriate for critically ill, hospitalized patients. Some authors adjust the RER using an illness factor based on the patient's underlying disease but, if this step is performed, the illness factor used should not be higher than 1.4 to avoid overfeeding.

Canine and feline cancer patients in the home environment are more likely to have energy requirements approximating maintenance. There is substantial disagreement regarding the equations that best estimate maintenance energy requirements, but the author has successfully used

$$MER = 60 \text{ to } 80(BW_{kg})$$

in feline patients, varying with activity level, and

$$MER = 132(BW_{kg})^{3/4}$$

in canine patients to estimate initial intake in kilocalories of energy required per day. Regardless of the equation used, food intake must always be adjusted up or down as necessary to maintain optimal body condition.

CONTROVERSIES

21. Should appetite stimulants be used in anorexic veterinary patients with cancer cachexia?
For: Pharmacologic appetite stimulation is a relatively simple and cost-effective measure that may increase voluntary food intake sufficiently to avoid the need for assisted enteral or

parenteral feeding in the veterinary cancer patient. It may also improve quality of life and allow the animal to remain in the home environment for a longer time. Megestrol acetate in particular has shown promise in clinical trials in human patients with cancer cachexia.

Against: There are no objective studies confirming the clinical efficacy of any appetite stimulant in canine or feline cancer patients, including megestrol acetate. Food intake is rarely measured carefully enough to confirm an adequate increase in food intake after initiation of appetite stimulant therapy. Furthermore, while the clinician awaits a response to therapy, the more appropriate placement of a feeding tube may be unnecessarily delayed.

22. Are diets high in n-3 fatty acids beneficial in veterinary cancer patients?

For: High-fat, low-carbohydrate diets enriched with n-3 fatty acids have been demonstrated to normalize various biochemical abnormalities in canine cancer patients, including hyperlactatemia and glucose intolerance. Improved survival times have been documented among dogs with World Health Organization stage III lymphoma also receiving chemotherapy. Other potential benefits include modulation of the immune response through altered eicosanoid production, decreased platelet aggregation resulting in lower rates of metastasis, stabilization of tumor-associated weight loss, and decreased acute radiation toxicity.

Against: Studies examining the efficacy of n-3 fatty acid enriched diets have been conducted primarily in canine cancer patients without documented weight loss, so the true significance of decreased hyperlactatemia and improved glucose intolerance is unknown. Products containing high concentrations of n-3 fatty acids are expensive, and greater improvements in remission duration and survival times can be obtained among dogs with lymphoma by using the financial resources of clients to intensify chemotherapy (i.e., a University of Wisconsin–Madison–type protocol). Diets excessively high in n-3 fatty acids may predispose patients to bleeding, decreased wound healing, and compromised immune function.

BIBLIOGRAPHY

1. Daniel HL, Mauldin GE: Body condition scoring in dogs and cats with and without malignant disease. Proc 19th Annu Vet Cancer Soc Conf, 1999, p 36.
2. DeWys WD: Weight loss and nutritional abnormalities in cancer patients: Incidence, severity and significance. Clin Oncol 5:251–261,1986.
3. Mauldin GE: Nutritional support of the cancer patient. In Bonagura JD (ed): Kirk's Current Veterinary Therapy XIII. Small Animal Practice. Philadelphia, WB Saunders, 2000, pp 458–462.
4. Ogilvie GK, Fettman MJ, Mallinckrodt CH, et al: Effect of fish oil, arginine, and doxorubicin chemotherapy on remission and survival time for dogs with lymphoma: A double-blind, randomized placebo-controlled study. Cancer 88:1916–1928, 2000.
5. Ogilvie GK, Walters LM, Fettman MJ, et al: Energy expenditure in dogs with lymphoma fed two specialized diets. Cancer 71:3146–3152, 1993.
6. Remillard RL, Armstrong PJ, Davenport DJ: Assisted feeding in hospitalized patients: Enteral and parenteral nutrition. In Hand MS, Thatcher CD, Remillard RL, et al (eds): Small Animal Clinical Nutrition, 4th ed. Topeka, KS, Mark Morris Institute, 2000, pp 351–399.
7. Tisdale MJ: Wasting in cancer. J Nutr 129:243S–246S, 1999.
8. Vail DM, Ogilvie GK, Wheeler SL, et al: Alterations in carbohydrate metabolism in canine lymphoma. J Vet Intern Med 4:8–11, 1990.

20. ONCOLOGIC EMERGENCIES AND CHEMOTHERAPEUTIC COMPLICATIONS

Gregory K. Ogilvie, DVM, Dipl ACVIM

1. What factors predispose patients with cancer to sepsis?

The most common factors that predispose cancer patients to infections are granulocytopenia, cellular immune dysfunction, humoral immune dysfunction, splenectomy, indwelling vascular catheters, prolonged hospitalization, poor nutrition, neurologic dysfunction, and the effects of cancer itself.

2. What are the most common causes of granulocytopenia?

Granulocytopenia may result from bone marrow destruction caused by leukemia or lymphoma or from the myelosuppressive effects of chemotherapy.

3. Do all anticancer drugs affect the bone marrow the same way?

Different drugs have different characteristic effects on the bone marrow. The myelosuppressive effects of anticancer drugs can be categorized as high, moderate, or mild. Doxorubicin, vinblastine, cyclophosphamide, and carboplatin are in the highly myelosuppressive category. Vincristine and asparaginase usually considered mildly myelosuppressive drugs but may cause a surprising degree of myelosuppression when used together.

4. Which specific bacteria are commonly associated with sepsis in patients with cancer?

The gram-negative bacteria most commonly associated with infection of patients with granulocytopenia include *Escherichia coli*, *Klebsiella pneumoniae*, *Pseudomonas* species, and *Enterobacteriaceae* species. The most common gram-positive bacteria include *Staphylococcus epidermidis* and *Staphylococcus aureus*.

5. What is the best way to recognize the septic patient?

Physical examination may reveal an animal with hyperdynamic septic shock, hallmarks of which include plethora (brick-red mucous membranes), tachycardia, and short capillary refill times. These symptoms may be followed by gastrointestinal signs, altered mentation, and decreased blood pressure. Endstage signs reflect a hypodynamic state and include hypothermia, pallor, mental depression, bloody diarrhea, and other signs of multiorgan failure. Hyperglycemia is an early finding, followed in many instances by hypoglycemia. Although bacterial cultures may be deceptively negative, a positive culture is common.

6. What is unusual about the results of diagnostic tests in a neutropenic patient with sepsis?

The absence of circulating neutrophils results in a urinalysis without pyuria and in thoracic radiographs that appear normal because of the lack of neutrophilic infiltrates. Neutrophils are responsible for the early radiographic changes associated with pneumonia. There, these conditions are often not identifiable by standard diagnostic tests.

7. What should be cultured in neutropenic septic patients?

At least two sets of aerobic and anaerobic blood cultures should be acquired. A cystocentesis specimen for urine culture should be acquired (after a platelet count of at least 60,000/µl has been assured). If neurologic signs are present, a cerebrospinal fluid (CSF) tap should be obtained and cultured appropriately. CSF should be sent for Gram stain, bacterial culture, cell count and differential, and glucose and protein determination. A cryptococcal antigen titer or india ink preparation should be performed in suspect cases. For animals with diarrhea, appropriate cultures should be done for clostridial organisms, including appropriate assays for endotoxin.

8. Should other diagnostic tests be considered?

A complete blood count, profile biochemical screen, and urinalysis should be performed on each patient. Thoracic radiographs should be taken when a site of infection is not obvious (caution on interpretation as above). Other diagnostic imaging studies including ultrasonography, especially echocardiography to identify valvular endocarditis. Invasive tests to consider include bronchoscopy, skin biopsy, bone marrow biopsy, percutaneous liver biopsy, and exploratory laparotomy as the case indicates.

9. What are the overall goals of treating septic neutropenic animals?

Treatment for septic neutropenic animals is directed primarily at restoring adequate tissue perfusion, improving alterations in metabolism, and controlling systemic infection.

10. What type, how much, and at what rate should fluids be administered to restore tissue perfusion?

Crystalloid solutions such as lactated Ringer's solution have been most commonly used. In critical situations, an initial intravenous infusion rate of 70 to 90 ml/kg for the first hour followed by 10 to 12 mg/kg/hr has been considered appropriate. The fluid rate should be adjusted to meet the needs of each patient as directed by monitoring of body weight, heart and respiratory rates, central venous pressure, and ongoing losses. For several reasons, it appears better to use normal saline or balanced, nonlactated, electrolyte solutions in septic hypermetabolic cancer patients. Dextrose (2.5% to 5%) should be included in fluids when systemic hypoglycemia is identified.

11. What type of antibiotic is used in neutropenic patients with or without sepsis?

Asymptomatic animals with fewer than 1000 to 1500 neutrophils/µl should be started on prophylactic antibiotics; orally administered trimethoprim-sulfa has been a common choice in this setting.

As soon as appropriate bacterial cultures have been obtained, neutropenic patients in septic shock should be supported with fluids and antibiotics administered intravenously. When a gram-negative infection is present, two antibiotics that are the most effective against the isolated organism are often recommended; gentamicin, cephalothin, and cefoxitin have been useful agents. Generally, gram-positive infections are treated with a single appropriate antibiotic; penicillin O sodium or penicillin O potassium, cephalothin, and cefoxitin have been useful agents. For anaerobic bacteria, cefoxitin and metronidazole have been useful. When a patient is seriously threatened by sepsis, the empiric use of imipenem has been useful.

12. What is the role of transfusions in an emergency situation?

Transfusions are frequently needed for veterinary patients as a result of various emergency situations, including blood loss, disseminated intravascular coagulation (DIC), clinical syndromes associated with the hypocoagulable state of malignancy and other diseases, and other hematologic abnormalities. In general, transfusions and blood components should be given only when specifically indicated. Other emergency support procedures, such as fluid therapy, should be used concurrently. The recent availability of blood components commercially makes this form of therapy practical for general practitioners.

13. What type of blood should be used to transfuse dogs or cats with acute blood loss?

Although there is a theoretical advantage to transfusing fresh whole blood, packed red blood cells may be administered with excellent results. Red blood cells stored for more than 2 weeks may have a depletion of 2,3-diphosphoglycerate, which may diminish red blood cell oxygen-carrying capacity. Transfusion should be performed to keep the hematocrit above 15% in dogs and above 10% in cats when possible.

14. What is bovine hemoglobin (Oxyglobin), and when should it be used in an emergency situation instead of blood?

Oxyglobin is the brand name of a product derived from bovine hemoglobin that acts to increase hemoglobin and arterial oxygen. Emergency treatment of the following conditions generally results in clinical improvement in up to 95% of the patients:
- Immune-mediated hemolysis
- Blood loss (from rodenticide, trauma, and surgical and gastrointestinal complications
- Ineffective erythropoiesis (red cell aplasia, ehrlichiosis).

15. How should Oxyglobin be administered?

Oxyglobin is given to dogs at 30 ml/kg intravenously at a rate of up to 10 ml/kg/hr. The product can be warmed to 37°C before administration. The half-life is 30 to 40 hours.

16. What are the adverse effects associated with the administration of Oxyglobin?
- Anaphylactic reactions
- Circulatory overload in cases of overdose (more than 10 ml/kg/hr) or in patients with preexisting cardiac disease. Monitor central venous pressure and clinical signs for circulatory overload.
- Discoloration of skin (yellow-orange), feces (red to dark green), and urine (brown-black).
- Vomiting
- Diarrhea and decreased skin elasticity can occur within 48 hours of transfusion.

17. What are the indications for treating a patient with thrombocytopenia?

Platelet counts greater than 30,000 to 40,000 are rarely associated with bleeding disorders. Indeed, a gradual reduction in platelet counts may result in healthy-appearing patients with only 2000 to 3000 platelets. Recently released platelets have much greater function than older platelets. Platelet transfusion should be used only in dogs or cats that exhibit clinical signs. Platelet-rich plasma may be considered in such patients; however, the half-life of platelets may last for only weeks or days or less, especially in the presence of immune-mediated conditions. One unit per 20 kg of body weight of platelet-rich plasma or fresh whole blood should be administered and repeated every hour until an adequate platelet count is reached.

18. What drug can be used to increase platelet numbers, assuming adequate megakaryocytes are present?

Vincristine (0.5 mg/m^2 intravenously every 1 to 3 weeks) may be administered to induce premature release of platelets from the bone marrow at other sites during this time. The platelet count usually increases 3 to 5 days after vincristine is administered.

19. What is disseminated intravascular coagulation?

DIC is a syndrome with severe bleeding and consumption of clotting factors and platelets.

20. How is DIC treated?

Because DIC is a syndrome and not a specific disease but secondary to some other problem, the ideal treatment is to control the underlying condition. Unfortunately, this is often frustrating, if not impossible in many cancer patients. Symptomatically, approximately one unit of fresh frozen plasma can be used and repeated as needed to maintain prothrombin and partial thromboplastin time at 1 to 1.5 times the normal bleeding time. Use of

heparin is controversial; however, if used in conjunction with platelets, it may have beneficial results. When all cell lines (red blood cells and platelets) are decreased, fresh whole
blood also can be used.

21. How do you determine how much blood or blood component to administer?

Animals with significant acute blood loss should be treated first for shock with crystalloid solutions. Hypertonic saline is also a reasonable choice in select patients. Packed red
blood cells may be given with crystalloid fluids or whole blood. As a general rule, one unit of
packed red blood cells is administered per 20 kg of body weight with close adjustments to
maintain the hematocrit above 15%. Dogs that require whole blood for either acute or chronic
anemias should be transfused using the general guidelines below:

General rule: amount to transfuse

ml donor blood = [(2.2 ´ wtkg) ´ (40dog or 30cat) ´ PCVdesired –
PCVrecipient)]PCVdonor

where PCV = packed cell volume; 2.2 ml of blood/kg raises PCV by 1% when transfused
blood has a PCV of 40.

General rule: rate of transfusion

Dogs: 0.25 ml/kg/30 min or faster (22 ml/kg/day) with close patient monitoring
Cats: 40 ml/30 min with close patient monitoring

Whenever plasma transfusions are considered, remember that 60% of the blood volume is
plasma. In addition, only 40% of the albumin in an animal is in the plasma. Therefore, it takes
six units of plasma to raise the albumin of a 66-pound dog from 1.8 g/dl to 3 g/dl.

22. What are the possible complications after transfusion?

Hemolysis is probably the most serious adverse effect; however, it is relatively rare. Fever
that develops during transfusion may indicate bacterial contamination of the blood, or the
fever may be related to leukocyte antigens that cause an elevation of endogenous pyrogens.
Elevation in body temperature is more commonly seen in cats than in dogs. Allergic reactions
may manifest as urticaria and angioneurotic edema. If such signs are noted, the transfusion
should be discontinued, and glucocorticoids should be administered.

**23. Are coagulation disorders an important oncologic emergency and a common cause
of death in animals with cancer?**

Disorders of hemostasis are a common cause of morbidity and mortality in animals with
cancer and may be loosely categorized as follows:

• DIC
• Malignancy-associated fibrinolysis
• Platelet abnormalities
• Clinical syndrome of the hypercoagulable state of malignancy (e.g., hemangiosarcoma,
  mast cell tumor)
• Chemotherapy-associated thromboembolism (e.g., L-asparaginase, prednisone)

24. What is the best way to diagnose DIC?

Clinical signs supportive of a diagnosis of DIC include but are not limited to oozing from
venipuncture sites, nosebleeds, oral bleeding, melena, ecchymoses and petechial hemorrhages
anywhere on the body, and hematuria. Widespread thrombosis may cause multiorgan failure
that results in various clinical signs, such as acute renal failure and acute onset of respiratory
distress. A diagnosis is best made by fulfilling at least three of the following criteria:

• Abnormal activated partial thromboplastin time (APTT), Prothrombin time (PT),
  thrombin clotting time
• Low plasma fibrinogen concentration
• Low plasma antithrombin III activity

• High serum fibrinogen-related antigen concentration
• Low platelet count.

The key is to identify the problem early in an emergency setting and to initiate therapy while the condition is clinically silent or before clinical signs become serious.

25. What laboratory abnormalities are associated with DIC?

Laboratory abnormalities associated with DIC vary depending on the organs involved and whether the DIC is acute or chronic; the chronic form of DIC is rarely associated with clinical signs. In addition, red blood cell fragmentation may result from microangiopathic events that are seen in DIC. Diagnosis is based on clinical findings and an elevated PT and APTT, thrombocytopenia, prolonged activated clotting time (ACT), decreased antithrombin III concentrations, hypofibrinogenemia, and increased fibrin degradation products. Many emergency facilities routinely screen patients for DIC by performing ACTs.

26. What is acute tumor lysis syndrome? Is it a life-threatening emergency?

Acute tumor lysis syndrome (ATLS) is a condition of acute collapse that may lead to death soon after administration of a chemotherapeutic agent to an animal with a chemosensitive tumor. Although uncommon, it certainly presents a urgent situation. In short, chemotherapy results in the acute death of large amounts of tumor and release of cellular contents that may be acutely toxic. This emergency situation is underrecognized in veterinary patients and is becoming more common with the widespread use of chemotherapeutic agents. Therefore, when a case is suspected, a complete history and physical examination is taken as an intravenous catheter is placed and blood samples are obtained for subsequent analysis.

In dogs and cats this syndrome has been associated with lymphoma and leukemia. ATLS may occur after effective chemotherapy in animals with rapidly growing, bulky, chemosensitive tumors. The patient often is presented with a history of acute decompensation over a short time—sometimes to the point of imminent death. Rapid diagnosis and therapy are essential to reduce mortality rates.

27. What factors predispose animals to ATLS?

Rapid tumor lysis may cause acute release of intracellular phosphate and potassium. This release of electrolytes causes hypocalcemia, hyperkalemia, and hyperphosphatemia. Hyperuricemia is also seen in people, but this is not a concern in veterinary patients.

ATLS is most common in animals with some degree of volume contraction and a large tumor mass that responds rapidly to cytotoxic therapy. In addition, septic animals or animals with extensive neoplastic disease that infiltrates the parenchyma are predisposed to ATLS. Veterinary patients at highest risk are volume-contracted dogs with stage IV or V lymphoma that are treated with chemotherapy and undergo rapid remission. ATLS is most often identified within 48 hours after the first treatment.

28. How is ATLS diagnosed?

When ATLS is suspected, the history should document the recent administration of chemotherapy to a pet with lymphoma, leukemia, or other chemoresponsive tumor. A rapid, thorough, and complete physical examination should be performed to identify telltale signs of cardiovascular collapse, vomiting, diarrhea, and ensuing shock. The accompanying hyperkalemia may result in a bradycardia and diminished P-wave amplitude, increased PR and QRS intervals and, rarely, spiked T waves on electrocardiogram. Biochemical analysis of blood may confirm the presence of hypocalcemia, hyperkalemia, and hyperphosphatemia. In the presence of elevated serum phosphate levels, hypocalcemia develops as a result of calcium and phosphate precipitation. Without effective treatment, renal failure may occur; therefore, concentrations of blood urea nitrogen and creatinine should be monitored closely. Fluid therapy should be initiated as soon as an intravenous catheter is placed.

29. What is the treatment for ATLS?

The ideal treatment is prevention. Identify predisposed patients that have heavy tumor burden, a chemoresponsive tumor, and volume contraction. Because the kidney is the main source of electrolyte excretion, metabolic abnormalities may be exacerbated in the presence of renal dysfunction. Identification of patients at risk and correction of volume depletion or azotemia may effectively reduce the risk of ATLS; chemotherapy should be delayed until metabolic disturbances such as azotemia are corrected.

If ATLS is identified, the animal should be treated with aggressive crystalloid fluid therapy. Further chemotherapy should be withheld until the animal is clinically normal and all biochemical parameters are within normal limits. The fluid rate should be adjusted to meet the needs of each patient, as directed by monitoring of body weight, heart and respiratory rates, central venous pressure, ongoing losses such as vomiting and diarrhea, and urine output.

30. Can anticancer drugs cause an emergency condition by inducing renal failure?

Absolutely! Cisplatin, piroxicam, and methotrexate have been associated with renal failure in veterinary patients.

31. How does cisplatin induce renal damage?

The most nephrotoxic chemotherapeutic agent is cisplatin. In dogs, 80% to 90% of the drug is eliminated in the urine within 48 hours. Nephrotoxicosis, characterized by reduced glomerular filtration rate and tubular injury, is the major dose-limiting toxicosis. Renal toxicosis may range from brief increases in serum urea nitrogen and creatinine concentrations to irreversible renal failure. However, renal damage generally is not a clinical problem if adequate hydration is maintained.

32. Do other chemotherapeutic agents induce renal disease?

Methotrexate, an antimetabolite, is eliminated primarily from the kidneys and also has been associated with development of nephrotoxicity. Piroxicam, a nonsteroidal antiinflammatory agent, shares the potential nephrotoxicity of other members of its class. Piroxicam is in quite common use presently, and its use requires regular monitoring of renal function.

33. What are the best ways to diagnose kidney damage induced by chemotherapeutic agents?

Acute or chronic renal failure results from decreased glomerular filtration rate with or without tubular damage; therefore, the parameters used for diagnosis are related to damage to these structures. Renal disease may have been significant for variable periods before clinical, hematologic, and biochemical abnormalities are identified, because at least two-thirds of kidney function must be abnormal before overt evidence of renal disease develops.

Acute renal failure may occur with nonoliguria, oliguria, or anuria. Regardless of the amount of urine, it is usually isothenuric or minimally concentrated with a high sodium content (more than 40 mEq/L). Glucose, protein, and renal epithelial cells also may be noted in the urine, along with an acute rise in serum urea nitrogen, creatinine, and phosphorus concentration.

34. What is the best treatment for dogs with chemotherapy-induced renal failure?

The best treatment for acute or chronic renal failure is prevention. Substantial data show that cisplatin nephrotoxicity can be reduced and almost eliminated with adequate hydration. The incidence of renal failure induced by other drugs can be reduced by eliminating dogs with preexisting renal disease and by increasing the duration of time the drug is administered.

35. How does the method of administering cisplatin influence the induction of renal failure?

The duration of saline diuresis may influence the induction of renal failure in dogs. For example, 24-, 6-, and 4-hour aggressive diuresis protocols have been shown to be effective for administering cisplatin with a low probability of inducing renal failure. Shorter diuresis protocols have been shown to be detrimental.

36. What is the best treatment for chemotherapy-induced renal failure?

The initial treatment maneuver of drug-related acute renal failure in dogs and cats is to discontinue all drugs that may be nephrotoxic; concurrently, it is important to document prerenal or postrenal abnormalities and to initiate fluid therapy. The primary objectives of fluid therapy are to correct deficits such as dehydration and excesses such as volume overload, as seen in oliguric renal failure; to supply maintenance needs; and to supplement ongoing losses, such as those due to vomiting and diarrhea. Each patient must be assessed carefully, and a treatment plan must be based on hydration status, cardiovascular performance, and biochemical data. In acute renal failure, potassium-containing fluids generally are not ideal because systemic hyperkalemia is often present. Until more is known about the systemic effects of sepsis, lactate-containing fluids should be avoided because sepsis and cancer are associated with hyperlactatemia, which worsens with administration of lactate-containing fluids.

If oliguric renal failure is present, a diligent and aggressive approach should be made to increase urine output, first by increasing glomerular filtration rate and renal blood flow. In addition, osmotic diuresis can be used to increase urine flow. If urine output is less than 0.5 to 2 ml/kg/hr despite aggressive fluid therapy, furosemide should be administered every 1 to 3 hours. Furosemide increases glomerular filtration rate and enhances diuresis in many patients. If furosemide is not effective, mannitol or 50% dextrose may be used as an osmotic diuretic to enhance urine production.

Treatment for acute renal failure should be continued until the patient is substantially improved and until abnormal biochemical parameters have been corrected or at least stabilized. Therapy then should be tapered over several days and a home treatment plan developed, including avoidance of nephrotoxic drugs; provision of a high-quality, low-quantity protein diet; maintenance of a low-stress environment, and provision of fresh, clean water at will.

37. What are the most common metabolic emergencies in patients with cancer?
- Hypercalcemia
- Hypoglycemia
- Hyponatremia

38. What are the most common cancers associated with hypercalcemia of malignancy?
- Lymphoma is the most common cause of hypercalcemia in dogs
- Apocrine gland/anal sac adenocarcinoma
- Mammary adenocarcinoma
- Primary hyperparathyroidism

39. What is the most common mechanism associated with hypercalcemia of nonparathyroid malignancies?

A parathormone-related peptide is most commonly associated with hypercalcemia of malignancy in dogs. Although it has been suggested that bone metastases may be associated with hypercalcemia, this mechanism is rare in veterinary medicine.

40. What are the most common clinical findings in animals with hypercalcemia of malignancy?

A hypercalcemic oncologic emergency has clinical signs associated with decreased sensitivity of the distal convoluted tubules and collecting ducts to antidiuretic hormone, noted clinically as polyuria and polydipsia. This initial sign may be followed by vomiting and dehydration. Calcium also may affect the gastrointestinal, cardiovascular, and neurologic systems directly and cause anorexia, vomiting, constipation, bradycardia, hypertension, skeletal muscle weakness, depression, stupor, coma, and seizures.

41. Does serum protein or albumin influence serum calcium values?

Yes, in both cases. It is important to interpret calcium in relation to serum albumin and blood pH. The following correction formula for dogs takes albumin into account:

Adjusted calcium (mg/dl) = [calcium (mg/dl) – albumin (g/dl)] + 3.5

Because no such formula has been shown to be accurate for cats, the correction for cats is not so precise but should be taken into account. Acidosis results in an increase in the free, ionized fraction of calcium and may magnify the observed clinical signs associated with hypocalcemia. An ionized calcium value does not have to be corrected for albumin or protein.

42. What intravenous fluids should be used to treat hypercalcemic animals?

Treatment of an emergency secondary to hypercalcemia depends on the severity of clinical signs and presence of renal disease. Treatment entails use of intravenous 0.9% saline in volumes that exceed daily maintenance requirements. Often, two to three times the maintenance needs, plus an amount to correct current dehydration and to account for ongoing losses, is needed. It will likely be necessary to supplement potassium when saline is administered at this rate.

43. How should potassium depletion be treated?

When potassium is administered intravenously, the rate should not exceed 0.5 mEq/kg/hr. In addition, the patient should be watched carefully for signs consistent with overhydration and congestive heart failure, and effective antitumor therapy should be initiated as soon as possible.

44. What additional drugs can be used to treat patients with hypercalcemia?

- Furosemide (1 to 4 mg/kg 2 times per day, intravenously or orally) and intravenous biphosphonates (e.g., etidronate, disodium pamidronate) also may be used in addition to saline diuresis.
- Mithramycin, a chemotherapeutic agent that decreases bone resorption by reducing osteoclast number and activity, also has been shown to be effective in people. Mithramycin has not been used extensively in dogs or cats; in refractory patients, it may require twice-weekly dosing.
- Salmon calcitonin (4 to 8 MRC U/kg subcutaneously) also may be used in refractory patients. Calcitonin inhibits bone resorption and thus causes a fall in serum calcium levels within hours of administration. When administered at approximately 40 U/kg, salmon calcitonin may result in hypocalcemia for several days.
- Corticosteroids are effective for treatment of hypercalcemia. Corticosteroids block bone resorption caused by osteoclast-activating factor, increase urinary calcium excretion, inhibit vitamin D metabolism, and increase calcium absorption after long-term use. To be effective, high doses are generally required for several days. Steroids should not be used until tissue diagnosis is made, primarily because lymphomas are the primary cause of malignancy-associated hypercalcemia.

Most patients are effectively managed with saline diuresis and antitumor therapy; treatment with hypocalcemia-inducing agents such as mithramycin and calcitonin is not commonly needed.

45. What drugs or vitamins are contraindicated in hypercalcemic animals?

Thiazide diuretics or vitamins A and D (which may elevate calcium levels) should not be used in hypercalcemic animals.

46. What tumors are most commonly associated with hypoglycemia?

Fasting hypoglycemia in the face of hyperinsulinemia occurs most commonly with insulinomas; however, other tumors of the liver (e.g., hepatomas, carcinomas) and large retroperitoneal masses also have been associated with hypoglycemia.

47. What are the most common clinical signs associated with malignancy-induced hypoglycemia?

Before being presented with seizures, coma, and impending death, most animals have a history of fatigue, weakness, dizziness, and confusion associated with paroxysmal lowering of the blood glucose levels. Hypoglycemic dogs with neurologic signs are presented like any other patient with a central nervous system abnormality, such as brain tumor, brain trauma, meningitis, or metabolic encephalopathy.

48. What is the best diagnostic plan to confirm the presence of malignancy-associated hypoglycemia and to identify the underlying cause?

Insulin-producing tumors can be diagnosed by identifying elevated insulin levels in association with low blood glucose concentrations. The diagnosis is made when the blood glucose is dramatically reduced but insulin levels are elevated.

49. What is the emergency treatment plan for animals with hypoglycemia of malignancy?

Glucose-containing fluids (2.5% to 5% dextrose in 0.9% NaCl or other isotonic crystalloid solution) should be administered to meet fluid requirements and to maintain blood glucose concentrations within acceptable limits. The administration of glucose, however, may trigger the tumor to release more insulin; therefore, a constant infusion of glucose to maintain normal serum glucose levels is preferred to intermittent high-dose bolusing. When the patient is stable and a diagnosis established, plans can be made for ongoing management.

50. What is the most common cause of hyponatremia that leads to an emergency?

An emergency condition related to the syndrome of inappropriate antidiuretic hormone secretion (SIADH) is a rare but underrecognized cause of true hyponatremia in patients with cancer.

51. What is SIADH?

SIADH is the presence of excessive quantities of antidiuretic hormone secondary to malignancy. The affected animal has low plasma osmolality despite inappropriate urine concentration (high sodium). Because this situation also may occur in renal disease, hypothyroidism, and adrenal insufficiency, these disorders must be excluded to confirm the diagnosis of SIADH.

52. What factors predispose an animal to hyponatremia due to SIADH?

The condition may be caused by a cancer or a drug that results in renal activation or enhanced release of antidiuretic hormone. SIADH has been identified in dogs with lymphoma. Drugs in veterinary medicine that may cause SIADH include but are not limited to the following:

- Chlorpropamide
- Vincristine
- Vinblastine
- Cyclophosphamide
- Opiates
- Thiazide diuretics
- Barbiturates
- Isoproterenol

53. What clinical signs are most commonly seen in animals with SIADH and hyponatremia?

When hyponatremia develops rapidly or sodium falls below 115 mg/dl, patients may develop mental status abnormalities, confusion, or coma. With profound hyponatremia, seizures also may occur. Serum and urine electrolytes, osmolality, and creatinine should be measured in suspect cases.

54. What is the best diagnostic plan to confirm SIADH?

The diagnosis of SIADH is initially made by the combination of hyponatremia on the biochemical profile and clinical signs. The diagnosis of SIADH is often missed. SIADH is associated with inappropriate sodium concentration in the urine for the level of hyponatremia in the serum. Urine osmolality is greater than plasma osmolality, but the urine specific gravity is not maximally dilute. With SIADH the urea nitrogen values in the serum are usually low because of volume expansion. Hypophosphatemia also may be noted. Adrenal and thyroid function should be normal.

55. What is the best treatment for animals with SIADH?

Initial treatment should be directed at resolution of the hyponatremia in an emergency setting. This includes:

- Fluids should be restricted to ensure that the patient receives only the amount needed to maintain normal hydration and to keep serum sodium concentration within normal levels.
- Demeclocycline may correct hyponatremia to reduce antidiuretic hormone stimulus for free water reabsorption at the collecting ducts in an emergency setting. The most common adverse effects of demeclocycline are nausea and vomiting.
- Lithium carbonate and phenytoin also have some use in treatment of SIADH.
- Hypertonic sodium chloride (3% to 5%) also may be used in an emergency situation; however, if not used carefully, it may result in fluid and circulatory overload.
- Furosemide may be used concurrently with the hypertonic saline to reduce volume overload. Rapid correction of hyponatremia may lead to neurologic damage. The following formula may help to determine approximate amounts of sodium to administer for correction of hyponatremia:

  Na for replacement (mEq) = [desired serum sodium (mEq/L) – observed serum sodium (mEq/L)] × observed serum sodium (mEq/L) × body weight (kg) × 0.6

56. What chemotherapeutic agent is most commonly associated with development of cardiac disease? Can chemotherapy-induced heart disease result in a life-threatening emergency?

Doxorubicin is the anthracycline commonly associated with development of cardiac disease. Cardiac disease secondary to anthracycline or anthracycline-like drugs is relatively common in dogs and may be life-threatening.

57. What are the most common cardiac abnormalities associated with doxorubicin-induced heart disease?

Doxorubicin is associated with development of tachyarrhythmias and dilated cardiomyopathy. Cardiomyopathy may occur in response to administration of any number of doses of doxorubicin, but the risk increases significantly after a dog receives a total cumulative dose exceeding 240 mg/m^2. The risk in cats appears to be minimal.

58. Can radiation induce heart disease?

Yes. The degree of radiation-induced heart disease is related to the number of fractions of radiation treatment, the dose per fraction, the type of radiation (photons vs electrons), and the total dosage.

59. What predisposing factors are associated with development of doxorubicin-induced cardiac disease?

Doxorubicin-induced cardiac disease may occur more frequently in animals with preexisting cardiac disease and in animals that cannot metabolize or eliminate the drug adequately after administration. Similarly, rapid infusion of the drug, which establishes high serum concentrations, may increase the prevalence of cardiac disease. Therefore, increased time for infusion of a dose of doxorubicin may reduce the prevalence of acute and chronic cardiac disease.

60. What are the most common clinical signs of doxorubicin-induced cardiomyopathy?

In an animal with cardiomyopathy and fulminant congestive heart failure, clinical signs vary from anorexia, lethargy, and weakness to more common signs associated specifically with decreased cardiac output and ensuing congestive heart failure.

61. If doxorubicin-induced cardiomyopathy is identified, can doxorubicin treatment be reinitiated in the future?

No. After doxorubicin cardiotoxicosis is identified, the drug should not be used in that patient again.

62. Is it possible to prevent doxorubicin-induced cardiac disease?

The use of liposome-encapsulated doxorubicin has been shown to limit cardiotoxicity, but the drug is expensive and will probably not find much use in veterinary medicine for some time. Other protective agents are presently beginning to reach the market, but their role is not yet clearly defined.

63. What is the preferred treatment for dogs with anthracycline-induced cardiomyopathy?

Treatment of cardiomyopathy begins with immediate discontinuation of the inciting cause (e.g., radiation or doxorubicin). Unfortunately, recovery from cardiomyopathy has not been documented in animal patients. Medical management of the cardiac dysfunction is indicated.

21. GASTROINTESTINAL TUMORS

Ruthanne Chun, DVM, Dipl ACVIM

1. What is the most common gastrointestinal tumor in the dog?

Throughout the entire gastrointestinal (GI) tract, the most common malignant tumors are epithelial in origin. Although they account for less than 1% of all reported neoplasms, gastric carcinomas and intestinal adenocarcinomas are the most frequent malignancies. Benign tumors such as adenomas or polyps are rare. Other neoplasms encountered in the canine GI tract include leiomyosarcoma, leiomyoma, lymphoma, plasmacytoma, and mast cell tumor.

2. What is the most common GI tumor in the cat?

Lymphoma. Interestingly, GI lymphoma in cats is not related to feline leukemic virus or feline immunodeficiency virus. Other reported malignancies include adenocarcinoma, mast cell tumor, and neuroendocrine tumors.

3. What might I find on history and physical examination that would support a suspicion of GI neoplasia?

Regardless of species and tumor type, the most common concerns are persistent anorexia, weight loss, vomiting, and diarrhea. Less commonly, animals will have tenesmus, hematochezia, melena, or hematemesis. Dogs are usually older (over 6 years), as are cats (over 10 years). Depending on the location of the primary tumor, an intra-abdominal mass may be palpable. Gastric tumors tend to be difficult to palpate in dogs; tumors in this site are easier to identify in cats.

4. Are there any good tumors of the GI tract?

Everything is relative. Polyps, though rare, are associated with an excellent prognosis following surgical resection. Plasma cell tumors are potentially curable with surgery alone. So long as no regional (e.g., lymph node) or distant (e.g., lungs, liver) metastases are present, dogs or cats with leiomyosarcoma and adenocarcinoma may do very well following complete surgical resection (3 to 5 cm of normal bowel on either side of the tumor and wide resection of the associated mesentery).

5. What diagnostic tests are most useful for GI tumors?

A number of tests are helpful in increasing the index of suspicion for and diagnosing a GI tumor. Because most animals present with vomiting and weight loss, a minimum database of a complete blood count, serum biochemistry profile, and urinalysis are essential to rule out differentials such as renal failure or liver disease. Rarely, leiomyomas and leiomyosarcomas may cause hypoglycemia as a paraneoplastic syndrome. Survey abdominal radiographs are always appropriate, and abdominal ultrasonography is useful in localizing and measuring the lesion, screening for regional lymph node enlargement and distant metastases, as well as in guiding fine-needle aspirates or Tru-cut biopsies of lesions. Endoscopy is another excellent test that allows for visualization and biopsy of the lesion so long as the tumor is gastric or within the proximal duodenum. Exploratory laparotomy is potentially the most thorough method by which to diagnose and stage GI tumors. During surgery, the mass should be resected, and regional lymph nodes and other sites such as the liver should be biopsied to evaluate for metastatic disease.

6. Do the treatment recommendations change depending on what the tumor is?

Yes, with the disclaimer that there are no good studies in dogs or cats that have compared survival and disease-free interval between animals treated with surgery alone with animals

121

treated with surgery and chemotherapy. All of our current knowledge is based on retrospective, rather than prospective, case analysis. For dogs with GI adenocarcinomas or leiomyosarcomas that have not metastasized, surgical excision is the current recommendation. Dogs with metastatic disease may require chemotherapy, but the most appropriate drug is not known. Cats with adenocarcinoma appear to have improved survival times with doxorubicin chemotherapy following complete surgical resection regardless of whether metastatic disease is identified. Chemotherapy, with or without surgery, is recommended for all animals with GI lymphoma or mast cell tumors.

7. In a patient that already has vomiting and diarrhea, how will I know if he or she is having adverse effects from chemotherapy or if the tumor is just causing problems?

There are two easy ways to solve this problem. First, is the animal in the proper window of time in which GI upset may occur (i.e., was chemotherapy given within the past week)? If not, reevaluate the patient with the original staging tests (i.e., radiographs and ultrasound) and compare the results with those of the initial staging tests. If there is obvious progression, the answer is straightforward. If there is not obvious progression, the answer is not so easy. In this case, one should be concerned about progression, and the patient should be closely monitored and treated symptomatically.

8. Are there any estimates of survival times for animals with GI tumors?

Although dogs with GI lymphoma do not do as well as dogs with stage 1 to 4 lymphoma, chemotherapy may prolong survival and provide an enhanced quality of life. Cats with GI lymphoma have a wide published range of survival times. For cats that respond to therapy, survival times approximate 10 months. Dogs with GI adenocarcinoma or leiomyosarcoma had a median survival of 10 months; when analyzed separately there was no difference in survival between these tumor types. Cats with colonic adenocarcinoma had longer survival times if they were free from metastatic lesions, had a subtotal colectomy, and had follow-up doxorubicin chemotherapy. In this scenario, median survival time was as high as 280 days. Dogs with GI mast cell tumors have a poor prognosis, with one study demonstrating survival times of up to 48 days.

9. Aside from neoplasia, what are the important differential diagnoses for primary GI disease?

The list is huge. However, given an older patient that presents with adult-onset chronic vomiting, weight loss, and diarrhea, some of the more common differentials should include inflammatory bowel disease, parasitism, or feline infectious peritonitis. The systematic use of diagnostic guidelines, such as the DAMNIT scheme (degenerative, anatomic, metabolic, neoplastic, infectious/inflammatory, traumatic/toxic), is helpful.

HEPATIC TUMORS

10. What primary tumors occur in the liver?

Primary liver tumors are rare; it is much more common to find hepatic involvement with systemic lymphoma or metastatic hemangiosarcoma. Primary malignant liver tumors in dogs and cats include hepatocellular carcinoma, biliary carcinoma, and biliary cyst adenocarcinoma. Benign liver masses include nodular regeneration, hepatoma, and biliary cyst adenoma.

11. If most hepatic neoplasms arise from tissue normally found in the liver, what about smooth muscle and connective tissues in the liver?

Malignancies of these tissues have been reported, but they are rare. Leiomyosarcoma and extraskeletal osteosarcoma, as well as neuroendocrine neoplasms, may arise within the liver. Only descriptive studies of these tumor types exist; no studies have documented appropriate therapeutic steps.

12. Are there any typical clinical signs that occur with hepatic tumors?

In dogs the most common signs reported for animals with hepatic tumors include vomiting and ascites. Cats more often present with anorexia and lethargy. Jaundice is relatively uncommon but, if present, certainly helps to focus the diagnostic evaluation. Abdominal palpation may reveal a cranial abdominal mass. Rarely, animals with liver tumors have been reported to be hypoglycemic secondary to factors released from their tumor.

13. Can I increase my index of suspicion for a liver tumor based on blood work?

Studies have found that there are no pathognomonic findings for hepatic cancer. Elevations in alkaline phosphatase, alanine transaminase, and bilirubin levels may be present, but they are not specific or prognostic for hepatic neoplasia. One study found that dogs with primary liver tumors had higher serum alpha-fetoprotein levels than dogs with other liver disease or nonhepatic neoplasia; no work has been published to corroborate this finding in dogs or cats.

14. What are the treatment options for liver tumors?

As with any other tumor type, the answer depends on the type of liver tumor. Hepatomas and biliary adenomas may be cured surgically. Dogs with hepatocellular carcinomas isolated to one liver lobe may have prolonged survival times after surgery alone. While the general belief is that animals with diffuse liver involvement or metastatic disease should be treated with systemic therapy, there is no standard of care regarding the medical management of animals with hepatic neoplasia.

PANCREATIC TUMORS

15. How common a problem is pancreatic neoplasia?

Pancreatic cancer is rare in dogs and cats. Neoplasms of the exocrine pancreas (i.e., pancreatic carcinoma) are very rare; the most commonly reported pancreatic tumor in dogs and cats is insulinoma.

16. Is pancreatic carcinoma a bad disease in dogs?

Unfortunately, pancreatic carcinoma in dogs appears to be a highly metastatic and painful neoplasm. No good treatment options have been reported.

17. Are there any typical clinical signs of pancreatic carcinoma?

No. Dogs may present with signs of pancreatitis such as vomiting and anorexia. Physical examination may reveal cranial abdominal pain and, potentially, a palpable mass. Ultrasound of the pancreas usually cannot differentiate between pancreatitis and neoplasia. Histopathology is necessary for diagnosis.

18. What is the best way to diagnose an insulinoma?

Document hypoglycemia concurrently with an inappropriately high (including midrange or high-normal) insulin concentration.

19. What signs might make me suspect that an animal has an insulinoma?

Clinical signs of insulinoma are related to hypoglycemia and include weakness, tremors, and seizures. Neoplasia should be suspected in any dog older than than 5 years old with an acute onset of seizures. Major differentials include a primary brain tumor, metastatic tumor to the brain, extension of a nasal tumor through the cribriform plate, and insulinoma. Other possibilities include paraneoplastic hypoglycemia secondary to a GI or hepatic tumor, lead intoxication, and trauma.

20. How can I stop a hypoglycemic seizure?

If placement of an intravenous catheter is not possible, dripping Karo syrup onto the oral mucous membranes may temporarily resolve hypoglycemia. Ideally, 50% dextrose can be given intravenously to effect. However, it is important to keep in mind that overzealous administration of oral or intravenous dextrose solutions may cause rebound insulin release from the tumor. A new approach using a constant-rate infusion of glucagon to control hypoglycemic seizures was recently reported. Glucagon has physiologic actions that are opposite to those of insulin. In the one animal in which use of this drug has been reported, this method was very successful in normalizing blood glucose values. To prevent seizures from recurring, the insulinoma must be removed.

21. What happens if the insulinoma is not resectable or the owner refuses surgery?

Medical management of insulinoma patients includes feeding frequent, small meals (preferably high in protein, fat, and complex carbohydrates), low-dose prednisone therapy (0.25 mg/kg twice daily), and minimal exercise. Diazoxide is a benzothiadiazide diuretic that inhibits the release of insulin, stimulates hepatic glyconeogenesis and glycogenolysis, and inhibits cellular uptake of glucose. There are few reports of the effectiveness of chemotherapy. Streptozocin is a drug that specifically kills pancreatic beta cells. Because this drug is nephrotoxic, it must be given in conjunction with a saline-induced diuresis. Currently, no case series or clinical trials discuss the effectiveness of this drug against canine insulinoma.

22. Do insulinomas occur in cats?

Yes. There is at least one case report discussing the diagnosis and management of a cat with insulinoma. This cat was treated surgically, died 18 months postoperatively, and had evidence of metastatic disease on necropsy.

BIBLIOGRAPHY

1. Crawshaw J, Berg J, Sardinas JC, et al: Prognosis for dogs with nonlymphomatous, small intestinal tumors treated by surgical excision. J Am Anim Hosp Assoc 34:451–456, 1998.
2. Feldman E, Nelson R: Beta-cell neoplasia: Insulinoma. In Canine and Feline Endocrinology and Reproduction. Philadelphia, WB Saunders, 1996, pp 422–441.
3. Fischer JR, Smith SA, Harkin DR: Glucagon constant-rate infusion: A novel strategy for the management for hyperinsulimenic-hypoglycemic crisis in the dog. J Am Anim Hosp Assoc 36:27–32, 2000.
4. Hawks D, Peterson ME, Hawkins KL, et al: Insulin-secreting pancreatic (islet cell) carcinoma in a cat. J Vet Intern Med 6:193–196, 1992.
5. Kapatkin AS, Mullen HS, Matthiesen DT, et al: Leiomyosarcoma in dogs: 44 cases (1983–1988). J Am Vet Med Assoc 201:1077–1079, 1992.
6. Lamb CR, Simpson KW, Boswood A, et al: Ultrasonography of pancreatic neoplasia in the dog: A retrospective review of 16 cases. Vet Rec 137:65–68, 1995.
7. Langenbach A, Anderson MA, Dambach DM, et al: Extraskeletal osteosarcomas in dogs: A retrospective study of 169 cases (1986–1996). J Am Anim Hosp Assoc 34:113–120, 1998.
8. Lowseth LA, Gillet MA, Chang I-Y, et al: Detection of serum α-fetoprotein in dogs with hepatic tumors. J Am Vet Med Assoc 199:735–741, 1991.
9. Mahony OM, Moore AS, Cotter SM, et al: Alimentary lymphoma in cats: 28 cases (1988–1993). J Am Vet Med Assoc 207:1593–1598, 1995.
10. Post G, Patnaik AK: Nonhematopoietic hepatic neoplasms in cats: 21 cases (1983–1988). J Am Vet Med Assoc 201:1080–1082, 1992.
11. Slawienski MJ, Mauldin GE, Mauldin GN, et al; Malignant colonic neoplasia in cats: 46 cases (1990–1996). J Am Vet Med Assoc 211:878–881, 1997.
12. Takahashi T, Kadosawa T, Nagase M, et al; Visceral mast cell tumors in dogs: 10 cases (1982–1997). J Am Vet Med Assoc 216:222–226, 2000.
13. Zwahlen CH, Lucroy MD, Kraegel SA, et al; Results of chemotherapy for cats with alimentary malignant lymphoma: 21 cases (1993–1997). J Am Vet Med Assoc 213:1144–1149, 1998.

22. TUMORS OF THE SKIN AND SUBCUTIS IN DOGS AND CATS

Linda S. Fineman, DVM, Dipl ACVIM

1. What percentage of skin tumors are benign in dogs and cats?
In dogs 80% are benign, in cats 59%.

2. What are the most common malignant skin tumors in dogs?
Mast cell tumors, hemangiosarcomas, squamous cell carcinomas, fibrosarcomas, melanomas, basal cell carcinomas, and cutaneous lymphomas.

3. What are the most common malignant skin tumors in cats?
Basal cell carcinomas, mast cell tumors, squamous cell carcinomas, and fibrosarcomas.

4. How are skin tumors diagnosed?
Fine-needle aspiration and cytology are useful to differentiate benign conditions from malignancies. Often, biopsy with histopathology will be necessary to make specific treatment recommendations for epithelial or mesenchymal tumors. Biopsies may be obtained with punch or Tru-cut instruments or via incisional or excisional surgery.

5. What types of tumors are seen in the skin?
Epithelial tumors, mesenchymal tumors, and round cell tumors.

6. What is the clinical presentation in animals with skin tumors?
Skin tumors are often found during grooming, petting, or routine physical examination. They are usually not painful. Some tumors can be ulcerated or pruritic, drawing the owner's attention to them.

EPITHELIAL TUMORS

7. What causes basal cell tumors?
No one knows. In human beings, these tumors are associated with chronic exposure to ultraviolet light. They do not appear to be solar-induced in dogs and cats.

8. What is the appearance of basal cell carcinoma?
The tumors are usually well-circumscribed, raised nodules, often forming around the head and neck in dogs. The tumors may be pigmented or have a bluish appearance and are usually nonhaired. It is not unusual for basal cell carcinomas to become ulcerated or fluid-filled. The tumors may be attached to the underlying subcutaneous tissues with an infiltrative growth pattern.

9. What is the biologic behavior of basal cell carcinoma?
In dogs and cats, the tumors are usually slow-growing and rarely exhibit aggressive behavior despite the frequent finding of a high mitotic index.

10. How are basal cell carcinomas treated?
Complete surgical excision is the treatment of choice. Local therapy with radiation or cryosurgery may be helpful if complete surgical excision is not possible.

11. What is the prognosis for animals diagnosed with basal cell carcinoma?

Metastasis is rare, and the prognosis is generally believed to be good in dogs and cats diagnosed with this tumor. However, in some patients, basal cell carcinoma may have very aggressive behavior leading to disseminated disease.

12. What causes cutaneous melanomas?

The cause is unknown, but there is an increased risk for melanomas in older, darkly pigmented dogs. Breed predispositions include chow chows, cocker spaniels, Airedales, Boston terriers, boxers, Chihuahuas, Doberman pinschers, golden retrievers, Irish setters, miniature schnauzers, Scottish terriers, and springer spaniels. There are no apparent breed predilections in cats, but the tumors are quite rare in that species.

13. What is the appearance of melanoma?

Melanomas are usually pigmented, firm masses occurring on the haired skin, most often on the head, trunk, or digits.

14. What is the biologic behavior of melanoma?

Melanomas can be benign or malignant. In dogs, the mitotic index seems to be the most reliable predictor of biologic behavior. A low mitotic index (below 3/10 hpf) is associated with a benign behavior. Up to 10% of histologically "benign" tumors will behave in a more aggressive fashion. Size of the tumor may be predictive of biologic behavior. Doberman pinschers and miniature schnauzers are more likely to have benign tumors than other breeds. Metastasis is usually to regional lymph nodes, with eventual spread to the lungs probable. Melanomas of the digits usually are subungual and have a 50% rate of metastasis. Data in the cat are scarce, but metastasis to regional lymph nodes occurred in half of the cats in one study.

15. How is melanoma best treated?

Benign and low-grade malignancies are best treated with wide surgical resection. Preventing metastasis remains the biggest hurdle to successful treatment of dogs and cats with cutaneous malignant melanoma. The role of chemotherapy has not been fully evaluated.

16. What is the prognosis for dogs and cats with malignant melanoma of the skin?

In dogs, the mitotic index and size and location of the tumor predict the likelihood of cure. Approximately 45% to 60% of dogs and 5% to 50% of cats with cutaneous malignant melanoma will develop metastasis. Dogs with malignant melanoma of the skin are reported to have an 8-month median survival time.

17. What causes cutaneous squamous cell carcinoma?

In light-skinned or poorly haired portions of the skin, exposure to ultraviolet radiation can induce squamous cell carcinoma. Solar-induced tumors are commonly seen in cats on the nasal planum, eyelids, pinnae, and preauricular areas. In dogs, they are most commonly seen in the inguinal areas and axillae. Not all cutaneous squamous cell carcinomas are solar-induced. In dogs, tumors may be found anywhere on the skin, with a predisposition for the nail bed.

18. What is the appearance of squamous cell carcinoma?

The tumors are frequently ulcerated and erosive, but the appearance may be proliferative or cauliflower-like. In cats with solar-induced tumors, the lesions are frequently crusty with ulcerated or erythemic tissue beneath the crusts.

19. What is the biologic behavior of cutaneous squamous cell carcinoma?

Solar-induced squamous cell carcinoma is usually preceded by a precancerous condition called actinic keratosis. Precancerous lesions consisting primarily of intermittent flaky or crusty skin may be present for years before progression to squamous cell carcinoma. Solar-induced squamous cell carcinoma is a slowly progressive disease that rarely metastasizes. If metastasis does occur, it is usually to regional lymph nodes. Subungual squamous cell carcinoma most commonly occurs in large, black dogs; giant schnauzers and standard poodles are predisposed. The disease usually only affects one digit, but multiple digits may be affected in some dogs. The tumor commonly destroys adjacent bone. Metastasis is uncommon, but metastasis to the regional lymph nodes and the lungs has been reported.

20. What is the treatment for squamous cell carcinoma?

Treatment of solar-induced squamous cell carcinoma consists of local therapy with wide surgical resection, cryosurgery, or radiation therapy. Intralesional carboplatin and photodynamic therapy have also been reported. Subungual squamous cell carcinoma is treated with digital amputation. Other cutaneous sites are treated with wide surgical excision. Follow-up radiation therapy may be of benefit in cases where complete excision is not possible.

21. What is the prognosis for dogs and cats with squamous cell carcinoma?

Solar-induced squamous cell carcinoma is generally associated with a fair to good prognosis with early detection and treatment. In one study of subungual squamous cell carcinoma in dogs treated with surgery alone, a 76.2% 1-year survival rate was reported, and only one dog had documented metastasis.

22. What is the appearance of sweat gland carcinoma?

These tumors appear in one of two ways. The first is a solitary, firm, well-circumscribed mass, which may be ulcerated. The second is a poorly circumscribed, diffuse, plaque-like lesion, which may be erythematous and ulcerated.

23. What is the biologic behavior of sweat gland carcinoma?

Metastasis is possible but uncommon with the well-circumscribed form. The diffuse form is characterized by invasion of dermal lymphatics, making local recurrence after surgery likely. Metastasis may occur to regional lymph nodes or to the lungs. In cats ceruminous gland carcinomas of the ear canal may occur. The tumors tend to be quite locally invasive but do not commonly metastasize.

24. What is the treatment for sweat gland carcinoma?

Wide surgical excision is the treatment of choice but may be difficult in the diffuse form of the disease. The role of adjuvant radiation therapy has not been defined. In cats with ceruminous gland adenocarcinomas, total ear canal ablation with bulla osteotomy is recommended because of the high risk of local recurrence following less aggressive surgical resection.

25. What is the prognosis for dogs and cats with sweat gland tumors?

A 20% metastatic rate has been reported for dogs and cats with sweat gland tumors.

Cats with ceruminous gland adenocarcinoma treated with total ear canal ablation and bulla osteotomy were reported to have a 42-month median remission time with a 25% recurrence rate compared with cats treated with lateral ear canal resection alone, which had a 10-month median remission time and a 67% recurrence rate.

26. What causes perianal adenomas?

Growth of perianal adenomas is stimulated by testosterone, usually in uncastrated male dogs. Female or male dogs with hyperadrenocorticism may develop perianal adenoma because of excess production of sex steroids by the adrenal gland.

27. What do these tumors look like?

Tumors are most commonly seen around the anus but may be located along the dorsal or ventral midline of the body, particularly in the caudal areas. Tumors are usually incidental findings on routine examination, and rarely will they become ulcerated or infected.

28. What is the biologic behavior of perianal gland adenoma?
These are benign, slow-growing tumors. The malignant counterpart, perianal gland carcinoma, frequently metastasizes to the internal iliac lymph nodes.

29. How are perianal gland adenomas and carcinomas treated?
Small adenomas may regress entirely following castration. Larger tumors may also require local resection following castration. Perianal gland adenocarcinomas are treated with surgical resection of the primary tumor and regional lymph nodes when possible. Removal of affected lymph nodes is not curative but may be palliative. The role and efficacy of adjuvant chemotherapy have not been fully evaluated.

30. What is the prognosis for dogs with perianal gland adenomas and carcinomas?
The prognosis for dogs with perianal gland adenomas is good with appropriate treatment. Perianal gland adenocarcinoma has a high rate of metastasis. Dogs with metastasis at the time of diagnosis have been reported to die of metastatic disease within about 7 months. Debulking the sublumbar lymph nodes surgically or with radiation therapy may result in significant palliation of clinical signs.

31. What causes apocrine gland adenocarcinoma of the anal sac?
Good question! The cause of anal sac adenocarcinoma is unknown. Some breed predisposition does occur, with English springer spaniels, English cocker spaniels, Alaskan malamutes, German shepherds and dachsunds reportedly being at risk. The tumor is rare in cats. These tumors are not believed to be hormone-dependent.

32. What is the appearance of the tumors?
Dogs typically have a firm, attached subcutaneous swelling in the perianal region.

33. What is the biologic behavior of anal sac adenocarcinoma?
Approximately 25% of dogs with anal sac adenocarcinoma will have hypercalcemia of malignancy. Elevated concentrations of parathormone hormone–related peptide are seen in the serum of affected dogs. Metastasis to the sublumbar lymph nodes occurs in more than 50% of cases, but distant metastasis is less common.

34. How is apocrine gland adenocarcinoma of the anal sac treated?
Surgical resection of the tumor usually results in a rapid reversal of the hypercalcemia. Wide surgical excision is the treatment of choice but may be difficult unless the tumors are very small. Debulking of the sublumbar lymph nodes may be palliative. Radiation therapy may be useful in temporarily shrinking the size of the primary tumor or affected lymph nodes, but optimal treatment protocols have not been established. Partial remissions have been reported with chemotherapy, including carboplatin, cisplatin, actinomycin, and doxorubicin. The role of chemotherapy in this disease has not been fully defined.

35. What is the prognosis for dogs with apocrine gland adenocarcinoma of the anal sac?
The prognosis depends on the size of the tumor, the presence of metastasis at the time of diagnosis, and whether hypercalcemia is present. Dogs with resectable tumors had a 50% local recurrence rate. Dogs with metastasis at the time of surgery had a median survival time of 6 months; dogs without metastasis had a median survival time of 15.5 months.

36. Are there other cutaneous epithelial tumors in dogs and cats?
Many. Other tumor types include papillomas, sebaceous adenomas, hair follicle tumors, and pilomatricomas.

MESENCHYMAL TUMORS

37. What three tumors are derived from adipocytes?

Lipoma, infiltrative lipoma, and liposarcoma.

38. What is the difference between the above three tumor types?

Lipomas are benign fatty tumors. Although they are usually unencapsulated, they are often easily resected. Infiltrative lipomas are benign tumors but have an infiltrative pattern of growth, with deep invasion into the surrounding soft tissues. Liposarcomas behave like other soft tissue sarcomas.

39. What is the difference between a histiocytoma and histiocytic sarcoma?

A histiocytoma is a benign round cell tumor usually seen in dogs younger than 2 years of age. They have a characteristic button-like appearance on the skin surface. These tumors often spontaneously regress, usually within 3 weeks to 3 months. Histiocytic sarcomas behave like other soft tissue sarcomas.

40. What are soft tissue sarcomas?

This is a large group of tumors that are characterized by a fairly similar pattern of behavior. The group includes fibrosarcomas, neurofibrosarcomas, peripheral nerve sheath tumors, hemangiopericytomas, myxofibrosarcomas, malignant fibrous histiocytomas, histiocytic sarcomas, liposarcomas, and lymphangiosarcomas.

41. What is the difference between a peripheral nerve sheath tumor and a hemangiopericytoma?

In the past few years, veterinary pathologists have clarified nomenclature for these tumors. Most pathologists currently use peripheral nerve sheath tumor as a general category to include neurofibrosarcomas and hemangiopericytomas.

42. What do soft tissue sarcomas look like?

These are typically subcutaneous masses that are often quite firm and frequently attached to the underlying tissues. Hemangiopericytomas may be fluctuant because of cystic fluid accumulations.

43. How do soft tissue sarcomas behave?

These tumors are characterized by infiltration of the tissue surrounding the main tumor mass, making local recurrence likely following incomplete resection. The tumors generally have a low metastatic potential. High-grade tumors are more likely to metastasize, most commonly to the lungs.

44. What treatments are recommended?

Most soft tissue sarcomas are best treated by wide surgical resection. Often, adjuvant radiation therapy is used when wide margins around the tumor cannot be achieved surgically. Chemotherapy is not usually needed unless the tumor is of a high histologic grade.

45. Is it acceptable to shell out soft tissue sarcomas from their capsule?

What appears to be a capsule around soft tissue sarcomas is really a pseudocapsule composed of compressed tumor cells; it is not a fibrous capsule formed as a host response. Soft tissue sarcomas should be excised with as wide a margin as possible.

46. What is the role of adjuvant therapy after surgery for soft tissue sarcomas?

Chemotherapy does not seem to be as helpful as adjuvant therapy for most soft tissue sarcomas in dogs, but adjuvant radiation therapy is beneficial. As many as 80% of dogs so treated are expected to live 5 years.

47. What is the prognosis?

This depends somewhat on the specific histologic features of the tumor. Location of the tumor is important in that the mainstay of successful therapy is the ability to do wide surgical excision.

48. Do hemangiosarcomas behave similarly?

No.

49. How do hemangiosarcomas of the skin and subcutis behave?

Solar-induced hemangiosarcomas are seen as superficial, purplish tumors arising from thinly haired, lightly pigmented skin. These tumors are treated with surgery or cryosurgery, and the prognosis is usually good. Subcutaneous hemangiosarcomas are much more aggressive. Deeply infiltrative or invasive subcutaneous hemangiosarcomas are not only likely to recur locally but also have a high metastatic rate. The prognosis for dogs with deep subcutaneous hemangiosarcoma is poor, with median survival times ranging from 5 to 10 months following surgical excision. Adjuvant chemotherapy with a doxorubicin-based protocol may be useful in dogs with subcutaneous hemangiosarcoma. Little is published about the biologic behavior of subcutaneous hemangiosarcoma in the cat, but in one series of 10 cats, 6 had local recurrence following surgery. Anecdotally, these tumors are believed to have the potential to be highly metastatic.

50. What are cutaneous round cell tumors?

This group includes histiocytoma, plasma cell tumors, lymphosarcoma, mast cell tumors, and transmissible venereal tumors.

51. What is the appearance of plasma cell tumors?

These tumors are commonly seen around the cartilage of the ear and on the feet. The tumors are typically smooth, pink and nonhaired. Cocker spaniels are predisposed.

52. What is the biologic behavior of cutaneous plasma cell tumors?

Cutaneous plasma cell tumors are usually benign, relatively slow-growing tumors. Surgical excision is often curative. In cases where complete surgical excision is not possible, follow-up treatment with radiation therapy or chemotherapy with prednisone and melphalan may be beneficial.

53. What causes transmissible venereal tumors?

The tumors are spread between dogs by whole-cell transfer, usually via direct implantation into the skin. Geographic regions where dogs commonly roam free are more likely to have reports of transmissible venereal tumor.

54. What is the appearance and biologic behavior of these tumors?

The tumors are well-encapsulated, moveable masses that may be cystic. Metastasis is rare but may occur at any site in the body. Regional lymph nodes, eye, and brain are the most likely areas for metastasis.

55. How are transmissible venereal tumors treated?

The tumors respond to a wide variety of treatments. Vincristine used once weekly until the tumor has regressed plus two additional treatments has been reported to be an effective treatment. Doxorubicin has been used in vincristine-resistant cases. Chemotherapy seems to be relatively ineffective to lesions in the eye or brain. Radiation therapy may be useful in these cases.

CONTROVERSIES

56. Do neurofibrosarcomas, hemangiopericytomas, and peripheral nerve sheath tumors share the same prognosis?

Because of the recent change in nomenclature by veterinary pathologists, earlier studies reporting metastatic potential of these tumors may no longer apply. Many clinicians believe there is a distinct behavior difference between these tumor types in that hemangiopericytomas tend to be slow-growing tumors with a low likelihood of metastasis, whereas neurofibrosarcomas tend to be more aggressive, particularly in young dogs.

BIBLIOGRAPHY

1. Kuntz CA, Dernell WS, Powers BE, et al: Prognostic factors for surgical treatment of soft-tissue sarcomas in dogs: 75 cases (1986–1996). J Am Vet Med Assoc 211:1147–1151, 1997.
2. Lana SE, Ogilvie GK, Withrow SJ, et al: Feline cutaneous squamous cell carcinoma of the nasal planum and the pinnae: 61 cases. J Am Anim Hosp Assoc 33:329–332, 1997.
3. MacEwan EG, Withrow SJ: Soft tissue sarcomas. In Withrow SJ, MacEwan EG (eds): Small Animal Clinical Oncology, 2nd ed. Philadelphia, WB Saunders, 1996, pp 211–226.
4. Madewell B: Treatment of skin cancer. In Bonagura JD, Kirk RW (eds): Current Veterinary Therapy XII, Small Animal Practice. Philadelphia, WB Saunders, 1995, pp 511–518.
5. Marino DJ, Matthiesen DT, Stefanacci JD, et al: Evaluation of dogs with digit masses: 117 cases (1981–1991). J Am Vet Med Assoc 207:726–728, 1995.
6. O'Brien MG, Berg J, Engler SJ: Treatment by digital amputation of subungual squamous cell carcinoma in dogs: 21 cases (1987–1988). J Am Vet Med Assoc 201:759–761, 1992.
7. Ogilvie GK, Moore AS: Tumors of the skin and surrounding structures. In Ogilvie GK, Moore AS (eds): Managing the Veterinary Cancer Patient: A Practice Manual. Trenton, NJ, Veterinary Learning Systems, 1995, pp 473–502.
8. Thomas RC, Fox LE: Tumors of the skin and subcutis. In Morrison WB (ed): Cancer in Dogs and Cats: Medical and Surgical Management. Baltimore, Lippincott Williams and Wilkins, 1998, pp 489–510.
9. Vail DM, Withrow SJ: Tumors of the skin and subcutaneous tissues. In Withrow SJ, MacEwan EG (eds): Small Animal Clinical Oncology, 2nd ed. Philadelphia, WB Saunders, 1996, pp 167–191.

23. ENDOCRINE AND NEUROENDOCRINE NEOPLASMS

Steven E. Crow, DVM, Dipl ACVIM

1. Why are diseases of the endocrine system of interest to oncologists?

Endocrinopathies present some of the most interesting paraneoplastic syndromes. Searching for the diagnosis is often a daunting challenge, but precise definition of the cause of the abnormality is key in treatment planning.

2. Which test(s) or procedure(s) is (are) most useful in diagnosing adrenal cortical tumors in dogs?

Although an endocrinologist would say the high-dose dexamethasone suppression test is one of the best tests, imaging techniques give a much clearer definition of size, location, and potential for resectability. Specifically, ultrasonography and computed tomography are useful tools to diagnose adrenal masses in dogs. Ultimately, open biopsy is necessary to prove whether the process is benign hyperplasia or adrenal cortical carcinoma.

3. What percentage of dogs with pituitary-dependent hyperadrenocorticism (PDH) have concurrent hypertension? Proteinuria? Urinary tract infections (UTIs)?

- Hypertension: In one small study, 12 of 12 dogs tested were hypertensive.
- Proteinuria: Studies document 44–75% prevalence of mild to severe proteinuria.
- Urinary tract infections: Although not clearly delineated in most studies, approximately 20–25% of dogs with PDH have a concurrent UTI at time of diagnosis. Among the 5–10% of dogs with PDH who are glucosuric, almost all show bacteruria.

4. What are the sensitivities and specificities of the adrenocorticotrophic hormone (ACTH) stimulation test, low-dose dexamethasone suppression test (LDDST), urine cortisol:creatinine ratio (UCCR), and plasma (endogenous) ACTH concentration in diagnosing the cause of canine hyperadrenocorticism?

Plasma ACTH concentration is not used as a screening test for diagnosing hyperadrenocorticism; it is useful for differentiating between pituitary and adrenal tumors. The following table shows the mean sensitivity, specificity, and diagnostic accuracy for the other three tests:

TEST NAME	SENSITIVITY	SPECIFICITY	DIAGNOSTIC ACCURACY
LDDST	95.3	65.0	80.5
ACTH stimulation	91.3	86.3	88.0
UCCR	81.0	55.8	65.8

5. What are the most common clinical signs in dogs with pheochromocytomas?

Although the clinical signs of pheochromocytomas are often profound and dramatic in humans, it is difficult to document headache, nausea, anxiety, and palpitations in dogs. The most commonly observed signs in dogs are weight loss, anorexia, panting, and weakness. Other signs may relate to tumor invasion of the caudal vena cava, including exercise intolerance and abdominal distention, or to cardiovascular effects of severe hypertension, such as epistaxis, retinal hemorrhages, and tachyarrhythmias.

6. How can pheochromocytomas be diagnosed biochemically?

Perform a 24-hour collection of urine for measurement of catecholamines and their metabolites (metanephrine, normetanephrine, and vanillylmandelic acid) in a metabolic cage.

7. How is phentolamine used to diagnose pheochromocytomas?

A phentolamine suppression test may be used in hypertensive dogs suspected for pheochromocytomas. Phentolamine, an alpha-1-receptor antagonist, is injected intravenously, and the blood pressure is measured at 1-minute intervals for 10 minutes. A decrease in systolic blood pressure > 35 mmHg for longer than 4 minutes is diagnostic for pheochromocytomas.

8. Describe the use of phentolamine in the treatment of pheochromocytomas.

Phentolamine is a short-acting alpha-1-receptor antagonist that is useful in controlling blood pressure during anesthesia induction and surgery. It is not appropriate for long-term treatment.

9. Which method(s) of diagnostic imaging is (are) most useful in diagnosing and staging pheochromocytomas?

Survey abdominal radiographs will reveal a perirenal mass in some cases, and the presence of dystrophic calcification supports the diagnosis of pheochromocytomas. Caudal vena cava angiography and ultrasonography may reveal the presence of tumor thrombi. CT is the method of choice to demonstrate primary adrenal masses and visceral metastases. Two of the most effective methods of imaging adrenal masses in human beings—magnetic resonance imaging (MRI) and metaiodobenzylguanidine (MIBG) scintigraphy—have yet to find widespread use in veterinary medicine, but MRI facilities are becoming more readily available to veterinarians.

10. What is an APUDoma?

APUDoma refers to a tumor arising from cells of neuroectodermal origin that share a common metabolic characteristic: amine-precursor uptake decarboxylation. Examples include islet cell tumors, pheochromocytomas, parathyroid tumors, and thyroid medullary carcinoma.

11. Which nonislet cell tumors have been associated with hypoglycemia in the dog?
- Hepatoma
- Hepatocellular carcinoma
- Leiomyoma
- Leiomyosarcoma
- Splenic hemangiosarcoma
- Metastatic melanoma
- Salivary gland adenocarcinoma.

12. What classes of drugs are used as palliative therapy for gastrinoma? Give examples of each class.

H2-receptor antagonists (cimetidine, ranitidine); proton pump inhibitors (omeprazole); and somatostatin analogues (octreotide).

13. Which clinical syndrome is most commonly seen in dogs with glucagonoma?

Although this tumor is very rarely diagnosed in dogs, most animals are presented with a history of chronic dermatitis. Lesions consist of hyperkeratosis of the footpads and planum nasale and crusting, erosive, or erythematous lesions involving the external genitalia, perineum, muzzle, and periocular skin.

14. What diagnostic criteria are used to differentiate glucagonoma from necrolytic migratory erythema?

Necrolytic migratory erythema is a dermatopathy that resembles the skin lesions associated with glucagon-secreting tumors. The former has more frequently been associated with liver disease, and almost half of the cases have concurrent diabetes mellitus. No pancreatic tumors have been found, and serum glucagon concentrations are normal.

Glucogonoma is diagnosed only when carcinoma cells positive for glucagon immunoreactivity are identified histopathologically.

15. Which of the multiple endocrine neoplasia (MEN) syndromes described in humans has also been reported in dogs?

MEN II (thyroid medullary carcinoma, parathyroid gland hyperplasia, and pheochromocytomas or parathyroid tumor and pheochromocytomas) has been reported in dogs. MEN I (tumors of the parathyroid, pancreatic islet cells, and pituitary gland) has not been described in dogs.

16. In feline hyperthyroidism, how can adenocarcinoma be differentiated from benign adenomatous hyperplasia?

Because benign adenomatous hyperplasia can occur bilaterally and in ectopic sites, it is difficult to determine whether the gland enlargement is benign or malignant solely on the basis of imaging techniques, including scintigraphy. Consequently, **histopathologic criteria** such as atypia, invasiveness, tumor embolization, and distant metastasis help make the diagnosis.

17. How are nuclear scintigraphy and high-resolution ultrasonography useful in the management of thyroid neoplasia?

Sodium pertechnetate (^{99m}Tc) is concentrated in thyroid tissue and can be used to show whether one or both thyroid lobes are involved and identify ectopic thyroid tissue. High-resolution ultrasonography (using a 10-MHz or greater probe) has good correlation with scintigraphy in identifying abnormal thyroid glands.

18. What are the advantages and disadvantages of surgery, iodine radiotherapy, and antithyroid drugs in the treatment of feline hyperthyroidism?

TYPE OF TREATMENT	ADVANTAGES	DISADVANTAGES
Surgery	Allows histopathologic diagnosis; cure possible with single treatment	Risk of anesthesia; life-threatening hypocalcemia, if bilateral
Iodine radiotherapy	Treats bilateral and metastatic lesions; no anesthesia needed	Expensive; long hospitalization if treating carcinoma; special license and facilities needed
Antithyroid drugs	Inexpensive (initially); easy and available everywhere	Many side effects, including vomiting, hepatic toxicity, hematologic disorders, and severe pruritus, and need for daily treatment for life of patient

19. True or false: Scintigraphy is more efficacious than thoracic radiography in the detection of pulmonary metastases in canine thyroid adenocarcinoma.

False. Because only 5–20% of canine thyroid carcinomas are hormonally functional, scintigraphy is no more sensitive in detecting pulmonary metastases than is thoracic radiography. However, nuclear medicine may be helpful in identifying which thyroid carcinomas should be treated with radioiodine rather than surgery.

20. Which method of treatment is most effective for canine thyroid carcinoma?

Functional thyroid carcinoma is probably best treated with radioiodine. Nonfunctional thyroid carcinomas should be treated by surgery followed by external beam irradiation.

Chemotherapy, especially protocols containing doxorubicin, is frequently effective in partially shrinking large neoplasms and in palliation of associated signs (dysphonia, dysphagia).

21. How can a parathyroid adenoma be differentiated from other common causes of hypercalcemia?

In a patient with a parathyroid adenoma, serum parathyroid hormone (PTH) concentration is increased, PTH-related peptide is decreased, serum total and ionized calcium concentrations are increased, and serum phosphorus and 25-hydroxycholecalciferol concentrations are normal. Profiles of these chemicals are different for hypercalcemia of malignancy, chronic renal failure, and hypervitaminosis D. Ultimately, demonstration of a parathyroid mass is the most definitive way to diagnosis primary hyperparathyroidism.

22. What are the advantages and disadvantages for using calcitriol in the management of hyperparathyroidism?

Several forms of vitamin D are available for treating dogs that develop hypocalcemia after surgical removal of parathyroid adenoma. Calcitriol, 1,25 dihydrocholecalciferol, has a faster onset of action and shorter half-life than ergocalciferol and dihydrotachysterol. Unfortunately, calcitriol is more expensive and must be reformulated to be used in cats or small dogs.

23. What are the common clinical features of feline acromegaly (hypersomatotrophism)?

Excessive secretion of growth hormone (somatotrophin) occurs most commonly in middle-aged or older cats. Males are more frequently affected than females. Many cats have concurrent diabetes mellitus, so that polyuria, polydipsia, polyphagia, and weight loss are often present. Insulin resistance is commonly observed in acromegalic cats. In addition, enlargement of the head (prognathism), tongue, heart, liver, and kidneys are documented. Joint pain and central nervous system signs are also seen in severe cases.

CONTROVERSIES

24. In the diagnosis of canine insulinoma, which of the following ratios has the greatest accuracy (sensitivity and specificity): insulin:glucose, glucose:insulin, or amended insulin:glucose?

Assuming that the glucose and insulin concentrations are determined in the same laboratory, all of the ratios will have the same sensitivity and specificity because they share a common relationship with one another (i.e., as in the algebraic equation $y = mx + b$, where the slope [m] is determined by the variables x and y). The accuracy of these methods can only be changed by assigning (statistically or arbitrarily) more or less appropriate reference values.

25. What is the best way to diagnose hyperadrenocorticism (HAC)?

If you hail from Pennsylvania, it's the LSDDT. If you're from Michigan State, it's probably the ACTH stimulation test. If you're from California, you may like the endogenous ACTH concentration. But if you're honest and experienced, you know that the answer is none (or all) of these tests. There is a study that statistically shows that the old combined ACTH-low dose dexamethasone suppression test (aka V test) may outperform any one of these tests as a screening test for HAC. The best advice may be to use any or all of the diagnostic tools available, including liver biopsies, response to therapy, or MRI, when your clinical index of suspicion is sufficiently high. A rule of thumb to go by: if you really believe a dog has HAC—it probably does!

BIBLIOGRAPHY

1. Berger B, Feldman EC: Primary hyperparathyroidism in dogs: 21 cases (1976-1986). J Am Vet Med Assoc 191:350–356, 1987.
2. Carver JR, Kapatkin A, Patnaik AK: A comparison of medullary thyroid carcinoma and thyroid adenocarcinoma in dogs: A retrospective study of 38 cases. Vet Surg 24:35–39, 1995.
3. Guptill L, Scott-Moncrief JC, Widmer WR: Diagnosis of canine hyperadrenocorticism. Vet Clin North Am Small Anim Pract 27:215–235, 1997.
4. Jeglum KA, Whereat A: Chemotherapy of canine thyroid carcinoma. Compend Contin Educ Pract Vet 5:96–98, 1983.
5. Johnson SE: Pancreatic APUDomas. Semin Vet Med Surg (Small Anim) 4:202–211, 1989.
6. Maher ER, McNeil EA: Pheochromocytomas in dogs and cats. Vet Clin North Am Small Anim Pract 27:359–380, 1997.
7. Peterson ME, Taylor RS, Greco DS, et al: Acromegaly in 14 cats. J Vet Intern Med 4:192–201, 1990.
8. von Dehn BJ, Nelson RW, Feldman EC: Pheochromocytomas and hyperadrenocorticism in dogs: six cases (1982-1992). J Am Vet Med Assoc 207:322–324, 1995.
9. Wright KN, Breitschwerdt EB, Feldman JM, et al: Diagnostic and therapeutic considerations in a hypercalcemic dog with multiple endocrine neoplasia. J Am Anim Hosp Assoc 31:156–162, 1995.
10. Zerbe CA: Screening tests to diagnose hyperadrenocorticism in cats and dogs. Compend Contin Educ Pract Vet 22:17–36, 2000.

24. BONE TUMORS

Gregory K. Ogilvie, DVM, Dipl ACVIM

OSTEOSARCOMA OF THE APPENDICULAR SKELETON IN DOGS

1. How common is appendicular osteosarcoma in the dog?

Osteosarcoma of the limbs is more common in dogs than in any other species and accounts for more than 80% of malignant bone tumors in dogs.

2. What is the most common signalment of dogs with osteosarcoma?

Large- to giant-breed dogs with a body weight of more than 20 kg are most often affected. Giant-breed dogs are 60 times more likely and large-breed dogs are eight times more likely to develop osteosarcoma than small dogs. Dogs with osteosarcoma are middle-aged to old animals with a median age of 8 years. There is no sex predilection.

3. Can surgical implants or radiation be associated with the development of osteosarcoma?

Osteosarcoma has been associated with sites of healed fractures or internal fixation devices, implying that chronic irritation may play a role in tumor development. High-, single-dose radiation (i.e., coarse fractionation) in one study increased the risk of the formation of tumors, including osteosaroma.

4. What is the most common anatomic location for the development of osteosarcoma in the dog?

Osteosarcoma most commonly affects the appendicular skeleton, particularly in the metaphyseal region. The most common sites are the distal radius and the proximal humerus. Less common sites are the proximal tibia and distal femur. This tumor has also been noted in any site of bone.

5. What is the optimal staging scheme for osteosarcoma?

Dogs with a suspected primary bone tumor should have high-quality radiographs of the lesion and chest. In addition, routine blood work and urinalysis as well as thoracic radiographs should be performed. A preoperative biopsy should be taken if it will change the client's willingness to treat or if it will change the way the lesion will be treated. A Jamshidi core needle biopsy instrument is the preferred method for doing a preoperative biopsy.

6. What is the most common radiographic pattern of appendicular osteosarcoma?

Primary bone tumors may have a lytic, productive, or mixed appearance on high-detail radiographs. The signs most suggestive of neoplasia include cortical bone lysis in a lesion that does not cross a joint space. Tumor extension and mineralization form periosteal spicules in the surrounding soft tissues, imparting a "sunburst" appearance on radiographs. Radiographs tend to underestimate the true extent of the lesion. Bone scintigraphy overestimates tumor margins.

7. How is a definitive diagnosis made?

Definitive diagnosis is confirmed by histopathology. For old animals with a large lytic metaphyseal bone lesion, osteosarcoma is the most common diagnosis. Differentials include other neoplastic conditions as well as fungal and bacterial infections. In each case, removal of the limb is an acceptable procedure. Therefore, biopsy at the time of amputation is advised. If there is significant doubt as to the cause of the lesion, a preoperative biopsy should be obtained.

8. Where should a Jamshidi biopsy be taken?

Unlike soft tissue tumors, in bone tumors diagnostic biopsy samples are best obtained from the center of the lesion. Multiple biopsy specimens increase the chance of diagnosis. Osteosarcoma frequently includes areas of cartilage and fibrous tissue as well as osteoid and is often surrounded by new bone.

9. What are important prognostic factors for predicting outcome?

Age at time of diagnosis was important for determining survival in dogs treated with amputation alone. Dogs between the ages of 7 and 10 years had the longest survival times; both old and young dogs fared less well. The higher the alkaline phosphatase levels, the poorer the prognosis. In studies of adjuvant therapy for appendicular osteosarcoma, the percentage of tumor necrosis following doxorubicin and cisplatin chemotherapy correlated with survival.

10. What is the most cost-effective treatment to control the local disease?

Amputation controls the primary tumor and provides pain relief with little to no reduction in mobility and quality of life for the dog. The procedure is also usually accepted by owners.

11. What surgical procedure is optimal for performing an amputation?

For lesions in the forelimbs, complete forequarter amputation, including the scapula, provides cosmetically and functionally good results. For distal hindlimb tumors, amputation at the proximal third of the femur is performed. For distal femoral tumors, a hip disarticulation is performed, and proximal femoral lesions are treated by hemipelvectomy.

12. Will amputation improve survival time?

Amputation is palliative but rarely increases survival. In one study, the median survival of 65 dogs treated with amputation was 126 days; only 10.7% of dogs were alive 1 year after surgery. A more recent study of 162 dogs treated with amputation corroborated these data. Chemotherapy should be administered to dogs after an amputation to help control metastatic disease.

13. Is limb-sparing surgery preferred over an amputation for the treatment of osteosarcoma?

No. Limb-sparing surgery may be ideal for dogs that are poor candidates for amputation, such as very large dogs or dogs with other orthopedic or neurologic problems, or for clients who refuse amputation.

14. How is limb-sparing surgery performed?

A cortical bone graft is used to replace the widely excised tumor, and arthrodesis of the nearby joint is usually performed. The best results are obtained with distal radial lesions or lesions of the ulna. It is possible to perform limb salvage for proximal humeral or scapular lesions, but function may be more impaired. Good functional results have been reported for partial or complete scapulectomy in dogs with osteosarcoma.

15. What are the limitations for limb-sparing surgery?

Limb salvage is not an option for large lesions that involve more than 50% of the bone, tumors that invade adjacent soft tissue, and tumors of the hind limb. Complications occurred in 55% of dogs treated with limb salvage. Recurrence rates of 17% to 27% are seen.

16. Which chemotherapeutic agents have been shown to be effective to help control metastatic disease?

Unquestionably for dogs with microscopic disease. Survival of dogs with osteosarcoma can be significantly prolonged by adjuvant chemotherapy. Cisplatin markedly improves survival rates to a median survival of between 180 and 400 days, and 1-year survival rates to between 30% and 62%; 2-year survival rates are between 7% and 21%. Preliminary evidence suggests that a polymer that slowly releases cisplatin (OPLA–Pt) may also influence survival, possibly by providing prolonged low plasma levels of cisplatin.

Doxorubicin (30 mg/m^2) has been used as an economically viable treatment for osteosarcoma; however, the results have been variable. In one study, 35 dogs with appendicular osteosarcoma were treated with five biweekly doses of doxorubicin (30 mg/ m^2). Median survival was 366 days; 50% of the dogs were alive at 1 year, and 10% were alive at 2 years, thereby approaching a similar efficacy to that of cisplatin.

A protocol alternating cisplatin (60 mg/m^2) with doxorubicin (30 mg/m^2) every 21 days for two cycles was delivered after amputation to 19 dogs with appendicular osteosarcoma. The median survival was 300 days.

Methotrexate was given intravenously to five dogs with osteosarcoma at doses ranging from 3 to 6 g/m^2. Myelosuppression was the dose-limiting toxicity, and no clinical response was seen.

Carboplatin (300 mg/m^2 intravenously) was given adjunctively after surgery to 48 dogs. Median survival was 321 days.

17. What is L-MTP-PE?

Liposome-encapsulated muramyltripeptide-phosphatidylethanolamine (L-MTP-PE) is a nonspecific activator of monocytes and macrophages that induces tumoricidal activity in these cells. Eleven dogs that had received four doses of cisplatin (70 mg/m^2 every 28 days) after amputation were treated with L-MTP-PE and had a median survival of 438 days.

18. Will dogs with metastatic disease respond to chemotherapy or radiation therapy?

Chemotherapy is ineffective for the treatment of metastatic disease. Osteosarcoma metastases were treated with cisplatin (70 mg/m^2 intravenously), doxorubicin (30 mg/m^2), mitoxantrone (5 mg/m^2 IV), or sequential combinations of these drugs every 3 weeks. Only one of 45 dogs experienced a partial remission for 21 days with doxorubicin.

Pulmonary metastasectomy seems to prolong survival in specific circumstances only if the animal develops clinically evident metastases more than 300 days after the initial diagnosis and if fewer than three nodules are radiographically apparent. Median survival time after metastasectomy was found to be 176 days.

19. How is palliative radiation therapy used to treat dogs with osteosaroma?

If clients refuse definitive treatment for their pet with osteosarcoma or if an animal is not considered an eligible candidate for amputation or limb sparing, consideration may be given to palliation of tumor pain with radiation therapy. This treatment can be given with many schedules such as on days 0, 7, and 21. The median duration of response was 130 days (range 17 ≈ 288 days). Chemotherapy has been shown to improve the duration of response.

20. What is samarium-153-EDTMP?

Samarium-153-EDTMP accumulates in areas of increased bony activity, thereby providing high-dose localized radiation therapy. When used to treat 28 dogs with appendicular osteosarcoma, the survival was 240 days.

OSTEOSARCOMA OF THE AXIAL SKELETON IN DOGS

Incidence, Signalment, and Etiology

21. What is the most common anatomic location of axial skeletal osteosarcomas in the dog?

In a large series of 116 dogs with osteosarcoma of the axial skeleton, the distribution of lesions was mandible (27%), maxilla (22%), spine (15%), cranium (12%), ribs (10%), nasal bones (9%), and pelvis (5%).

22. What is the most common signalment?

These tumors are more common in female dogs than in males; the trend is most pronounced for maxillary and pelvic osteosarcoma, which occur primarily in female dogs.

23. Is metastatic disease commonly found at the time of original diagnosis?

At the time of presentation, few dogs have evidence of pulmonary metastasis.

24. What is the treatment of choice for these tumors?

Surgery. In most dogs with axial osteosarcoma, tumors recur after surgery and before metastases are clinically evident. This contrasts with appendicular osteosarcoma, where surgical margins are easily obtained but the metastatic rate is very high.

25. What is the survival time with or without surgery?

Overall median survival for 38 dogs that underwent attempted surgical removal of an axial osteosarcoma was 22 weeks; 25% of the dogs were alive at 1 year, and nearly 20% were alive at 2 years. Untreated dogs died within 1 month.

MULTILOBULAR OSTEOCHONDROSARCOMA

26. How common is multilobular osteochondrosarcoma?

Multilobular osteochondrosarcoma (MLO) is considered the most common tumor of the canine skull and has been described using several names, including chondroma rodens, multilobular osteoma/osteosarcoma/chondroma, and multilobular tumor of bone.

27. What is the most common signalment associated with this tumor?

MLO is a tumor of middle-aged dogs that are usually middle to large dogs of either sex.

28. What is the most common location of these tumors?

The most common sites are the parietal crest, temporo-occipital region, and zygomatic arch, from which tumors may extend into the sinuses, orbit, or cranial vault.

29. What are the most common clinical signs associated with this tumor?

Dogs may also be presented for dysphagia and pain in opening the mouth, exophthalmia, or neurologic signs. Radiographically, the lesion is sharply delineated with a lobulated "popcorn ball" appearance.

30. How common are metastases?

Metastasis at the time of presentation is common; however, metastasis occurred a median of 14 months after surgical excision in 7 of 12 dogs. Interestingly, the median time from detection of metastasis to death was 11 months (range 5 to 33 months), which concurs with other reports of long survival of dogs even after they have metastatic disease.

31. What is the optimum staging scheme?

Radiographs of the thorax and tumor site are recommended prior to treatment, and thoracic radiographs should be used to monitor patients after surgery. A computed tomography (CT) scan may assist the surgeon in planning surgery. Blood work is essential to document the general health of the patient.

32. What is the treatment of choice for MLO?

Surgery, but complete excision is rarely accomplished. In one study, wide resection was accomplished in nine dogs with MLO, and there was no recurrence in four dogs that had histologically complete resection. Treatment of MLO with radiation therapy as an adjunct to surgical excision seems justified on the basis of limited data. Although cisplatin seems to give the best chance of preventing metastasis, there are only preliminary data at this time.

EXTRASKELETAL OSTEOSARCOMA IN DOGS

33. How common is extraskeletal osteosarcoma in the dog?
It is extremely rare.

34. Where do extraskeletal osteosarcomas occur?
They most often have been reported in the spleen but also occur in the adrenal gland, eye, testicle, vagina, kidney, intestine, mesentery, and liver.

35. What is the most common age, breed, and sex for this tumor type?
Dogs with extraskeletal osteosarcoma are old (mean 11 years; range 9 to 15 years). There may be a higher incidence in female dogs. There is no breed predilection.

36. What is the metastatic rate of this disease?
Metastatic disease is common. Metastases have been reported for extraskeletal osteosarcoma of the eye, testicle, vagina, intestine, and liver, principally to regional lymph nodes. Splenic osteosarcoma metastasizes to the liver and omentum.

37. What is the optimum treatment for this disease?
Surgery. Splenectomy for splenic osteosarcoma has not resulted in good survival times. Survival in three dogs with extraskeletal osteosarcomas of other sites ranged from 15 to 124 days. Adjuvant chemotherapy has not been commonly reported for this disease.

NONOSTEOSARCOMA BONE TUMORS IN DOGS

38. What other tumors can involve the skeletal system?
Primary bone tumors that are not osteosarcomas are rare but include chondrosarcomas, fibrosarcomas, hemangiosarcomas, giant cell tumors, liposarcomas, and synovial cell sarcomas. In a series of 26 nonosteosarcoma appendicular bone tumors, the most frequently recognized was fibrosarcoma. Hemangiosarcoma and chondrosarcoma were less frequently noted. Chondrosarcoma probably predominates in the axial skeleton. Affected dogs are mostly large breeds. There is no gender predilection, and old dogs are most often affected.

39. What is the optimal treatment for nonosteosarcoma tumors of the bone?
Surgery. Chemotherapy and radiation therapy have been tried with variable results. Chemotherapy using doxorubicin (30 mg/m^2 intravenously) has been reported to provide long-term response in dogs with synovial sarcoma.

40. Do cats get osteosarcoma?
Osteosarcoma is the most common primary bone tumor in cats and occurs in old cats (median age 11 years), with a predilection for male cats in the United Kingdom and for female cats in the United States. In four series of cases totalling 106 cats with osteosarcoma, 30 occurred in the skull, 56 occurred in the appendicular skeleton (38 in the hindlimb and 18 in the forelimb), and the remaining 20 involved either vertebrae (8 cats), scapula (2 cats), rib (5 cats), or pelvis (5 cats).

Parosteal (juxtacortical) osteosarcomas have also been reported.

41. What is the metastatic potential of osteosaroma in the cat?
Metastasis is uncommon in cats with osteosarcoma.

42. How should disease in cats with osteosarcoma be staged?
Thoracic radiographs should be performed in all cats with primary bone lesions; however, it is unusual for these cats to develop metastases even long after surgery. A hemogram,

biochemical profile, urinalysis, tests for feline leukemia virus and feline immunodeficiency virus, thyroxine analysis, and a preoperative biopsy is optimal.

43. Is surgery effective for the treatment of osteosarcoma?

The prognosis with surgical removal of osteosarcoma is good. In 12 cats with appendicular osteosarcoma treated by amputation, pulmonary metastasis occurred in only one cat; more than half of the cats were alive 64 months after surgery.

44. How effective is radiation therapy?

The low rate of metastasis implies that radiation therapy may play an important role in the control of incompletely excised osteosarcoma.

45. Is adjunctive chemotherapy warranted in this disease?

Adjunctive chemotherapy is rarely warranted for the treatment of feline osteosarcoma because of the low rate of metastasis.

BIBLIOGRAPHY

1. Tjalma RA: Canine bone sarcoma: Estimation of relative risk as a function of body size. J Natl Cancer Inst 36:1137–1150, 1966.
2. Spodnick GJ, Berg J, Rand WM, et al: Prognosis for dogs with appendicular osteosarcoma treated by amputation alone: 162 cases (1978–1988). J Am Vet Med Assoc 200:995–999, 1992.
3. Misdorp W, Hart AAM: Some prognostic and epidemiologic factors in canine osteosarcoma. J Natl Cancer Inst 62:537–545, 1979.
4. Brodey RS, Riser WH: Canine osteosarcoma: A clinicopathologic study of 194 cases. Clin Orthop Rel Res 62:54–64, 1969.
5. Gillette-McChesney S, Gillette EL, Powers BE, Withrow SJ: Radiation-induced osteosarcoma in dogs after external beam or intraoperative radiation therapy. Cancer Res:54–57, 1990.
6. Lamb CR, Berg J, Bengston AE: Preoperative measurement of canine primary bone tumors, using radiography and bone scintigraphy. J Am Vet Med Assoc 196:1474–1478, 1990.
7. Berg J, Lamb CR, O'Callaghan MW: Bone scintigraphy in the initial evaluation of dogs with primary bone tumors. J Am Vet Med Assoc 196:917–920, 1990.
8. Weinstein MJ, Berg J, Kusazaki K, et al: In vitro assay of nuclear uptake of doxorubicin hydrochloride in osteosarcoma cells of dogs. Am J Vet Res 52:1951–1955, 1991.
9. Powers BE, Withrow SJ, Thrall DE, et al: Percent tumor necrosis as a predictor of treatment response in canine osteosarcoma. Cancer 67:126–134, 1991.
10. Carberry CA, Harvey HJ: Owner satisfaction with limb amputation in dogs and cats. J Am Anim Hosp Assoc 23:227–232, 1987.
11. Brodey RS: Results of surgical treatment in 65 dogs with osteosarcoma. J Am Vet Med Assoc 168:1032–1035, 1976.
12. Trout NJ, Pavletic MM, Kraus KH: Partial scapulectomy in the treatment of malignant sarcomas in three dogs and two cats. Vet Surg, 1994.
13. O'Brien MG, Straw RC, Withrow SJ: Recent advances in the treatment of canine appendicular osteosarcoma. Compend Contin Educ Pract Vet 15:939–947, 1993.
14. Withrow SJ, Thrall DE, Straw RS: Intra-arterial cisplatin with or without radiation in limb sparing for canine osteosarcoma. Cancer 71:2484–2490, 1993.
15. Shapiro W, Fossum TW, Kitchell BE, et al: Use of cisplatin for treatment of appendicular osteosarcoma in dogs. J Am Vet Med Assoc 192:507–511, 1988.
16. Straw RC, Withrow SJ, Richter SL, et al: Amputation and cisplatin for treatment of canine osteosarcoma. J Vet Intern Med 5:205–210, 1991.
17. Thompson JP, Fugent MJ: Evaluation of survival time after limb amputation, with and without subsequent administration of cisplatin, for treatment of appendicular osteosarcoma in dogs: 30 cases (1979–1990). J Am Vet Med Assoc 200:531–533, 1992.
18. Kraegel SA, Madewell BR, Simonson E, Gregory CR: Osteogenic sarcoma and cisplatin chemotherapy in dogs: 16 cases (1986–1989). J Am Vet Med Assoc 199:1057–1059, 1991.
19. Berg J, Weinstein J, Schelling SH, Rand WM: Treatment of dogs with osteosarcoma by administration of cisplatin after amputation or limb-sparing surgery: 22 cases (1987–1990). J Am Vet Med Assoc 200:2005–2008, 1992.

20. Madewell BR, Leighton RL, Theilen GH: Amputation and doxorubicin for treatment of canine and feline osteogenic sarcoma. Eur J Cancer 14:287–293, 1978.

21. Berg J, Weinstein MJ, Springfield DS: Response of osteosarcoma in dogs to surgery and chemotherapy with doxorubicin. J Am Vet Med Assoc, 1994, in press.

22. Mauldin GN, Matus RE, Withrow SJ, Patnaik AK: Canine osteosarcoma. Treatment by amputation versus amputation plus adjuvant chemotherapy using doxorubicin and cisplatin. J Vet Intern Med 2:177–180, 1988.

23. Cotter SM, Parker LM: High-dose methotrexate and leucovorin rescue in dogs with osteogenic sarcoma. Am J Vet Res 39:1943–1945, 1978.

24. Bergman PJ, MacEwen EG, Kurzman ID, et al: Amputation and carboplatin for treatment of dogs with osteosarcoma: 48 cases (1991–1993). J Am Vet Med Assoc, 1994, in press.

25. MacEwen EG, Kurzman TD, Rosenthal RC, et al: Therapy for osteosarcoma in dogs with intravenous injection of liposome encapsulated muramyl tripeptide. J Natl Cancer Inst 81:935–938, 1989.

26. MacEwen EG, Helfand SC: Recent advances in the biologic therapy of cancer. Compend Contin Educ Pract Vet 15:909–922, 1993.

27. Knapp DW, Richardson RC, Booney PL, Hahn K: Cisplatin therapy in 41 dogs with malignant tumors. J Vet Intern Med 2:41–46, 1988.

28. Ogilvie GK, Straw RC, Jameson VJ: Evaluation of single-agent chemotherapy for treatment of clinically evident osteosarcoma metastasis in dogs: 45 cases (1987–1991). J Am Vet Med Assoc 202:304–306, 1993.

29. O'Brien MG, Straw RC, Withrow SJ, et al: Resection of pulmonary metastases in canine osteosarcoma: Thirty-one cases (1983–1992). Vet Surg 22:105–109, 1993.

30. Lattimer JC, Corwin LA, Stapleton J, et al: Clinical and clinicopathologic response of canine bone tumor patients to treatment with samarium-153-EDTMP. J Nucl Med 31:1316–1325, 1990.

31. Heymann SJ, Diefender DL, Goldschmidt MH, Newton CD: Canine axial skeletal osteosarcoma. A retrospective study of 116 cases (1986 to 1989). Vet Surg 21:304–310, 1992.

32. Patnaik AK, Lieberman PH, Erlandson RA, Liu SK: Canine sinonasal skeletal neoplasms: Chondrosarcomas and osteosarcomas. Vet Pathol 21:475–482, 1984.

33. Wallace J, Matthiesen DT, Patnaik AK: Hemimaxillectomy for the treatment of oral tumors in 69 dogs. Vet Surg 21:337–341, 1992.

34. White RAS: Mandibulectomy and maxillectomy in the dog: Long-term survival in 100 cases. J Small Anim Pract 32:69–74, 1991.

35. Withrow SJ, Doige CE: En bloc resection of a juxtacortical and three intraosseous osteosarcoma of the zygomatic arch in dogs. J Am Anim Hosp Assoc 16:867–872, 1980.

36. Straw RC, Withrow SJ, Powers BE: Partial or total hemipelvectomy in the management of sarcomas in nine dogs and two cats. Vet Surg 21:183–188, 1992.

37. Straw RC, Powers BE, Henderson RA, et al: Canine mandibular osteosarcoma. Forty-five cases (1980–1991). Proc 11th Ann Conf Vet Cancer Soc pp 79–80, 1991.

38. Pirkey-Ehrhart N, Straw RC, Withrow SJ, et al: Primary rib tumors in 54 dogs. J Am Anim Hosp Assoc, 1994, in press.

39. Feeney DA, Johnston GR, Grindem CB, et al: Malignant neoplasia of canine ribs: Clinical, radiographic, and pathologic findings. J Am Vet Med Assoc 180:927–933, 1982.

40. Matthiesen DT, Clark GN, Orsher RJ, et al: En bloc resection of primary rib tumors in 40 dogs. Vet Surg 21:201–204, 1992.

41. Straw RC, LeCouteur RA, Powers BE, Withrow SJ: Multilobular osteochondrosarcoma of the canine skull: 16 cases (1978–1988). J Am Vet Med Assoc 195:1764–1769, 1989.

42. Pool RR: Tumors of bone and cartilage. In Moulton JE (ed): Tumors in Domestic Animals, 3rd ed. Berkeley, CA, University of California Press, 1990, pp 157–230.

43. Johnston TC: Osteosarcoma of the canine skull (a case report). Vet Med Small Anim Clin 71:629–631, 1976.

44. McLain DL, Hill JR, Pulley LT: Multilobular osteoma and chondroma (chondroma rodens) with pulmonary metastasis in a dog. J Am Anim Hosp Assoc 19:359–362, 1983.

45. Losco PE, Diters RW, Walsh KM: Canine multilobar osteosarcoma of the skull with metastasis. J Comp Pathol 94:621–624, 1984.

46. Pletcher JM, Koch SA, Stedham MA: Orbital chondroma rodens in a dog. J Am Vet Med Assoc 175:187–190, 1979.

47. Weinstein MJ, Carpenter JL, Schunk-Mehlaff, CJ: Nonangiogenic and nonlymphomatous sarcomas of the canine spleen: 57 cases (1975–1987). J Am Vet Med Assoc 195:784–788, 1989.

48. Patnaik AK: Canine extraskeletal osteosarcoma and chondrosarcoma: A clinicopathologic study of 14 cases. Vet Pathol 27:46–55, 1990.

49. Gibbs C, Denny HR, Lucke VM: The radiological features of nonosteogenic malignant tumors of bone in the appendicular skeleton of the dog. J Small Anim Pract 26:537–553, 1985.
50. Brodey RS, Misdorp W, Riser WH, Heul van der RO: Canine skeletal chondrosarcoma: A clinico-pathological study of 35 cases. J Am Vet Med Assoc 165:68–78, 1974.
51. Wesselhoeft-Ablin L, Berg J, Schelling SH: Fibrosarcoma of the canine appendicular skeleton. J Am Anim Hosp Assoc 27:303–309, 1991.
52. Salisbury SK, Lantz GC: Long-term results of partial mandibulectomy for treatment of oral tumors in 30 dogs. J Am Anim Hosp Assoc 24:285–294, 1988.
53. McChesney SL, Withrow SJ, Gillette EL, et al: Radiotherapy of soft tissue sarcomas in dogs. J Am Vet Med Assoc 194:60–63, 1989.
54. Mauldin GN, Meleo KA, Burk RL: Radiation therapy for the treatment of incompletely resected soft tissue sarcomas in dogs: 21 cases. Proc Vet Cancer Soc 13th Ann Conf p 111, 1993.
55. Liu SK, Dorfman HD, Huruitz AI, Patnaik AK: Primary and secondary bone tumors in the dog. J Small Anim Pract 18:313–326, 1977.
56. Popovitch CA, Weinstein MJ, Goldschmidt MH, Shofer FS: Chondrosarcoma: A retrospective study of 97 dogs (1987–1990). J Am Anim Hosp Assoc 30:81–85, 1994.
57. Obradovich JE, Straw RC, Powers BE, Withrow SJ: Canine chondrosarcoma: A clinicopathologic review of 55 cases (1983–1990). Proc 10th Ann Conf Vet Cancer Soc pp 29–30, 1990.
58. Matthiesen DT, Clark GN, Orsher RJ, et al: En bloc resection of primary rib tumors in 40 dogs. Vet Surg 21:201–204, 1992.
59. Montgomery RD, Henderson RA, Powers RD: Retrospective study of 26 primary tumors of the osseous wall in dogs. J Am Anim Hosp Assoc 29:68–72, 1993.
60. Hammer AS, Couto CG, Filppi J, et al: Efficacy and toxicity of VAC chemotherapy (vincristine, doxorubicin and cyclophosphamide) in dogs with hemangiosarcoma. J Vet Intern Med 5:160–166, 1991.
61. McGlennon NJ, Houlton JEF, Gorman NT: Synovial sarcoma in the dog: A review. J Small Anim Pract 29:139–152, 1988.
62. Vail DM, Powers B, Morrison WB, et al: Clinical aspects of synovial cell sarcoma (SCS) in the canine: A retrospective study of 35 cases. Proc 10th Ann Vet Cancer Soc Conf pp 31–32, 1990.
63. Vail DM, Powers BE, Getsy D, et al: Prognostic importance of histological grade and cytochemical staining patterns for canine synovial cell sarcoma: Preliminary results of a VCOG study. Vet Cancer Soc Newsletter 17(1):1–4, 1993.
64. Tilmant LL, Gorman NT, Ackerman N, et al: Chemotherapy of synovial cell sarcoma in a dog. J Am Vet Med Assoc 188:530–532, 1986.
65. Ogilvie GK, Reynolds HA, Richardson RC, et al: Phase II evaluation of doxorubicin for treatment of various canine neoplasms. J Am Vet Med Assoc 195:1580–1583, 1989.
66. Quigley PJ, Leedale AH: Tumors involving bone in the domestic cat: A review of fifty-eight cases. Vet Pathol 20:670–686, 1983.
67. Liu SK, Dorfman HD, Patnaik AK. Primary and secondary bone tumors in the cat. J Small Anim Pract 15:141–156, 1974.
68. Carpenter JL, Andrews LK, Holzworth J: Tumors and tumor-like lesions. In Holzworth J (ed): Diseases of the Cat. Medicine and Surgery. Philadelphia, WB Saunders, 1987, pp 406–596.
69. Bitetto WV, Patnaik AK, Schrader SC, Mooney SC: Osteosarcoma in cats: 22 cases (1974–1984). J Am Vet Med Assoc 190:91–93, 1987.
70. Turrel JM, Pool RR: Primary bone tumors in the cat: A retrospective study of 15 cats and literature review. Vet Radiol 23:152–166, 1982.
71. Easton CB: Extraskeletal osteosarcoma in a cat. J Am Anim Hosp Asoc 30:59–61, 1994.

25. TUMORS OF THE RESPIRATORY TRACT

Kevin A. Hahn, DVM, PhD, Dipl ACVIM

TUMORS OF THE NASAL PLANE

1. What is the incidence of tumors of the nasal plane?
Malignant tumors of the nasal plane are common in the cat and rare in the dog.

2. Describe the natural behavior of tumors of the nasal plane.
Squamous cell carcinoma is by far the most frequent malignant diagnosis and is the result of prolonged exposure of the nonpigmented planum to ultraviolet light. Solar-induced dermatitis followed by erythema, crusting, or ulceration of the planum is considered a preneoplastic process. While regional and distant metastases have not been reported, extensive local invasion of the nasal cavity with destruction of underlying soft-tissue structures and bone is common to all types of tumors of the nasal plane, and explains their poor response to most conventional therapeutic approaches (e.g., superficial excision, localized irradiation).

3. What is the diagnostic approach to tumors of the nasal plane?
With erosive or proliferative lesions, a deep wedge biopsy should be performed to determine the degree of invasion and the histologic type of disease. These superficial lesions tend to be inflammatory owing to tumor necrosis and bacterial contamination; thus, cytologic scrapings or superficial biopsies are of little value. Lymph nodes are rarely involved except in very advanced disease, and thoracic radiographs are invariably negative for metastasis.

4. Describe the therapeutic approach to tumors of the nasal plane.
Nasal plane tumors can be cured with aggressive surgical resection. The entire non-haired nasal plane, deep cartilage, and turbinates should be removed, and any areas where deeper tumor invasion is suspected should be biopsied selectively or removed. Careful case selection is imperative, and advanced imaging procedures such as computed tomography, if available, may be helpful prior to definitive therapy to delineate more clearly the extent of tumor. Accurate assessment of the extent of the tumor is essential for determining whether clean surgical margins can be expected with resection of the nasal plane, as well as for planning appropriate fields if radiation therapy is to be applied.

5. What is the prognosis?
In one series of cases in which nine cats and five dogs were treated with aggressive resection of the nasal plane, the median postoperative, tumor-free survival period was 16 months (1–27+ months) for cats and 24 months (14–48+ months) for dogs. Radiation protocols involving higher doses and modified dose-fractionation schemes have led to improvements in the survival times of cats with deeply invasive squamous cell carcinomas of the nasal plane. Following irradiation, 1- and 5-year progression–free survival rates were 60.1% and 10.3%, respectively.

TUMORS OF THE NASAL CAVITY AND PARANASAL SINUS

6. What is the clinical presentation of nasal and paranasal sinus tumors?
Intranasal tumors are locally aggressive and most animals are presented with signs referable to the upper respiratory system (e.g., epistaxis, nasal discharge, sneezing, reverse sneezing,

dyspnea). However, some animals are presented with facial swelling (with or without exophthalmos) and neurologic signs (e.g., seizures, behavioral changes), suggesting extension beyond the nasal cavity and paranasal sinuses (i.e., brain involvement).

7. Which tumor types occur in the nasal and paranasal sinuses?

In dogs, approximately two-thirds of intranasal tumors are epithelial in origin; slightly fewer than one-third are mesenchymal in origin; and only a few are of neuroendocrine origin. In cats, epithelial tumors predominate, mostly squamous cell carcinomas and adenocarcinomas. Mesenchymal tumors and lymphoma may also be seen in cats.

8. Outline the biological behavior of nasal and paranasal tumors.

Intranasal tumor metastasis is infrequently reported at presentation; however, it appears that **micrometastases** do occur and can remain subclinical for 12 to 36 months following presumed definitive treatment. Metastatic sites may include the regional lymph nodes (e.g., medial retropharyngeal, submandibular, prescapular, hilar lymph nodes), lungs, liver, kidneys, and bone. The extremely rare canine patient with a neuroendocrine tumor usually presents with metastatic lesions (> 86%) and has a poor prognosis.

Although intranasal lymphomas and carcinomas occur more commonly in the cat than in the dog, the results of a retrospective study of 16 cats with intranasal neoplasia suggest that cats and dogs with intranasal tumors have similar biologic courses. In that study, metastasis was uncommon (i.e., lymph node metastasis occurred in only two cats—one with olfactory neuroblastoma, one with undifferentiated carcinoma), and local extension to the brain occurred in two cats (one with neuroblastoma, one with undifferentiated carcinoma).

9. What is the diagnostic approach to nasal and paranasal tumors?

When presented with a dog or cat with an intranasal neoplasm, perform a thorough **head and neck palpation** and obtain **radiographs** of the thorax to identify any metastatic lesions. Destruction of the nasal turbinates, evidence of septal deviation, and soft-tissue or fluid-density lesions are common abnormalities observed radiographically in dogs and cats with intranasal neoplasia. However, advanced images such as those obtained with the use of CT or MRI techniques, if available, are far better than conventional radiographic images to determine whether disease has extended beyond the nasal cavity and paranasal sinuses.

A definitive diagnosis of intranasal neoplasia requires **biopsy**. Various biopsy methods such as core catheter biopsy or punch biopsy can effectively be combined with antegrade or retrograde rhinoscopy to attain an accurate diagnosis in about 80% of cases. Rhinoscopy-assisted biopsy is less invasive, less expensive, and has less morbidity than an exploratory rhinotomy, which may be necessary if rhinoscopy-assisted biopsy fails to yield a diagnosis.

10. What is the prognosis and therapeutic approach to nasal and paranasal sinus tumors?

Intranasal neoplasms generally have a short clinical course following diagnosis. With or without turbinectomy, **localized irradiation** of the nasal cavity and paranasal sinuses is the accepted therapeutic approach. It substantially improves the median survival time of dogs and cats with intranasal neoplasms. Median survival times in the dog are 8–36 months with the use of teletherapy (i.e., fractionated external beam) or brachytherapy (i.e., short-term implantation) protocols. The median survival time of dogs receiving no therapy is usually less than 6 months and does not improve after surgery alone. **Systemic chemotherapy** using cisplatin (cis-diamminedichloroplatinum II; Platinol, Bristol-Myers-Squibb, Syracuse, NY) at a dosage of 60 mg/m^2 IV once every 4 weeks resulted in the palliation of clinical signs (e.g., epistaxis, pain secondary to facial deformity) in some dogs for as long as 12 months.

Few reports regarding the treatment of intranasal neoplasms in cats exist; however, in one study survival times after 48 Gy of telecobalt or orthovoltage irradiation were 1–36 months. The 1- and 2-year overall survival rates were 44.3% and 16.6%, respectively. Histologic type

(10 carcinomas, 6 sarcomas) and clinical stage did not have prognostic value in this limited study.

TUMORS OF THE LARYNX AND TRACHEA

11. How common are tumors of the larynx and trachea?

Tumors arising from the laryngeal, perilaryngeal, and tracheal tissues are rarely encounterd in dogs and cats. In both, males are affected more commonly than females. No breed predilection has been identified in dogs or cats.

12. What are some of the larynx and trachea tumor types observed in dogs and cats?

Dogs. *Tracheal tumors:* Benign osteocartilaginous tumors are common in young dogs with active osteochondral ossification. The most common tracheal tumor appears to be osteochondroma, which routinely arises in dogs < 1 year of age, and may be amenable to complete resection. Most other canine tracheal tumors are malignant epithelial or mesenchymal tumors. *Laryngeal tumors:* Benign oncocytomas also occur in young dogs. Epithelial tumors and rhabdomyomas (oncocytomas) are the most frequently reported malignant tumors of the canine larynx.

Cats. Malignant epithelial and lymphoid tracheal tumors, though rare, have been reported. Malignant epithelial tumors and lymphomas are more common.

13. List the clinical signs of a tracheal or laryngeal tumor.

Clinical signs for tracheal and laryngeal tumors are similar. Dyspnea, wheezing, coughing, and stridor are common complaints. Voice change may be noted in some animals affected by laryngeal tumors.

14. What is the diagnostic approach to a tracheal or laryngeal tumor?

Radiographically, most animals have evidence of a distinct mass, although some show only a narrowing of the lumen at the tracheal laryngeal area. The veterinarian uses biopsy to make the definitive diagnosis after first performing laryngoscopy and tracheoscopy to assess the function and structure of the larynx and trachea.

15. What is the prognosis and therapeutic approach to laryngeal and tracheal tumors?

The prognosis for malignant tracheal tumors, although difficult to assess from historical information, is likely to be poor, especially if the tumor involves the adventitial surface of the trachea. Radiation therapy may be valuable as an adjunct to surgery or alone in the treatment of lymphoreticular tumors. Only tracheal osteochondromas appear to be amenable to complete resection.

LUNG TUMORS

16. Describe the natural behavior of lung tumors in the dog or cat.

Tumors originating within the lung parenchyma (primary lung neoplasia) are rare in dogs and cats. The average age at presentation in dogs and cats with primary lung tumors is 10 to 12 years. No breed or sex predisposition has been observed. The majority of primary lung tumors arise from the airways (e.g., bronchial adenocarcinomas). Fewer cases are classified as originating from the terminal airways or alveoli (bronchiolar-alveolar), and rarely are tumors identified as arising from the bronchial glands. Primary lung tumors of connective tissue origin are uncommon in the dog or cat (i.e., < 2.5% of all primary lung tumors reported). Primary nonepithelial tumors of the lung are uncommonly reported in other domestic species as well.

17. What are the clinical signs of lung neoplasia?

Weight loss, lethargy, dyspnea, and coughing are common owner complaints at the time of presentation to a veterinarian; however, such signs may not manifest until quite late in the course of the disease. Lameness has been reported to be a presenting sign in cats and may be associated with musculoskeletal metastases or with hypertrophic osteopathy.

18. True or false: Thoracocentesis is unnecessary in the diagnostic approach to tumors of the lung.

False. Accumulation of thoracic fluid is an important factor contributing to dyspnea in many cases of primary lung neoplasia. If there is extensive accumulation of clear thoracic fluid, thoracocentesis may be necessary to allow radiographic pulmonary detail to be assessed accurately and to determine whether exfoliated neoplastic cells are present. Cytologic evaluation of effusive material can be helpful in differentiating primary lung neoplasia from other causes of clear fluids, such as cranial mediastinal lymphoma and cardiomyopathy.

19. What is the radiographic appearance of primary lung neoplasia?

Radiographic findings that justify a high index of suspicion for a primary lung tumor include the finding of a **single circumscribed mass**, **marked lobar consolidation**, or **diffuse patterns containing severe peribronchial infiltration**, a **reticulonodular pattern**, and **alveolar filling**. There is no correlation between the interpretation of thoracic radiographic images and the histologic type of tumor. The right caudal lung lobe and accessory lung lobe in dogs and the left caudal lung lobe in cats are the preferred sites of occurrence for primary lung tumors. The list of possibilities in the differential diagnosis of radiopaque lung lesions includes metastatic neoplasia, granuloma, cysts, infarcts, localized hemorrhage, localized pneumonia, torsion, and abscess.

If a mass is identified radiographically, consider cytologic evaluation of **fine-needle aspiration** (FNA) material obtained from a pulmonary mass to resolved the diagnosis. Since the vast majority of primary lung tumors are epithelial in origin, carcinoma cells are likely to be observed. In one series of cats with primary lung tumors, a diagnosis was obtained in 80% of cases, prior to surgery or necropsy, when an FNA biopsy procedure was performed.

20. True or false: The treatment of choice for primary lung tumors is surgical resection.

True. Lung lobectomy is the preferred treatment for lung tumors in dogs and cats. Significant morbidity and mortality are associated with the surgical treatment of lung cancer; thus, it is important to identify and to exclude from primary surgical therapy the patient who will not benefit from attempts at resection.

21. What is the prognosis for lung tumors?

Dogs and cats without enlarged tracheobronchial lymph nodes observed radiographically or at the time of surgery have a significantly longer survival time compared with dogs and cats with enlarged lymph nodes (345 versus 60 days in the dog; 335 days versus 54 days in the cat). The presence of pleural effusion or distant metastatic disease, including the dissemination to tracheobronchial lymph nodes, is a contraindication to pulmonary resection for cure in dogs and cats.

BIBLIOGRAPHY

1. Hahn KA, Anderson TA: Tumors of the respiratory tract. In Bonagura JD (ed): Kirk's Veterinary Therapy XIII. Philadelphia, W.B. Saunders Co, 2000.
2. Hahn KA, Knapp DW, Richardson RC, Matlock C: The clinical response of nasal adenocarcinoma to cisplatin chemotherapy in 11 dogs. J Am Vet Med Assoc 1992;200:355.
3. Hahn KA, McEntee MF, Patterson MM, et al: Prognostic factors for tumor remission and survival in cats after surgery for primary lung tumor: 21 cases (1979–1994). Vet Surgery 1998; 27:307.
4. Hahn KA, McEntee MF: Feline lung primary lung tumors: A retrospective review of 86 cases (1979-1994). J Am Vet Med Assoc 1997;211:1257.

5. O'Brien RT, Evans SM, Workman JA, et al: Radiographic findings in cats with intranasal neoplasia or chronic rhinitis: 29 cases (1982–1988). J Am Vet Med Assoc 1996; 208:385.
6. Ogilvie GK, Haschek WM, Withrow SJ, et al: Classification of primary lung tumors in dogs: 210 cases (1975–1985). J Am Vet Med Assoc 1989; 195:106.
7. Ogilvie GK, Weigel RM, Haschek WM, et al: Prognostic factors for tumor remission and survival in dogs after surgery for primary lung tumor: 76 cases (1975–1985). J Am Vet Med Assoc 1989; 195:109.
8. Patnaik AK: Canine sinonasal neoplasms: Clinicopathological study of 285 cases. J Am Anim Hosp Assoc 1989; 25:103.
9. Theon AP, Madewell BR, Harb MF, et al: Megavoltage irradiation of neoplasms of the nasal and paranasal cavities in 77 dogs. J Am Vet Med Assoc 1993; 202:1469.
10. Theon AP, Madewell BR, Shearn VI, et al: Prognostic factors associated with radiotherapy of squamous cell carcinoma of the nasal plane in cats. J Am Vet Med Assoc 1995; 206:991.
11. Theon AP, Peaston AE, Madewell BR, et al: Irradiation of nonlymphoproliferative neoplasms of the nasal cavity and paranasal sinues in 16 cats. J Am Vet Med Assoc 1994; 204:78.
12. Withrow SJ, Straw RC: Resection of the nasal planum in nine cats and five dogs. J Am Anim Hosp Assoc 1990; 26:219.

26. TUMORS OF THE REPRODUCTIVE TRACT

Jeffrey C. Philibert, DVM

1. What is the incidence rate of ovarian tumors?

Ovarian tumors account for less than 5% of the tumors seen in dogs and cats. This is undoubtedly a reflection of most animals being spayed at an early age. These tumors occur in older dogs and cats, with the exception of teratomas, which can been seen in young animals. An interesting point of comparative oncology is that the incidence rate of ovarian tumors in dogs is similar to the incidence rate in people (approximately 1.5%). The tumors also occur in older women with a median age of 59 years.

2. How do dogs with ovarian tumors present?

The tumors are usually associated with signs of a space-occupying mass or abdominal distention due to malignant effusion. Sex cord stromal tumors (granulosa cell tumors) can produce excessive estrogens, leading to signs of vulvar enlargement, persistent estrus, endocrine alopecia and, in severe cases, bone marrow suppression and resultant pancytopenia. Sex cord stromal tumors can produce progesterone as well as cause cystic endometrial hyperplasia and/or pyometra.

3. What are the classifications of ovarian tumors?

- *Epithelial malignancies* (papillary adenomas/adenocarcinomas, undifferentiated carcinomas, cystadenomas) account for 40% to 50% of the cases.
- *Sex cord stromal tumors* (granulosa cell tumors) account for 50% of the cases.
- *Germ cell tumors* (dysgerminomas, teratomas, teratocarinomas) account for 6% to 10% of all cases.

4. What is the best treatment for ovarian tumors?

Surgery is the mainstay of treatment for these tumors. Most are unilateral, but a few carcinomas and sex cord stromal tumors can be bilateral. Survival averages longer than 1 year in cases without overt metastasis.

5. What is the metastatic rate of ovarian tumors?

- *Epithelial tumors* are the most common to metastasize, occurring in 50% of cases. Metastasis occurs to the renal, para-aortic, and mesenteric lymph nodes; liver; and lung. Local seeding (carcinomatosis) of the abdomen when tumors rupture or have malignant effusions may also occur.
- *Sex cord stromal tumors:* 20% of these tumors will metastasize, most commonly to the local lymph nodes, liver, pancreas, lung, and abdomen.
- *Germ cell tumors:* 30% of these tumors will metastasize, most commonly to the abdomen, liver, kidney, pancreas, and lung. Teratomas are the most aggressive biologically.

6. What is the best option for treatment for metastatic ovarian carcinoma?

Because most result in carcinomatosis when they metastasize, local treatment seems to work the best. Reports cite intracavitary cisplatin (50 mg/m^2 every 3 weeks for five to six treatments) as having survival times ranging from 6 months up to 5 years.

7. Are there any tumor-like conditions that can mimic neoplasia?

Yes, ovarian cysts are quite common and can appear as large masses that are easily confused with ovarian tumors. Less commonly, cystic rete tubules, vascular hematomas, or adenomatous hyperplasia of the rete ovarii can mimic an ovarian tumor. All of these conditions are benign, and surgery would be curative.

8. How common are uterine tumors in dogs and cats?

In both species they account for less than 1% of all tumors seen. Most tumors in dogs are benign mesenchymal tumors and are usually incidental findings. Some patients are presented when the tumor becomes big enough to cause space-occupying effects in the abdomen. Remember, though, that German shepherds can have multiple uterine leiomyomas accompanying bilateral renal cystadenocarcinomas. Except in the latter group, surgery is usually very successful. Cats, on the other hand, usually have adenocarcinomas arising from the endometrium. Unfortunately, these are also silent in their clinical behavior and are advanced locally or metastatic at the time of diagnosis, making surgery impossible in most cases.

9. How common are vaginal and vulvar tumors in dogs and cats?

They are actually quite common, accounting for 2% to 3% of all tumors in the dog. Most are also benign leiomyomas seen in older intact dogs. Interestingly, their incidence is highest in nulliparous bitches, suggesting a relationship to hormones. Simple surgical excision through a transvaginal approach is usually curative. Ovariohysterectomy can be performed at the same time, and the author has anecdotally seen some dogs have partial regression of vaginal masses when they were spayed prior to primary surgery. This allowed a less aggressive surgery to be performed in these cases.

10. What is the incidence of mammary gland tumors in dogs and cats?

They are seen in both intact (nonneutered/spayed/fixed) as well as neutered dogs and cats. They are most common in females and rare in males. These tumors are the most common cancer of female dogs; 0.2% of dogs are at risk, constituting more than 50% of all cancers. They represent the third most common type of cancer in cats. Average age at development is 10 to 12 years in dogs and cats. They can affect any breed of dog or cat, but breeds that appear to be at increased risk are poodles, terrier breeds, cocker spaniels, German shepherds, and Siamese cats.

11. What percentage of canine and feline mammary gland tumors are malignant?

Canine 50%, feline more than 90%.

12. What are the important clinical prognostic factors for canine mammary gland tumors?

Poor prognostic signs for canine mammary gland tumors include:
- Size 3 cm or larger
- Ulceration
- Invasion into local tissues (i.e., the property of being fixed versus being mobile)
- Nodal involvement
- Histology: sarcomas are worse than carcinomas
- A lack of lymphoid cellular reactivity within the tumor, indicating poor immune response to the tumor's presence
- Lymphatic and vascular invasion by the tumor
- Degree of differentiation (i.e., histologic grade): poorly differentiated tumors have a poor prognosis
- Inflammatory carcinoma (10% of malignant mammary gland tumors)

13. What prognostic factors exist but are not routinely available?

- Hormone receptors: tumors that are estrogen– and progesterone-receptor–positive carry a better prognosis.

- Microvessel density: a reflection of angiogenic activity. High microvessel density per a given tumor has been linked to a poorer prognosis.
- E-cadherin status: a cellular adhesion molecule that is lost with progression to malignancy, allowing cells to break free from one another and metastasize.
- DNA ploidy status: aneuploid tumors (abnormal number of chromosomes) have a worse prognosis than diploid tumors (normal complement of chromosomes).
- S-phase rate: a marker of cellular proliferation; the higher the rate, the more aggressive tumor growth.

14. What type of surgery should be done for mammary gland tumors?

This is an area for debate. Less extensive surgery appears to be adequate for dogs, although convention is still to perform regional mastectomies. For cats, more extensive surgery is better and it is suggested to perform at least a unilateral radical mastectomy of the involved chain with the possibility of bilateral mastectomy. The recommendation for cats differs from that for dogs because cats seem to have a high propensity to have other microscopic tumors (i.e., carcinoma in situ) in the apparently normal breast tissues.

15. Which animals should receive adjuvant chemotherapy?

This is also an area of debate, but all of the factors listed above that carry a poor prognosis should be used as a guideline for deciding which patients should receive chemotherapy. Given the poor prognosis for cats, it is the author's opinion that all cats should receive chemotherapy.

16. What is the best protocol to use?

Doxorubicin (Adriamycin) with or without cyclophosphamide seems to be the most popular choice. Doxorubicin is given at a dose of 30 mg/m^2 intravenously every 3 weeks (or 1 mg/kg in cats and dogs weighing less than 15 pounds). Cyclophosphamide is given orally at a dose of 200 mg/m^2 divided on days 4 to 7 of the first week of each treatment cycle. For cats, the author has routinely used 25 mg orally on days 2 and 4 of the first week of each cycle to avoid breaking any tablets. Many other drugs have been tried, such as mitoxantrone, cisplatin, carboplatin, and paclitaxel. If we follow the human trend, polychemotherapy yields a higher response than monotherapy, and anthracycline- (doxorubicin) containing protocols show an overall 44% increase in response rate over traditional methotrexate-containing protocols. The taxanes (paclitaxel and docetaxel) have also been promoted in recent years, with their combination with doxorubicin generating statistically significant improvement in response rates.

17. How effective are these treatments?

Good question! No large studies have been established to examine the efficacy of adjuvant chemotherapy in dogs and cats with mammary gland cancer. What exists in the literature are a number of case reports and data extracted from phase I clinical trials looking at various drugs that included patients with mammary gland tumors. The interesting point when reviewing the human oncology experience is that, as the shift has gone toward polychemotherapy protocols, the response rates have shot up but, when comparing survival in advanced breast cancer, rates have stayed about the same. In veterinary medicine we must wait until the time comes when larger clinical trials may elucidate more information on the best way to treat advanced breast cancer.

18. What role does ovariohysterectomy play?

Hormonal ablation is an important part of managing breast cancers in women and therefore warrants attention in our domestic animal patients as well. Because the measurement of hormone receptors is rarely performed in veterinary oncology, the true incidence of hormonally active disease is unknown. Two recent abstracts have shown that dogs that were spayed at or near the time of diagnosis had improved survival over dogs that remained intact. In intact ıuthor recommends ovariohysterectomy at the time of diagnosis and primary tumor ⟩ capitalize on any chance of this protective effect.

19. Can we use antiestrogens such as tamoxifen?

Unlike in human breast cancer where the use of tamoxifen (and, more recently, other antiestrogens such as raloxifene) has significantly improved 5-year survival rates, its use in dogs does not appear to be as effective. Conflicting reports exist in the literature, with one claiming a modest tumor response rate in 5 of 7 dogs with metastatic or nonoperable tumors and another having 0 of 18 responders. Both of these studies reported a high incidence of estrogenic adverse effects such as vulvar swelling, vaginal discharge, incontinence, urinary tract infections and, most seriously, stump pyometra. To the best of the author's knowledge no one has tried the newer antiestrogens in dogs or cats; they were designed to have fewer adverse effects in humans and therefore may be a useful adjuvant to therapy in dogs and cats with mammary gland cancer.

20. What is the incidence of testicular tumors?

They constitute 5% to 15% of all tumors in the dog, which makes them the second most common tumor in the male dog. Testicular tumors are more common in the dog than in any other species, including humans. Multiple tumor types can be present in one testicle at the same time. Dogs who are cryptorchid have a 14-fold increased risk of developing testicular tumors. In the dog the distribution of histologic types is about equal between Sertoli's cell tumors, seminomas, and interstitial cell tumors. Because most male cats are neutered at a young age, these tumors are very rare, but carcinomas, interstitial cell tumors, Sertoli's cell tumors, and malignant seminomas have been reported.

21. Are there any known risk factors for testicular tumors?

Etiology generally is unknown, but there is a strong association between an extrascrotal location and development of seminomas and Sertoli's cell tumors.

22. What are the common clinical signs for testicular tumors?

The most common finding is a scrotal, inguinal, or abdominal mass that is detected on physical examination, radiographs, or ultrasound. About 20% to 30% of Sertoli's cell tumor patients present for signs due to hyperestrogenism (gynecomastia, penduolus penile sheath, attracting other male dogs, alopecia, prostatic hyperplasia due to squamous metaplasia and, in severe cases, bone marrow suppression). The incidence of these signs is higher with tumors that occur in an extrascrotal location. Hyperestrogenism has also been reported with seminomas and interstitial cell tumors. Clinical signs of prostatic hypertrophy, perineal hernia, and perianal adenoma or adenocarcinoma can occur with interstitial cell tumors and are due to increased testosterone levels.

23. What is the reported metastatic rate of testicular tumors?

- Sertoli's cell tumors: 2% to 15%; usually to the local lymph nodes
- Seminomas: 5% to 10%; can occur to multiple locations
- Interstitial cell tumors: fewer than 1% of cases; essentially nonmetastatic

24. What are the options for treatment of testicular tumors?

The mainstay is castration with removal of a generous portion of the spermatic cord in cases with local extension. Dogs with clinical signs of hormone excess will usually have resolution of these signs in 2 to 6 weeks. Metastatic seminoma can be treated with good success using cisplatin chemotherapy or radiation therapy.

25. What is the incidence rate for prostate cancer in dogs?

It is an extremely rare form of cancer, with a reported incidence of 0.29 to 0.6%. Adenocarcinoma is the most frequent neoplasm of the prostate gland with transitional cell carcinoma, and leiomyosarcomas are also reported at lower percentages. It occurs most commonly in aged sexually intact dogs and dogs castrated after sexual maturity.

26. What role does castration play in the development and progression of prostate cancer?

Castration has long been debated as a prevention for prostate cancer. The bottom line is that it does not prevent its development, but there is a protective effect if dogs are castrated prior to sexual maturity. In a study by Obradovich et al., only 7 of 43 (16%) dogs diagnosed with prostatic carcinoma had been castrated at younger than 1 year of age. In a study conducted at Purdue University Veterinary Teaching Hospital, only 6 of 76 (8%) dogs castrated at younger than 6 months of age developed the disease.

27. What clinical signs are most likely to be seen with prostate cancer?

Signs associated with the urinary tract are most frequent, including hematuria, stranguria, and dysuria. Signs associated with colonic or rectal obstruction are also seen, causing tenesmus and ribbon-like stools. Other signs, such as pelvic limb lameness or neurologic abnormalities, are seen with fair frequency (35% to 50%) in association with vertebral metastasis of carcinoma.

28. What are potential differential diagnoses for prostate cancer?

Abscess, paraprostatic cysts, acute or chronic prostatitis, benign prostatic hyperplasia, and urothelial carcinoma.

29. What is the metastatic rate of prostatic carcinoma?

This is a very aggressive disease, with most dogs presenting with metastatic disease. This is corroborated by the reported studies in which 80% to 100% of dogs had evidence of metastasis at necropsy, with a mean time from diagnosis to necropsy of 2 to 3 weeks. Metastasis occurs most frequently to the regional (iliac/sublumbar) lymph nodes (50% to 75%), lung (50% to 65%), and bone (15% to 35%).

30. Given the high rate of metastasis, what is the prognosis for a dog with prostate cancer?

Poor in most cases. Median survivals are less than 4 months in most reported studies. Given its relatively silent clinical behavior (i.e., clinical signs that most owners do not pick up on right away), which can result in advanced disease at the time of diagnosis, many dogs are euthanized shortly after initial presentation.

31. Are there any effective therapies for prostate cancer?

Most are palliative at best. Castration may at least cause some regression of the gland and may relieve clinical signs. Prostate cancer in humans and dogs seems to be a nonresponsive disease to existing chemotherapy regimes. Attempts at surgical total or subtotal prostatectomy have been reported but are fraught with complications associated with trauma to the urethral/bladder enervation and resultant urinary incontinence. A variety of experimental approaches such as interstitial implants, hyperthermia, and laser ablation are reported in the literature. Most of these treatments are not widely available or economical for veterinary patients. Radiotherapy has been used in a palliative fashion. Turrel reported on 10 dogs treated with intraoperative orthovoltage radiotherapy with doses ranging from 20 to 30 Gy. One dog received a dose of 15 Gy and then a boost of 40 Gy using cobalt 60 radiotherapy. Seven of these dogs had disease confined to the prostate, and three had regional lymph node metastasis. Median survival time was 114 days, with a range of 41 to 750 days. Treatment was tolerated well by all dogs. Although five dogs had a complete response, median survival was not significantly different than for dogs that were untreated. Based on this information and personal communication with radiotherapists that have used external beam radiation therapy for the palliation of canine prostate cancer with modest success, this approach warrants further investigation and would be recommended as a means of palliation in these patients.

BIBLIOGRAPHY

1. Ahern RP, Smith IE, Ebbs SR: Chemotherapy and survival in advanced breast cancer: The inclusion of doxorubicin in Cooper type regimens. Br J Cancer 67:801–805, 1993.
2. Cornell KK, et al: Canine prostate carcinoma: Clinicopathologic findings in 168 cases. Proc Vet Canc Soc 1997, p 86.
3. Dhaliwal RS; Kitchell BE, Knight BL, Schmidt BR: Treatment of aggressive testicular tumors in four dogs. J Am Anim Hosp Assoc 35:311–318, 1999.
4. Fossati R, Confalonieri C, Torri V, et al: Cytotoxic and hormonal treatment for metastatic breast cancer: A systematic review of published randomized trials involving 31,510 women. J Clin Oncol 16:3439–3460, 1998.
5. Kitchell BE, Fidel JL: Tamoxifen as a potential therapy for canine mammary carcinoma. Proc Vet Canc Soc 1991, p 91.
6. Moore AS, Kirk C, Cardona A: Intracavitary cisplatin chemotherapy experience with six dogs. J Vet Intern Med 5:227–231, 1989.
7. Morris JS, Dobson JM, Bostock DE: Use of tamoxifen in the control of mammary neoplasia. Vet Rec 133:539–542, 1993.
8. Obradovich J, Walshaw R, Goullaud E: The influence of castration on the development of prostatic carcinoma in the dog. J Vet Intern Med 1:183–187, 1987.
9. Philibert JC, Snyder PW, Glickman N, et al: Influence of host factors and biomarker expression on prognosis in canine malignant mammary gland tumors. Proc Vet Canc Soc 1999, p 27.
10. Sorenmo K, Shofer F, Goldschmidt M, et al: Effects of spaying and timing of spaying on survival in dogs with mammary carcinoma. J Vet Intern Med 14:266–270, 2000.
11. Turell JM: Intraoperative radiotherapy of carcinoma of the prostate gland in ten dogs. J Am Vet Med Assoc 190:48–52, 1987.

27. TUMORS OF THE URINARY TRACT

Jeffrey C. Philibert, DVM

1. Tumors of the urinary tract are reportedly rare. How much do I need to know about them?

Yes, they are rare, but they are important differentials when dealing with diseases of the urinary tract. For example, many cases of transitional cell carcinoma (TCC) of the bladder go undiagnosed and mistreated as urinary tract infections until they are at an advanced stage, resulting in a poor likelihood of treatment success.

2. What is the most common tumor of the urinary tract?

In dogs, it is undoubtedly bladder and urethral tumors, with most being TCC (90% to 95%) and the remainder being split between other epithelial tumors (squamous cell carcinoma, adenocarcinoma, and papilloma) and mesenchymal tumors (leiomyosarcoma, fibrosarcoma, hemangiosarcoma, and rhabdomyosarcoma). Renal tumors are rare in dogs; the most common types are carcinomas and adenocarcinomas. In cats, lower urinary tract tumors are extremely rare, and lymphosarcoma accounts for the highest percentage of renal tumors. Nephroblastoma, a tumor that arises from primordial cells in the kidney, is rare in both species, as are primary renal sarcomas.

3. What are the typical clinical signs and presentation for a dog with bladder cancer?
- Mean age at diagnosis: 11 years.
- Mean body weight: 16 kg.
- Female to male ratio: Some estimates show a 1.7:1 increased risk up to a 2:1 risk.
- Typical presentation: with hematuria, stranguria, pollakiuria and, less commonly, lethargy, weight loss, and bone pain due to metastasis.

4. Are there any known risk factors for TCC?
- Breed predisposition. Scottish terriers (18.09 odds ratio in one study), Shetland sheepdogs, West Highland white terriers, and beagles are the prevalent breeds in most studies.
- Female dogs are at an increased risk over male dogs.
- Neutered dogs are at an increased risk over intact dogs, possibly related to changes in urethral diameter associated with loss of hormonal influence.
- Obesity has been linked to an increased rate of occurrence, probably through an increased deposition of carcinogens in the fat over an animal's life and, therefore, increased release and exposure to the body.
- In one study, dogs who had been dipped with insecticide compounds for fleas and ticks more than twice per year were at a 3.5-fold increased risk of development than dogs dipped only once or twice per year, which had a 1.6-fold increased risk. This is most likely related to the inert ingredients like benzene in these insecticides. Inert chemicals have been linked to human TCC.
- Obese female dogs that lived in areas containing marshes that were sprayed for insect control had an odds ratio of 13.2 of developing TCC in comparison with dogs not living in marshy areas.
- A small number of cases of TCC have been linked to the use of cyclophosphamide (Cytoxan). One of the metabolites of Cytoxan is a compound called acrolein, which is known to induce hemorrhagic cystitis and could result in malignant transformation of the bladder epithelium in a process called field carcinogenesis.

5. What constitutes a complete staging work-up for a suspected bladder tumor?

A complete physical examination, complete blood cell count, biochemistry profile, urinalysis with culture and sensitivity, thoracic and abdominal radiographs, and bladder imaging, including cystography, ultrasound, and cystoscopy.

6. Because animals with bladder cancer often present with nonspecific signs of urinary tract disease such as hematuria, stranguria, and pollakiuria, what clinical signs raise your suspicion of cancer?

It is true that these clinical signs can mimic what is seen with urolithiasis and urinary tract infection. It is therefore important to rule out these far more common diseases first. But if signs persist in the face of negative urine sediment, urine culture, and normal radiographs, additional diagnostic tests should be performed. Contrast cystography was once considered the gold standard but has largely been replaced by ultrasonography and, where available, cystoscopy. The latter provides the best means of determining the extent of disease, especially in cases with urethral involvement, as well as allowing for biopsy for histopathology. The author has even used cystoscopy in a somewhat therapeutic manner on a few dogs with severe obstruction in which repeated biopsy through the cystoscope has temporarily relieved lower urinary tract obstruction. One of the most frustrating dilemmas is differentiating TCC from prostate carcinoma. In one study of 102 dogs evaluated at Purdue University, TCC involved the urethra as well as the bladder in 56% of the cases. Of 38 male dogs in this study, 11 (29%) had involvement of the prostate. Given its relative rarity and much poorer prognosis, any male dog with a diagnosis of prostate carcinoma should be screened carefully to rule out involvement of the urethra and bladder with TCC.

7. Is measurement of urine basic fibroblastic growth factor a good screening test for TCC?

Basic fibroblastic growth factor (b-FGF) is a potent proangiogenic (i.e., pro–blood vessel growth) peptide found in high concentration in human cases of bladder cancer. In a study by Allen et al., it was predictive, with the cases of TCC having the highest levels, but there was overlap in the midrange with cases of urinary tract infection. It is therefore a screening tool but not a means of definitive diagnosis. High urine concentrations of b-FGF with a positive cytology examination would support the diagnosis. The test kit is available commercially for benchtop use, but the test is not run by any commercial laboratory. It likely may play a role in early detection as a screening test and to follow treated cases to detect minimally residual disease.

8. What is the best way to treat TCC?

The jury is still out on this question. Surgery is rarely effective because this tumor is usually diagnosed at an advanced stage. Out of a series of 70 dogs seen at Purdue University Veterinary Teaching Hospital, only two had resection performed; one had a complete remission without relapse, and one had a complete remission but developed lymph node metastasis and an abdominal wall mass suspected to be due to seeding of tumor cells at the time of surgery. Many of these dogs also are likely to develop other lesions in the bladder because of the concept of field carcinogenesis. However, in this series 25 dogs that underwent debulking surgery followed by medical therapy (with chemotherapy or piroxicam) had a median survival of 272 days, compared with 195 days for 42 dogs undergoing surgery for biopsy only and medical therapy, and 150 days for 36 dogs undergoing medical therapy only (chi-square test, $P < .06$). Although this did not achieve statistical significance, the difference in clinical signs and quality of life for these dogs may warrant this approach.

Radiation therapy historically was used intraoperatively, with the main disadvantages being total dose deliverable and complications with bladder fibrosis.

Chemotherapy seems to be the mainstay of treatment. Various drugs have been analyzed in phase I and phase II clinical trials, including cisplatin, carboplatin, doxorubicin, gemcitabine, and mitoxantrone. The nonsteroidal antiinflammatory drug piroxicam (Feldene) has antineo-plastic activity and has been used alone or in combination with these various chemotherapeutics. However, it is reported to cause treatment-limiting renal failure when combined with cisplatin and is therefore not recommended. Disease-free interval and therefore, in most instances, survival averages 150 to 200 days for these treatments. Recent retrospective studies suggest that if the tumor responds to piroxicam, it seems to have the best long-term control— more than 180 days.

9. Is combination therapy effective?

Multimodal therapy may hold promise for being the best treatment. Recently, external beam radiation therapy has been revisited in treating bladder lesions. Ten dogs with TCC of the bladder were treated with a combination of six weekly 5.75-Gy fractions of cobalt 60 radiotherapy, 5 mg/m^2 of mitoxantrone every 3 weeks, and standard-dose piroxicam (0.3 mg/kg once daily) until progressive disease was noted. All dogs but one completed radiotherapy and received a mean of 3 doses of mitoxantrone. Reported adverse effects were mild and consisted of dermatitis, hyperpigmentation, and mild urinary incontinence. Seven dogs experienced stable disease with clinical improvement for a median of 90 days (range 47 to 320 days). The other three experienced progressive disease during treatment and went on to other therapies. Overall median survival for the group was 240 days (range 21 to 607 days). This information warrants more investigation into this multimodal approach to TCC.

10. How does piroxicam work?

The exact mechanism is unknown, but tumor cells overproduce cyclooxygenase (COX-1 and COX-2), the enzymes responsible for the production of the arachidonic acid metabolite prostaglandin E_2 (PGE_2). PGE_2 is proinflammatory, immunosuppressive, angiogenic, and may have direct effects on cell growth. Piroxicam is a nonselective cyclooxygenase inhibitor and therefore may retard production of these procancer effects. Dogs that go into remission on piroxicam have decreased PGE_2 concentrations, but dogs with progressive disease have increased levels.

11. How metastatic is TCC?

In a study done at Purdue University School of Veterinary Medicine of 102 dogs diagnosed with TCC, 16% had nodal metastasis, 14% had distant metastasis, and 10% had evidence of both at diagnosis. This percentage rose to 49% having distant metastasis at the time of death. The cause of death was known for 85 of these dogs and was due to the primary tumor in 52 dogs (61%), metastatic disease in 12 (14%), and nontumor-related causes in 21 (25%). If dogs were not euthanized because of urinary tract obstruction, distant metastasis was more common. In the 50 dogs that were necropsied, the distribution of sites of metastasis was as follows: lung (28%), iliac nodes (26%), liver (18%), kidney (4%), spleen (4%), other nodes (4%), uterus (4%), and sites such as the vertebrae, ileum, colon, abdominal wall, diaphragm, and oral mucosa (about 2% each).

12. What are the known prognostic factors for TCC?

- Factors associated with the development of metastasis include clinical involvement of the urethra and vascular involvement histologically.
- Factors associated with a better response include lower tumor stage in the WHO tumor node metastasis scheme, while the histopathologic subclassification of glandular differentiation carries a poor likelihood of response. Of 12 cases with this diagnosis, none experienced remission.
- A more advanced stage at diagnosis is associated with male gender, prostatic involvement, and younger age at diagnosis.
- Factors associated with a decreased survival include advanced TNM (tumor node metastasis) stage at diagnosis and prostatic involvement.

13. What can be done for the obstructed dog or cat?

Options include intermittent catheterization (which owners can be taught to perform at home for male dogs), a permanent indwelling catheter with a closed collection system (which would require hospitalization), or a tube cystotomy.

14. Isn't the rate of urinary tract infection higher with these options?

Sure, but fighting a urinary tract infection is the lesser of two evils! Furthermore, if the animal responds even minimally to the primary treatment, catheters can be removed. The nice thing about tube cystotomy is that it provides a means to empty the urine without obstructing normal urine flow.

15. What is the next most common tumor of the urinary tract?

Renal tumors. More than 90% of renal tumors in dogs and cats are malignant, with more than 50% being carcinomas, 20% mesenchymal, 10% arising from the pluripotential stem cells (i.e., Wilms' tumors, nephroblastomas, embryonal nephroma), and a spattering of renal lymphomas in both dogs and cats.

16. What is nodular dermatofibrosis, and how does it relate to renal tumors?

This is an autosomal dominant hereditary disorder seen concurrently with renal cystadenocarcinoma in German shepherd dogs. These dogs present with diffuse, firm, dermal nodules—many times affecting the limbs—which represent an increase in dermal collagen. This is a very uncommon condition but one that allows the oncologist to diagnose a kidney tumor with a fair degree of certainty just by looking at the dog! Female dogs can also present with multiple uterine leiomyomas.

17. How common is it for renal tumors to metastasize?

Very common. In most studies more than 50% of dogs and cats with carcinomas will have metastasis at diagnosis. Sarcomas are less likely to metastasize, but most of them will have locally extensive or invasive disease.

18. Should nephrectomy be performed for renal tumors?

If it can! Because of their silent clinical behavior, most are advanced at the time of diagnosis. Ideally, function of the unaffected kidney should be determined through glomerular filtration rate nuclear studies or, at the least, an excretory urogram, which is a crude test of the contralateral kidney's ability to concentrate and excrete urine. The advantage of the latter is that it does not require the expense and limited availability of glomerular filtration rate studies and can therefore be performed in most veterinary hospitals.

19. Is chemotherapy an option for metastatic disease?

It has not proved to be helpful. An exception is lymphoma, which can respond to systemic combination chemotherapy and, in the author's experience, in particular protocols using cytosine arabinoside (Cytosar-U). In humans, renal tumors carry a high concentration of the transmembrane chemotherapy pump p-glycoprotein that makes them resistant to wide groups of chemotherapeutic agents.

CONTROVERSY

20. Do I need to concurrently prescribe misoprostol (Cytotec) or other gastric protectants when prescribing piroxicam?

Although gastric ulceration is a possibility with the use of any nonsteroidal antiinflammatory drug, it is not always necessary to prescribe gastric protectants when using piroxicam to treat TCC. Most dogs seem to tolerate piroxicam monotherapy fine and, in those that do develop signs (i.e., melena, hematemesis), discontinue piroxicam for a few days, start a gastric protectant, and then restart the piroxicam. If dogs tolerate this approach, it saves the owner the expense of the gastric protectant and the inconvenience of two- to three-times daily dosing of these drugs.

Use of piroxicam can lead to renal vasoconstriction and decreased GFR. This is uncommon at the recommended doses, but renal papillary necrosis has been reported at higher doses. Therefore, it is important to monitor the patient's renal function while on piroxicam therapy.

BIBLIOGRAPHY

1. Allen DK, Waters DJ, Knapp DW, Kuczek T: High urine concentrations of basic fibroblastic growth factor in dogs with bladder cancer. J Vet Intern Med 10:231–234, 1996.
2. Chun R, Knapp DW, Widmer WR, et al: Cisplatin treatment of transitional cell carcinoma of the urinary bladder in dogs: 18 cases (1983–1993). J Am Vet Med Assoc 209:1588–1591, 1996.
3. Glickman LT, Schofer FS, Mc Kee LJ: Epidemiology study of insecticide exposures, obesity, and risk of bladder cancer in household dogs. J Toxicol Environ Health 28:407–414, 1989.
4. Knapp DW, Glickman NW, DeNicola DB, et al: Naturally-occurring canine transitional cell carcinoma of the urinary bladder: A relevant model of human invasive bladder cancer. Urol Oncol 5:47–59, 2000.
5. Knapp DW, Richardson RC, Chan TCK, et al: Piroxicam therapy in 34 dogs with transitional cell carcinoma of the urinary bladder. J Vet Intern Med 8:273–278, 1994.
6. McCaw DL, Lattimer JC: Radiation and cisplatin for treatment of canine urinary bladder carcinoma, a report of two case histories. Vet Radiol 29:264–268, 1988.
7. Poirier VJ, Vail DM, Forrest LJ: Pilot study evaluating palliative radiotherapy in combination with mitoxantrone/piroxicam in the treatment of transitional cell carcinoma—10 cases. Proc Vet Canc Soc 1999, p 18.
8. Walker M, Brieder M: Intraoperative radiotherapy of canine bladder cancer. Vet Radiol 28:200–204, 1987.

28. NEOPLASIA OF THE NERVOUS SYSTEM

John Speciale, DVM, Dipl ACVIM

1. How common is neoplasia of the nervous system?

As many as 3% of necropsied dogs were found to have intracranial neoplasia. In immature dogs, only hematopoietic neoplasia occurred more frequently than brain neoplasia. The incidence of nervous system tumors in cats is uncertain. Enumeration of intracranial neoplasia in cats is complicated by the high incidence of asymptomatic cats with brain tumors. Post mortem examinations have revealed brain tumors in up to 6% of asymptomatic cats. Tumors of canine and feline spinal cords and peripheral nerves occur less frequently.

2. What kinds of tumors are likely to affect the brain?

Meningiomas are the most common nervous system tumor in dogs and cats. Neuroectodermal tumors (tumors of astrocytes or oligodendrocytes) are the next most common in dogs, but they occur infrequently in cats. Choroid plexus tumors, ependymomas, and pituitary, nasal, and metastatic tumors (including hemangiosarcoma, adenocarcinoma, and malignant melanoma) are less common. Rare tumors include craniopharyngioma, pineal gland tumors, and germ cell tumors.

Cystic structures and malformations act as space-occupying lesions, and the signs are most often indistinguishable from neoplasia. Cystic structures include hemangiomas, epidermoids, and dermoid and arachnoid cysts.

Most tumors of dog and cat brains are extra-axial tumors, including meningiomas. The most common locations are the dorsal surfaces of the hemispheres and the falx. Cat meningiomas are often multiple. As few as 50% of cat meningiomas are likely to cause clinical signs. Meningiomas in dogs often cause seizures, but seizures are much less common in cats with meningiomas.

Intra-axial tumors are most frequently astroglial cell tumors, including astrocyte tumors (most common), glioblastoma, and oligodendroglioma (often bloody). Glial cell tumors are uncommon in cats. Unlike cats with meningeal tumors, seizures are the most common sign in cats with glial cell tumors.

Intraventricular tumors include ependymomas and choroid plexus tumors. Choroid plexus tumors most often originate in the fourth ventricle or choroid plexus. These tumors may be multifocal because they spread via cerebrospinal fluid (CSF). Ependymomas are rarer than choroid plexus tumor and, for that reason, characterization of the clinical behavior is incomplete. Other rare and poorly characterized tumors in dogs and cats are tumors of nerve cells, of the pineal gland, and medulloblastoma.

Determination of benign versus malignant tumors within the central nervous system (CNS) may not be as pressing a concern as it is in other organs. Some histopathologically malignant tumors slowly infiltrate the brain, and signs may progress slowly or be controlled for years. In other instances, a benign cyst may cause signs that progress rapidly and relentlessly. Rarely, brain tumors metastasize to the lungs.

3. What kinds of tumors are likely to affect the spinal cord?

Spinal tumors are classified as extramedullary, intradural extramedullary, or intramedullary.

Extramedullary spinal tumors, including bone tumors, are the tumors that most often cause spinal cord disease. Osteosarcoma is the most common spinal tumor of dogs, but other sarcomas and various metastatic carcinomas are also reported. Extradural lymphoma is the most common spinal tumor of cats. Feline spinal lymphoma may be considered a metastasis because most cats with spinal lymphoma have disseminated lymphosarcoma that can be documented with positive feline leukemia antigen or identification of malignant lymphocytes in bone marrow.

Intradural extramedullary spinal tumors are most often nerve root tumors. Classification of these tumors is complex, but they include neurofibrosarcoma, neurofibroma, and schwannoma. They invade the spinal cord by infiltration along nerve roots and, in this way, even histologically benign tumors can be devastating. Meningioma is the second most common intradural extramedullary spinal cord tumor. Neuroepithelioma is a rare spinal tumor of dogs younger than 1 year old that is invariably located within the T10–L2 vertebrae.

Intramedullary tumors, including glial cell tumors, ependymomas, choroid plexus tumors, and spinal metastasis of hemangiosarcoma or lymphosarcoma are the least common, occurring in less than 25% of spinal tumors.

4. What kinds of tumors are likely to affect the peripheral nerves?

Peripheral nerve tumors are less common than central nervous system tumors but, nevertheless, they account for more than 25% of all nervous system tumors. Peripheral nerve tumors are much more common in dogs than cats. Nerve root tumors (dogs) and lymphoma (cats) are most prevalent. The brachial plexus and nerve roots of the cervical spine are a common site for peripheral nerve neoplasia. Neoplasia of cranial nerves usually involves the trigeminal nerve and infrequently involves the eighth nerve. Other cranial nerves are less likely sites of neoplasia.

Tumors of the Nervous System

		COMMON	UNCOMMON
Primary tumors	Brain	Meningioma Astroglial Choroid plexus Sarcoma Pituitary adenoma	Neuroma Ependymoma Pineal gland tumor Craniopharyngioma
	Spinal cord	Nerve sheath tumor	Neuroepithelioma Meningioma Astroglial Lymphosarcoma
	Peripheral nerves	Nerve sheath tumor	

Secondary tumors	Brain and spine	Osteosarcoma
		Metastasis, including
		  hemangiosarcoma,
		  mammary gland tumor,
		  fibrosarcoma, and
		  lymphosarcoma	

	Peripheral nerves	Lymphosarcoma	

5. What clinical criteria suggest nervous system neoplasia?

Three criteria are used to characterize nervous system neoplasia: signalment, history, and localization.

• Signalment

Most animals with nervous system neoplasia are aged. Meningiomas are most common in aged dogs and cats (average age above 9 years). Glial cell tumors are also most common in mature dogs but the age incidence (average age above 6 years) may be somewhat less than that of animals with meningioma. Other tumors, including ependymomas, choroid plexus tumors, and pituitary and nerve root tumors are often diagnosed in dogs younger than 6 years of age. Vascular malformations and germ cell tumors of the brain are most often diagnosed in young and young adult animals.

Brachycephalic breeds of dogs, including boxers, Boston terriers, and bulldogs, have an increased incidence of neuroectodermal tumors. Golden retrievers and German shepherd dogs appear to have an increased incidence of meningiomas. Germ cell tumors are most common in Doberman pinschers.

Spinal tumors are more often seen in large dogs (90%). Dogs with spinal cord tumors are often younger than dogs with brain tumors, and more than a third of the dogs with spinal tumors were younger than 3 years of age.

• History

Signs of nervous system neoplasia usually progress slowly. However, brain tumors can cause hemorrhage, hydrocephalus, ischemia, or brain stem distortion that may cause acute signs.

• Localization

Signs of CNS neoplasia usually relate to a single neuroanatomic region. Exceptions include ependymomas and choroid plexus tumors, which can spread via the ventricular system, and sarcoidosis and basal meningiomas, which may spread along meninges and cause diffuse peripheral or cranial nerve signs.

6. What neurologic signs are most likely to result from tumors of the nervous system?

Three groups of signs necessarily result from a lesion within a particular region of the nervous system.

If the signs include seizures or behavioral changes, a lesion **necessarily** lies within the **anterior** or **middle fossae**, which house the prosencephalon (thalamus and cerebrum).

If the signs include coma, other severe alteration of consciousness, or cranial nerve deficits, a lesion **necessarily** lies within the **caudal fossa**, which houses the **brain stem** and cranial nerves.

If the signs include decreased stretch reflex or decreased flexion reflex, a lesion **necessarily** lies within segmental **spinal cord** (the region of spinal cord from which peripheral nerves originate) or peripheral nerve roots or nerves.

Presence of signs from more than one of these areas suggests that there is more than a single lesion, and CNS neoplasia is less likely.

Neither postural deficits nor gait abnormalities specifically indicate the location of a lesion. A single consistent exception to this rule is that severe alteration of gait is **unlikely** to result from cerebral disease. Thus, a gait abnormality suggests that there is a neurologic lesion in some region **other than** the prosencephalon.

	SEIZURE	BEHAVIORAL CHANGE	COMA	CRANIAL NERVE DEFICIT	ABSENT REFLEX	ABSENT FLEXION	POSTURAL DEFICIT	GAIT DEFICIT
Prosencephalon	Yes	Yes	No	No	No	No	Possibly	No
Brain stem	No	No	Yes	Yes	No	No	Possibly	Often
Segmental spinal cord	No	No	No	No	Yes	Yes	Possibly	Often
Nonsegmental spinal cord	No	No	No	No	No	No	Possibly	Often
Cerebellum	No	No	No	Possibly	No	No	Unlikely	Usually

7. Do brain tumors necessarily cause disease?

Signs result from the location of the lesion. Many tumors are incidental and cause no signs. The severity of signs may be associated with hemorrhage, pressure, metabolism, vascular compromise, or lateral brain-stem distortion. This last condition may be very important in the pathogenesis of feline meningioma.

The most common site of asymptomatic feline meningiomas was the tela choroidea, a midline structure where space occupying lesions were unlikely to cause lateral distortion. Cats with bilateral meningiomas were three times more likely to be asymptomatic than those with a single tumor that, presumably, caused lateral distortion or displacement.

8. What aids are available for diagnosis of brain tumors?

Clinical signs, history, and signalment, as outlined above, are most important in raising the index of suspicion for initial diagnosis.

Computed tomography (CT) and magnetic resonance imaging (MRI) are superior to conventional radiographs for detection of CNS lesions, but neither is completely reliable for diagnosis. Abnormalities that may be seen with either mode of imaging include mass effect and contrast enhancement. Signs of mass effect include effacement of ventricles and shift of midline structures. Contrast enhancement of the brain occurs because growth of tumors and inflammatory processes are accompanied by new blood vessels that do not form *tight junctions* between endothelial cells to prevent leakage of intravenously injected radiopaque (CT) or paramagnetic (MRI) contrast agents.

CT images of brain tissue are less detailed than MRI images. CT relies on vascular contrast enhancement to visualize the lesion. MRI images are based on the brain tissue's water content.

CSF analysis is rarely diagnostic for CNS disease but, nevertheless, it can be useful to characterize the nature of a CNS disease process.

9. What aids are available to diagnose tumors of the spinal cord?

Myelography is useful to detect spinal tumors. Radiographic contrast fills the subarachnoid space. Areas of the subarachnoid space that fail to be filled with radiographic contrast are abnormal. Intramedullary lesions are less likely to be visualized than extramedullary lesions. CT is excellent for viewing bone and, if used along with myelography, can greatly aid diagnosis.

MRI is most sensitive for detection of spinal cord disease.

CSF is unlikely to provide a specific diagnosis of spinal cord disease. Nevertheless, if spinal fluid contains many cells or high protein, chronic disc displacement or vertebral instability is less likely. Acute disc herniation can result in abnormal spinal fluid.

10. What aids are available to diagnose tumors of the peripheral nervous system?

MRI can visualize nerve roots, and the most common peripheral tumors (nerve root tumors and lymphoma) readily enhance with paramagnetic contrast.

Myelography and CT myelography are useful to demonstrate nerve root tumors.

CSF is often normal with peripheral nerve tumors, but increased protein is often found with neoplasia of the nerve roots.

Electromyography is helpful to determine distribution of lesion. Denervation causes the membranes of muscle fibers to depolarize spontaneously. Sensitive electromyography electrodes can detect the small depolarizing potentials and, in this way, affected muscles can be plotted for neuroanatomic localization.

11. Is there a "gold standard" for diagnosis of the nervous system tumors?

Definitive diagnosis of nervous system tumors requires biopsy. All other tests merely suggest a diagnosis.

12. Is surgery useful for treatment of brain tumors?

Reports of successful brain surgery in dogs are anecdotal. There are no good controlled studies. Evaluation of the patient's quality of life should be emphasized in such studies because many patients do not die but, rather, are euthanized at the discretion of the pet owner.

This precludes consistent and objective evaluation of survival and therapeutic success. Surgical debulking of brain tumors has been suggested as a palliative treatment, but this has not been evaluated objectively.

Cat meningiomas have been routinely treated with surgery. However, recent studies cast some doubt on the benefit of surgical treatment for cat meningioma. Feline meningiomas are more easily resected when compared with those of dogs, which often infiltrate the brain parenchyma along the Virchow-Robin spaces.

13. Is radiation a useful treatment for brain tumors?

There is evidence of increased survival of dogs with brain tumors that were treated with radiation. Like studies of brain surgery, studies of radiation treatment are uncontrolled, but they are more numerous and the bulk of evidence points toward benefits. Moreover, unlike surgical treatment, the morbidity of radiation treatment is low. It has also been shown that radiation is advantageous for treatment of inflammatory brain disease. This is a substantial advantage for radiation treatment because neither CT nor MRI can necessarily differentiate neoplastic from focal inflammatory lesions.

14. What is boron neutron capture treatment, and does it have any benefit?

Boron neutron capture treatment is an experimental treatment for brain tumors that takes advantage of the high metabolic index of brain tumor cells and their greater affinity for boron than normal brain tissue. Intravenous solutions of boron are given to dogs with brain tumors. Neutron irradiation induces a fission reaction of boron to lithium and an alpha particle that may lethally damage neoplastic cells. It appears to be useful, especially as postoperative therapy.

15. What treatments are there for spinal tumors?

Surgery can be beneficial for extradural spinal neoplasms. However, surgery may not be useful for vertebral osteosarcoma or intramedullary tumors. The efficacy of radiation for treatment of intramedullary spinal tumors has not been widely reported but appears to be very useful.

16. What treatments are there for peripheral nerve tumors?

Surgery is reported to be useful, but complete resection of the tumor is not routine. Tumors that involve the nerve root and grow into the spinal cord parenchyma have a poor prognosis.

CONTROVERSIES

17. Is chemotherapy a useful treatment for brain tumors?

The normal blood-brain barrier resists penetration of chemotherapeutic drugs. However, lipophilic drugs such as nitrosoureas may be able to penetrate the intact blood-brain barrier. Furthermore, the vessels of CNS neoplasms are more porous than normal brain blood vessels and may allow penetration by chemotherapeutic agents. A clinical report of lomustine treatment for brain tumors is uncontrolled but suggests that there may be substantial benefit to treatment.

18. What is the diagnostic value in evaluation of CSF?

Evaluation of CSF is rarely diagnostic but, along with physical examination and advanced imaging, CSF evaluation helps to determine diagnosis. Similarly, evaluation of complete blood count alone is unlikely to be diagnostic but, nevertheless, it is necessary to characterize a disease process.

CSF from animals with brain neoplasia may be normal or have increased protein, cells, or both. However, certain types of tumors often have a characteristic CSF pattern.

	NORMAL CSF	NORMAL PROTEIN	WBC > 50/µl	PROTEIN > 100 mg/dl
Astroglial	Often	Often	Rare → never	Rare → never
Choroid plexus	Rare	Very unlikely	Unlikely	Often → usually
Ependymoma	Uncertain	Unlikely	Unlikely	Often
Meningioma	Rare	Unlikely	Often	Unlikely

19. Is there high risk of brain herniation when collecting CSF from patients with brain tumors?

The admonition that patients with brain tumors or increased intracranial pressure are at greater risk for brain herniation and sudden death is poorly documented. Two series of brain herniation in the veterinary literature failed to show correlation between brain herniation and collection of CSF.

Evidence suggests that the benefits of CSF collection outweigh the risk:

- Clinical reports document that the incidence of brain herniation (with or without CSF collection) is much more frequent with infectious or inflammatory diseases than with neoplasia.
- Brain herniation is essentially unknown in a group of human patients with extremely high intracranial pressures (psuedotumor cerebri). CSF is routinely and repeatedly collected from these patients without mishap.
- The survival rate for dogs and humans with neurologic disease is greater when CSF is evaluated.

BIBLIOGRAPHY

1. Bagley RS, Bavin PR, Moore MP, et al: Boron neutron capture therapy (BNCT) for brain tumors in dogs: Experience of the past 14 years. Proc 17th ACVIM Forum, 1999.
2. Bailey CS, Higgins RJ: Characteristics of cisternal cerebrospinal fluid associated with primary brain tumors in the dog: A retrospective study. J Am Vet Med Assoc 188:414–417, 1986.
3. Braund KG: Neurologic diseases. In Braund KG (ed): Clinical Syndromes in Veterinary Neurology, 2nd ed. St. Louis, Mosby, 1994, pp 198–211.
4. Fingeroth JM, Prata RG, Patnaik AK: Spinal meningiomas in dogs: 13 cases (1972–1987). J Am Vet Med Assoc 191:720–726, 1987.
5. Fulton L: The use of lomustine in the treatment of brain masses. Proc 9th ACVIM Forum 827–828, 1991.
6. Lobetti RG, Pearson J: Magnetic resonance imaging in the diagnosis of focal granulomatous meningoencephalitis in two dogs. Vet Radiat Ultrasound 37:424–427, 1996.
7. Lugenbuhl H: Studies on meningomas in cats. Am J Vet Res 22:1030–1040, 1961.
8. Luttgen PJ, Braund KG, Brawner WR, et al: A retrospective study of 29 spinal tumors in the dog and cat. J Small Anim Pract 21:213–226, 1980.
9. Moore MP, Bagley RS, Harrington ML, et al: Intracranial tumors. Proc 14th ACVIM Forum 331–334, 1996.
10. Nafe LA: Meningiomas in cats: A retrospective clinical study of 36 cases. J Am Vet Med Assoc 174:1224–1226, 1979.
11. Patnaik AK, Kay WJ, Hurvitz: Intracranial meningioma: A comparative pathologic study of 28 dogs. Vet Pathol 23:369–373, 1986.
12. Rosin A: Neurologic disease associated with lymphosarcoma in ten dogs. J Am Vet Med Assoc 181:50–53, 1982.
13. Speciale J: Brain herniation. Proc 14th ACVIM Forum 673–675, 1996.
14. Speciale J, Koffman BM, Bashirelahi N, et al: Identification of gonadal steroid receptors in meningiomas from dogs and cats. Am J Vet Res 51:833–835, 1990.
15. Speciale J, Van Winkle TJ, Steinberg SA, et al: Computed tomography in the diagnosis of focal granulomatous meningoencephalitis: Retrospective evaluation of three cases. J Am Amin Hosp Assoc 28:327–332, 1992.
16. Spodnick GJ, Berg J, Moore FM, et al: Spinal lymphoma in cats: 21 cases (1976–1989). J Am Vet Med Assoc 200:373–376, 1992.

17. Summers BA, Cummings JF, deLahunta AD: Diseases of the peripheral nervous system. In Veterinary Neuropathology. St. Louis, Mosby, 1995, pp 473–481.
18. Summers BA, Cummings JF, deLahunta AD: Tumors of the central nervous system. In Veterinary Neuropathology. St. Louis, Mosby, 1995, pp 351–402.
19. Turrel JM, Fike JR, LeCouteur RA, et al: Radiotherapy of brain tumors in dogs. J Am Vet Med Assoc 184:82–86, 1984.
20. Zaki FA, Nave LA: Choroid plexus tumors in the dog. J Am Vet Med Assoc 176:328–330, 1980.

29. OCULAR TUMORS

Kimberly M. Stanz, DVM, DACVO

EYELID/CONJUNCTIVA

1. What is the most common tumor of the eyelid in dogs?

The most common tumor is the meibomian gland adenoma, which tends to occur in older dogs. Squamous papillomas are the most common lid tumor in young dogs. Most lid tumors in dogs are benign. Surveys indicate that only 8.2% to 24.7% of eyelid tumors in dogs are malignant. Tumors that are malignant tend only to be locally invasive and rarely metastasize. Examples include malignant melanoma, mastocytoma, basal cell carcinoma, and squamous cell carcinoma.

2. What is the recommended course of therapy for eyelid tumors?

The presence of a lid tumor is not only of cosmetic concern, but treatment becomes essential when there is evidence of corneal irritation, hemorrhaging, or malignancy. Generally, eyelid tumors should be surgically removed and a histopathologic diagnosis obtained. Small tumors should be completely removed. Larger, more invasive masses are better treated after an initial biopsy because knowledge of the specific tumor type is necessary in planning an appropriate therapeutic strategy. Impression smears are rarely helpful.

3. What factors influence the choice of surgical technique?

Size and location. The breed can also play a factor. In general, the smaller the neoplasm, the more likely it can be excised without additional plastic surgical techniques. *Up to one-third of the eyelid margin can be removed during a simple full-thickness wedge resection.* However, the maximum removed during this procedure may be less in brachycephalics and breeds with "tight-fitting" eyelids, such as collies and poodles. Removal can be complicated if the tumor involves the canthus or lacrimal puncta. Surgical techniques have been recently reviewed (see bibliography). Additional or alternative treatment modalities include cryosurgery, radiation therapy, hyperthermia, and laser ablation. Cryosurgery following partial debulking is very effective for papillomas and meibomian adenomas. Cosmetic outcome is excellent. This technique is useful for larger tumors and those involving the canthus because complicated reconstructive surgeries can often be avoided.

4. What is the most common tumor of the eyelid and conjunctiva of the cat?

Squamous cell carcinoma.

5. Describe the typical appearance of an eyelid squamous cell carcinoma.

It is often either a slightly raised or depressed ulcerative lesion. It can have a crusty or scabby surface. There seems to be a predilection for white cats.

6. What is the treatment and prognosis of adnexal squamous cell carcinoma?

Squamous cell carcinoma is treatable by the same surgical options as for other eyelid tumors. It is locally invasive, and metastasis does not occur until late in the disease process. Therefore, early diagnosis and removal are key to providing an excellent prognosis. Wide surgical excision is usually curative. The main difficulty with treatment is visually identifying the margins of the tumor. Cryosurgery is an effective, simple, and inexpensive way to treat this tumor because the surgeon can include a wide area of "normal" tissue in the treatment site.

7. During cryosurgery, how far should the iceball extend past visible tumor?
Three to five millimeters.

PRIMARY INTRAOCULAR TUMORS

8. What part of the eye is most commonly affected by neoplasia?
The anterior uveal tract (iris and ciliary body).

9. What is the most common primary uveal tumor in the dog?
Benign melanoma (melanocytoma).

10. What is the typical appearance of this tumor?
Melanocytomas are typically nodular (versus diffuse infiltration). Pigmentation is generally heavier than the rest of the iris, but amelanotic melanomas do occur.

11. What is the second most common uveal tumor in the dog?
Ciliary body adenoma and adenocarcinoma. The incidence of adenoma (benign) is approximately equal to that of adenocarcinoma (potentially malignant).

12. What is the typical appearance of this tumor?
This tumor is often a nodular, cream or pink-colored mass that can be seen bulging through the pupil. However, it can be pigmented and appear very similar to a melanocytoma.

13. What are the most common clinical signs associated with a tumor involving the iris or ciliary body?
Anterior uveitis can occur with any intraocular neoplasm. Hyphema is the most common sign that catches the owners' attention. Other changes include secondary glaucoma with buphthalmos, retinal detachment, lens subluxation, scleral distortion, and dyscoria (pupil distortion).

14. What is the prognosis for primary anterior uveal tumors in the dog?
In general, distant metastasis for melanocytoma or ciliary body tumors is rare. The metastatic rate for uveal melanomas has been reported to be approximately 4%. Prognosis may be less favorable in melanomas with high mitotic indices. Melanoma can also metastasize to the eye from cutaneous or oral sites, thus making the primary tumor site difficult to determine. For ciliary body tumors, metastasis is rare, even for adenocarcinoma. When metastasis has occurred, it is usually late in the disease course.

15. What are the treatment options for an iris or ciliary body tumor?
Eyes with intraocular tumors, especially those associated with secondary ocular disease, should be enucleated as soon as possible. Globe salvaging procedures can be considered for small tumors localized to the iris and not invading the filtration angle. However, iridectomy or iridocyclectomy is extremely challenging because hemorrhage can be particularly profuse. Less invasive procedures include photodynamic or laser therapy. These procedures are controversial, and current data are limited. Because preoperative histopathology is not feasible, diagnosis is presumptive in cases treated by these methods. From a practical standpoint, enucleation or exenteration is the recommended treatment because it allows histopathologic confirmation and has a high curative potential.

16. What is the typical behavior of a limbal (epibulbar) melanoma?
This is usually a slow-growing, well-delineated, raised, heavily pigmented mass beneath the conjunctiva near or at the limbus in dogs. It may invade the cornea secondarily, but it does

not typically extend inward toward intraocular structures. Limbal melanomas are always benign and have never been documented to metastasize. A limbal melanoma must be differentiated from external extension of an intraocular melanoma. Gonioscopy is helpful to determine involvement of the drainage angle and iris base.

17. What are the treatment options for a limbal melanoma?
In older dogs with a nonprogressive limbal melanoma, "benign neglect" would be appropriate, with periodic observation for any sudden change. In younger dogs (2 to 4 years old), the tumor can have a more rapid growth pattern. Treatment would be warranted in this situation to avoid invasion of the cornea. Full-thickness corneal and scleral resection and placement of freehand corneoscleral grafts can be done to maintain a functional eye. Nd:YAG or diode laser has been used successfully. Surgical debulking and cryosurgery is another commonly used option. With cryosurgery, the tumor may not regress completely, but it seems to be "stunned" so that growth is inhibited or slowed significantly.

18. How do pigmented iris tumors in cats differ from those in dogs?
As in dogs, melanoma is the most common primary intraocular neoplasm in the cat. However, this is where the similarities between the two species end. This tumor develops as a progressive pigmentation of the iris; hence the name diffuse iris melanoma (DIM). This tumor can appear simultaneously in several areas on the iris surface or as a focal lesion. Nodular growth is rarely observed. As the amount of pigmentation increases across the surface, the tumor cells become invasive and can exfoliate into the aqueous and drainage angle. Unlike its behavior in dogs, this tumor in cats has morphologic features of malignancy, and metastasis does occur.

19. What is the prognosis of feline DIM?
DIM has histopathologic features of malignancy. Attempts have been made to develop clinical and histologic parameters to help determine the appropriate treatment course and prognosis. A recent study correlated histopathologic findings with survival times in cats with DIM. This study found that cats with tumor confined to the iris or with moderate spread (including spread into the drainage angle, with or without glaucoma) had survival times similar to those in the control group. Cats with more advanced melanoma (infiltration of the iris, its posterior epithelium, and ciliary body) had shortened survival times. The cause of death in these patients was usually suggestive of metastatic disease.

20. What is the treatment for DIM?
Enucleation of the affected eye. This tumor rarely occurs bilaterally. The dilemma for clinicians is when to recommend removal of the eye. It is difficult to differentiate benign iris pigmentation (i.e., iris freckle or nevus) from early DIM. Based on the survival study just discussed, enucleation seems to be justified when there is an increase in the amount of pigmentation, involvement of the drainage angle, changes in pupil shape and motility, or glaucoma. With an early potential lesion, it is difficult to recommend removal of a sighted, nonpainful eye. Therefore, it is important to discuss the information known about this tumor with the owner so that an informed decision can be made.

21. Can a preoperative diagnosis be made for a pigmented iris lesion in a cat?
Realistically, no. A needle "vacuuming" procedure via aqueous paracentesis has been described for use as an attempt to differentiate a benign pigmented lesion from DIM. However, the results are inconsistent and probably not reliable.

22. What is the second most common primary intraocular tumor in the cat?
Post-traumatic sarcoma (PTS).

23. What is an essential part of the history in cats that develop this tumor?

Ocular trauma seems to be the antecedent event. In particular, trauma to the lens is a feature associated with this tumor in all cases studied to date. The time between ocular trauma and tumor development is 1 to 10 years.

24. What is the prognosis for PTS?

This is an aggressive tumor, and most cats will die of tumor-related causes within several months of diagnosis. The tumor tends to line the globe circumferentially and then extend down the optic nerve to invade the central nervous system. Local lymph node and distant metastasis can occur. Early enucleation, with exenteration of the orbit, should be performed in cats suspected of having PTS. Care should be taken to remove as much of the optic nerve as possible and to submit it for histopathologic examination. The prognosis is mainly dependent on whether the neoplasm has extended beyond the cut end of the optic nerve. Blindness and central nervous system disease due to optic nerve invasion is usually the most common reason for euthanasia postoperatively.

25. Should all traumatized, blind, phthisical or buphthalmic eyes in cats be enucleated in an attempt to prevent this tumor?

Yes! (This is the author's opinion.)

SECONDARY TUMORS

26. What is the most common neoplasm to metastasize to the canine and feline eye?
Lymphosarcoma.

27. What percentage of dogs diagnosed with lymphosarcoma have ocular involvement?
In one prospective study, 37% of dogs had ocular lesions.

28. What ocular signs are associated with lymphosarcoma in dogs?

Anterior uveitis is most common. Posterior uveitis, panuveitis with retinal detachment, retinal hemorrhages, and infiltration of the cornea, conjunctiva, nictitans, or orbit can also be seen.

29. Ocular involvement with lymphosarcoma is often indicative of what stage?
Stage V.

30. What systemic signs are associated with ocular lymphosarcoma in cats?

Typically, cats do not exhibit signs of systemic disease at the time ocular lymphosarcoma is diagnosed. This makes differentiating ocular lymphosarcoma from severe idiopathic anterior uveitis difficult, and routine blood work is typically unremarkable. A question proposed is whether ocular lymphosarcoma in the cat is primary, with anterior uveitis as an initiating cause for malignant transformation of inflammatory lymphocytes. A recent retrospective study attempted to determine factors influencing survival after enucleation in cats with ocular lymphosarcoma. Over half the cats with this tumor had coexisting uveitis. Of these cats, 73% died an average of 110 days after enucleation. In cats without coexisting uveitis, 50% died an average of 30 days after enucleation. Only 7 of 36 (19%) cats were positive for feline leukemia virus. Interestingly, 7 of 21(33%) cats were positive for feline immunodeficiency virus. The conclusion was made that cats with concurrent uveitis and lymphosarcoma appear more likely to present with further systemic disease if positive for feline immunodeficiency virus.

ORBITAL NEOPLASIA

31. What are the classic signs of orbital neoplasia?

Orbital tumors typically cause a unilateral, slowly progressive exophthalmos with variable displacement of the globe. Retropulsion of the globe is nonpainful. Enophthalmos can occur with tumors involving the rostral part of the orbit. The eye often remains visual, depending on the tumor type and optic nerve involvement. Blindness tends to occur early in the disease process for optic nerve meningioma (usually before significant exophthalmos develops).

32. What are the most common orbital tumors in the dog?

In general, orbital tumors are primary and malignant. All types of tumors occur; they can arise from any orbital tissue. Secondary neoplasms occur from either invasion of the orbit from adjacent structures or as metastasis from another site. The most common tumors reported, depending on the study, were osteosarcoma, fibroma, meningioma, lymphosarcoma, multilobular osteochondrosarcoma, and mastocytoma. In the author's practice, invasion of the orbit by nasal adenocarcinoma is the most frequently encountered orbital tumor in the dog.

33. What are the most common orbital tumors in the cat?

Most feline orbital tumors are malignant and usually of epithelial origin. The most common is squamous cell carcinoma. Orbital lymphosarcoma is a common metastatic tumor that can occur unilaterally or bilaterally.

34. What are the most useful diagnostic procedures for animals with suspected orbital neoplasia?

In addition to routine blood work, thoracic radiographs are a good start to identify potential metastatic disease. Ocular ultrasound and skull radiographs are helpful but often cannot determine the full extent of tumor involvement. Computed tomography scans and magnetic resonance imaging provide the most information and should be considered whenever possible to help define treatment plans and the most accurate prognosis. Retrobulbar aspirates are often a high-yield diagnostic procedure and are most helpful to differentiate among other orbital diseases. These procedures should be considered before attempting surgical biopsy.

35. What is the general prognosis with orbital neoplasia?

Prognosis is guarded to poor. Unfortunately, most orbital tumors are identified in an advanced stage, and treatment options therefore are limited. A retrospective study in cats found the mean survival time after diagnosis was 1.9 months. Most dogs with orbital tumors are euthanized shortly after diagnosis. Survival time tends to increase with early diagnosis and surgical therapy. Enucleation with orbital exenteration can be offered as palliative therapy to keep animals comfortable as long as possible. It is important to explain to the owner that a cure is unlikely and that this surgery usually does not increase survival time.

BIBLIOGRAPHY

1. Bussanich NM, et al: Canine uveal melanomas: series and literature review. J Am Anim Hosp Assoc 23:415–424, 1987.
2. Dubeilzig RR, Everitt J, Shadduck JA, Albert DM: Clinical and morphological features of post-traumatic sarcomas in cats. Vet Pathol 27:62–66, 1990.
3. Fischer BL, Vail DM, Dubeilzig RR: A study of factors influencing survival after enucleation in feline ocular lymphosarcoma [abstract No. 26]. 30th annual meeting of the American College of Veterinary Ophthalmologists, Chicago. Vet Ophthalmol 2: 259, 1999.
4. Gilger BC, et al: Orbital neoplasms in cats: 21 cases (1974–1990). J Am Vet Med Assoc 201:1083–1086, 1992.
5. Kalishman JB, Chappell R, Flood LA, Dubielzig RR: A matched observational study of survival in cats with enucleation due to diffuse iris melanoma. Vet Ophthalmol 1:25–30, 1998.

6. Krohne SG, Henderson NM, Richardson RC, Vestre WA: Prevalence of ocular involvement in dogs with multicentric lymphoma: prospective evaluation of 94 cases. Vet Comp Ophthalmol 4:127–134, 1994.
7. Moore CP, Constantinescu GM: Surgery of the adnexa. Vet Clin North Am Small Anim Pract 27:1011–1066, 1997.
8. Roberts SM, Severin GA, Lavach JD: Prevalence and treatment of palpebral neoplasms in the dog: 200 cases (1975–1983). J Am Vet Med Assoc 189:1355–1359, 1986.
9. Spiess BM, Wallin-Håkanson N: Diseases of the canine orbit. In Gelatt KN (ed): Veterinary Ophthalmology, 3rd ed. Baltimore, Lippincott Williams & Wilkins, 1999, pp 511–533.
10. Sullivan TC, Nasisse MP, Davidson MG, Glover TL: Photocoagulation of limbal melanomas in dogs and cats: 15 cases (1989–1993). J Am Vet Med Assoc 208:891–894, 1996.

30. HEMOLYMPHATIC DISORDERS

30.1 LYMPHOMA IN DOGS

Robert C. Rosenthal, DVM, PhD, Dipl ACVIM, Dipl ACVR

1. What is lymphoma?

Lymphoma is a neoplasm that arises from the lymphoreticular cells, usually in lymph nodes, spleen, or bone marrow, but perhaps other tissues as well.

2. What is the difference between lymphoma, malignant lymphoma, and lymphosarcoma?

All of these terms refer to the same disease. Lymphoma is the current preferred terminology.

3. What is the cause of lymphoma in dogs?

The cause of lymphoma in dogs is unknown. There has been speculation that a viral etiology, as in cats, may be found, but the finding of reverse transcriptase and other viral footprints in canine lymphoma cells has not led to the isolation of any virus that could be implicated. Currently, there is a good deal of interest in elucidating the role of genetic factors. As the canine genome is better understood, it may be possible to find crucial genetic control points.

4. Do herbicides cause lymphoma in dogs? Should dogs be kept off treated lawns?

The role of herbicides, particularly 2,4-dichlorophenoxyacetic acid (2,4-D), is a matter of some controversy. Studies in people pointing to up to a sixfold increased risk with frequent exposure led to investigations in dogs. The studies in dogs have also pointed to a possible association, but not definitively a causal association. Review of the pertinent papers has concluded that 2,4-D is not implicated. It may be prudent to limit dogs' exposure to recently treated lawns.

5. Dogs of what ages are affected?

Dogs of almost any age may be diagnosed with lymphoma, but the disease is most common in dogs of middle and older ages.

6. Is gender implicated? Is there a protective effect of neutering?

There is a bit of evidence that intact females may have a decreased risk for lymphoma. In a practical sense, any difference seems to be very small, and male and female, intact and neutered dogs should all be considered susceptible.

7. With lymphoma, do breed predilections exist?

Any breed may be affected, but golden retrievers presently seem to be the breed most diagnosed with lymphoma. To what extent that finding reflects the current popularity of that breed versus some not-as-yet understood genetic factors is unclear. In various reports, breeds at high risk for the development of lymphoma have included Airedale terriers, basset hounds, boxers, bulldogs, Saint Bernards, and Scottish terriers; pomeranians and dachshunds may be at low risk.

8. What is the incidence of lymphoma in dogs?

Epidemiology questions in veterinary medicine are difficult to answer precisely because the denominator for the various rates involved is usually not known. There is no national reporting system, and local or regional tumor registries of various types are likely to see a

skewed population. However, the annual incidence of lymphoma in dogs has long been believed to be about, and is widely quoted as, 24/100,000 overall; the rate may be three times
higher for dogs 10 to 11 years old. A more recent report suggests an overall annual incidence
approaching 110/100,000.

9. Is the incidence of lymphoma really increasing?
It is difficult to know for sure. Thirty years have elapsed since the studies mentioned
above. It is possible that incidence has truly changed, but other factors may exist, such as
overall improved health care (vaccinations, nutrition, control of other diseases) and increased
awareness of cancer by the pet-owning public and veterinarians.

10. What are the common presenting signs in dogs with lymphoma?
Many dogs with lymphoma seem to feel well when they are presented for veterinary attention. It is not unusual to find painless generalized lymphadenopathy on routine annual
physical examination; indeed, owners frequently report that they or the groomer noticed enlarged lymph nodes while petting the dog. There may be a variety of signs depending on what
tissues are involved, and the clinician needs to maintain an index of suspicion. Lymphoma
may look like other diseases initially. Dogs may have vague nonspecific signs, including a
poor appetite and lethargy. Polyuria and polydipsia may be the first signs to alert the owner.

11. Should enlarged lymph nodes be aspirated? Which nodes are best?
Fine-needle aspiration cytology is an excellent consideration for any dog with lymphadenopathy. It is a safe, easy, and very rewarding diagnostic technique. It is best to avoid
the submandibular lymph nodes because the cytologic picture from that site can be con-
founded by the tendency for reactivity because of oral disease and exposure to many antigens;
it is better to sample the prescapular or other accessible nodes. The popliteal nodes may
appear a bit more reactive than other nodes, but this does not seem to be a big problem.

12. What is the utility of aspiration cytology?
Cytologic evaluation of enlarged nodes is used primarily to differentiate neoplastic from
inflammatory disease. In some cases, other infectious diseases may be recognized as well.
Cytology is very good for diagnosing lymphoma, especially for the classical immunoblastic
type, but there can be some confusion between intermediate types and reactive nodes. Part of
the problem in this regard is that there is no well-defined cytologic grading system. (In fact, a
lack of consistent terminology also plagues histologic reports.) Nonetheless, many dogs have
been successfully treated on the basis of cytologic diagnosis alone.

13. What is meant by clinical staging for lymphoma?
Clinical staging is the process by which the patient is evaluated and a numeric or alpha-
betic designation (stage) assigned. Ideally, the clinical stage defines therapy and correlates
with prognosis but, in veterinary medicine, this goal has not yet been achieved for dogs with
lymphoma. Staging does, however, provide a useful shorthand that allows clinicians to com-
municate in a brief form the extent of the patient's disease. In addition, clinical staging has
become a standard that researchers use in randomization schemes in clinical trials.

14. How is a stage assigned?
The results of a standard set of tests define the patient's stage. These tests include a physical examination, complete blood count, profile biochemical screen, urinalysis, thoracic and
abdominal radiographs, abdominal ultrasound, (lymph node and) bone marrow aspiration cytology, and lymph node biopsy.

15. Must all these tests be done?
It is advisable to stage the patient as fully as possible, but many patients have been accurately diagnosed on the basis of fine-needle aspiration cytology and successfully treated with

limited additional staging information. Of course, there is always a trade-off anytime an owner elects to proceed with less, rather than more, information. With less information there is always added uncertainty, and this lack of information may be particularly important in predicting and responding to adverse effects of chemotherapy.

16. Can other tests be done to understand lymphoma better?

In addition to the standard tests mentioned above, there will likely soon be widely available new means of evaluation. Immunophenotyping to determine the lymphocyte lineage of the cells should offer important prognostic information; B-cell lymphomas seem to respond better than T-cell lymphomas. Argyrophilic nucleolar organizer region staining or other tests to determine proliferative activity of the neoplastic cells also seem to have prognostic value, but these have yet to become standard.

17. Are there tumor markers for lymphoma in dogs?

No lymphoma-specific tumor marker is presently available for lymphoma in dogs. Hypercalcemia is found in dogs with lymphoma in perhaps 10% to 30% of cases, but it is by no means specific for lymphoma and can be seen in other neoplastic and nonneoplastic conditions as well. α_1-acid glycoprotein (AAGP) has been suggested as a useful marker for monitoring canine lymphoma patients.

18. What is AAGP testing used for? Is it reliable?

AAGP is an acute-phase protein found in elevated concentrations in dogs with lymphoma. In dogs that are successfully put into remission, AAGP concentrations return to normal reference ranges. Elevation of AAGP reportedly occurs 3 to 6 weeks prior to clinically recognizable relapse. AAGP cannot be considered a standard procedure at this time. Some dogs will have low AAGP concentrations at the time of diagnosis, and whether these will increase later is unknown. Some dogs will have high AAGP concentrations at diagnosis and retain these high concentrations despite having a clear clinical response for long periods. However, in the dog that fits the expected pattern, AAGP may indicate when dose intensification or reinstitution of chemotherapy is in order. Of course, to monitor AAGP in a meaningful way, it would seem necessary to monitor concentrations approximately at 6-week intervals.

19. What do the various stages describe?

In its strictest form, the World Health Organization's staging protocol calls for an anatomic designation, mostly ignored by veterinary clinicians, as well as a description of the lymph node and other tissue involvement, and a substage. Nodal distribution/tissue involvement is as follows:

I — solitary node involved
II — nodes in one region involved
III — nodes on both sides of the diaphragm involved
IV — splenic/hepatic involvement (± III)
V — bone marrow, other non-lymphoid tissue involvement (± III, IV)

Substage *a* applies to patients who are feeling well and are not clinically or biochemically affected by the disease. Substage *b* applies to patients who are feeling sick, have lost weight, are anorexic, or have marked biochemical abnormalities.

20. What is the most common finding indicating a *b* substage?

Clinically, anorexia, unexplained weight loss, and polyuria/polydipsia are the most common signs. Biochemically, hypercalcemia is the classic *b* change.

21. Does clinical staging have prognostic significance?

Most oncologists agree that stages I and II, which are seen less often than the higher stages, carry a better prognosis. However, with stages III, IV, and V there is less agreement.

Some studies indicate a worse prognosis for dogs with stage V disease, but these differences may reflect the degree of marrow infiltration more than anything else.

There does appear to be prognostic significance to the substage. Substage *b* patients are as likely to respond to chemotherapy initially as substage *a* patients, but overall survival seems to be a bit less—perhaps a few months.

22. Why don't substage *b* patients survive as long?

It is difficult to generalize, but one explanation for hypercalcemic patients might include the development of chronic renal disease. Other substage *b* signs could be related to marrow problems that might affect survival time.

23. How common is hypercalcemia in dogs with lymphoma?

Various studies indicate that 10% to 40% of dogs with lymphoma will be hypercalcemic. The most common site involved seems to be the anterior mediastinum, with perhaps 50% of patients also having hypercalcemia.

24. In addition to lymphoma, what other diagnoses should be considered for a dog with hypercalcemia?

Laboratory error, especially in lipidemic samples; young, growing dogs; hyperalbuminemia; granulomatous disease; other malignancies; other osseous disease; acute renal failure; hypoadrenocorticism; vitamin D toxicity.

25. What is the mechanism of hypercalcemia in canine lymphoma patients?

Several mechanisms have been proposed, including localized osteolysis and humoral hypercalcemia of malignancy. Tumor cells may produce products (interleukins, tumor necrosis factor, colony-stimulating factors, or interferons) that activate osteoclasts, leading to bone resorption locally. Humoral hypercalcemia is believed to occur following tumor-induced elaboration of a parathormone hormone–related peptide (PTHrP) that stimulates osteoclastic bone resorption at sites remote from the tumor. PTHrP is found in the circulation of about 20% of dogs with lymphoma.

26. Why is hypercalcemia of such concern?

Initially, hypercalcemia causes functional polyuria with secondary polydipsia, which is reversible if promptly treated. If hypercalcemia is severe or persistent, the deposition of calcium along the basement membrane of renal tubules will lead to azotemia and irreversible renal failure. There is no good formula including duration, severity, and rate of progression of hypercalcemia that will predict which patients will have permanent renal damage.

27. How should hypercalcemia be treated?

Hypercalcemia is not a disease itself—it is a secondary manifestation of some other problem. Therefore, the key to successful management of hypercalcemia is to treat the underlying problem. In most cases, the diagnosis of lymphoma in dogs is fairly straightforward. If effective therapy is initiated in a timely fashion, it is unlikely that hypercalcemia will persist as a problem. While the diagnosis is being secured, saline diruesis is usually an effective initial approach. The addition of furosemide and other medications has been suggested, but these measures usually are not critical.

28. How long will a lymphoma patient live if untreated?

The literature suggests that a survival time of only 30 to 60 days is expected. Although that range might seem pessimistic, it is found in the literature and is what most oncologists will offer.

29. What is the best treatment for lymphoma?

Lymphoma in dogs is very responsive to chemotherapeutic intervention. It should be considered a medical, not a surgical, disease. There have been several investigations into the role of radiation therapy (half-body studies), and hyperthermia has also been considered but, at this time, cytotoxic chemotherapy is the approach of choice.

30. Is there a role for immunotherapy (biologic response modification) for lymphoma?

Interestingly, when chemotherapy and biologic response modification (BRM) have been compared concurrently, the approaches using BRM have usually had more favorable outcomes. However, those studies usually used products or techniques that are not readily available, and none became standard therapy. Currently, the most popular form of BRM for lymphoma in dogs includes chemotherapy and monoclonal antibody 231. Monoclonal antibody 231 seems to react against the malignant cells of about 75% of canine lymphoma patients. Initial reports were encouraging, but there has not been follow-up that has convinced most oncologists.

31. Specifically, what protocol is best?

There is no single answer to this question because each owner and clinician will have personal considerations and biases about therapy. A variety of combination chemotherapy protocols have been shown to be effective. In any event, clinicians should use drugs that they can use safely while being prepared to respond to any adverse effects.

32. What should a clinician tell the owner of a dog with lymphoma about therapy and prognosis?

It is best to discuss with the owner a range of options and to outline expected response rates, remission times, survival times, and costs for each. It is important to remember that the diagnosis of cancer carries with it a great deal of anxiety and uncertainty. The clinician must be sure that the owner has the emotional and intellectual capacity to understand the important questions at hand. At the time of these discussions, many owners are not listening carefully. The clinician should have the owner paraphrase to assure there is an appropriate level of comprehension.

33. What drugs are effective in the therapy of lymphoma?

Many drugs have been used successfully in combination to treat lymphoma in dogs. Ideally, each drug would have well-defined characteristics as a single agent, but that has not always been the case. The drugs most often used in first-line combinations include prednisone, vincristine, cyclophosphamide, doxorubicin, and L-asparaginase. Other drugs with a putative role (most often mentioned in the rescue setting) include DTIC, chlorambucil, methotrexate, vinblastine, CCNU, actinomycin D, mitoxantrone, mechlorethamine, procarbazine, cisplatin, and cytosine arabinoside.

34. Is single-agent therapy as good as multidrug therapy?

No. In theory and in practice, multidrug protocols are better. As a general rule, it seems that the more drugs you use, the better the outcome. However, costs and risks are likely to increase as well.

35. What about single-agent prednisone?

Treatment with prednisone alone will result in an objective response in perhaps 50% of patients so treated, but no one has demonstrated any survival advantage to such treatment. For some owners, the transient improvement in quality of life experienced by some patients may be exactly what they are seeking.

36. Is there a downside to treating with prednisone alone?

Yes. Prednisone used as a single agent may induce drug resistance. In theory, such induction may take place in as little as a few days, but some evidence suggests that dogs treated for fewer than 10 days have not shown such a response, although dogs treated for more than 30 days did. If an owner opts to try prednisone alone first and asks for combination therapy later, the results may not be as good as usually expected.

37. Are there any helpful single-agent protocols?

Doxorubicin seems to be the best single agent. It is reasonable to expect that about 60% to 65% of patients so treated will have a good response, with resolution of nodes. The median first remission time seems to range from 6 to 7 months.

Early on, cyclophosphamide was evaluated as a single agent. No improvement in survival time compared with untreated dogs was reported.

38. Can oral therapy alone be effective, or must drugs be delivered intravenously?

In general, drugs administered intravenously offer the best results. The combination of oral prednisone and cyclophosphamide seems attractive as an easy option. These drugs are not particularly effective as single agents, however, and this combination has not been an effective one.

39. Are multidrug protocols effective?

Many multidrug protocols have been investigated, with most offering high response rates (80% to more than 90%) and median first remission times in the range of 7 to 11 months. The inclusion of doxorubicin, the best single agent, seems to strengthen a protocol.

40. How long should therapy continue?

Various protocols have called for different treatment periods. In general, treatment times are tending to become shorter (6 to 12 months versus 24 to 36 months), but this is a question that is by no means resolved.

41. What should I feed my lymphoma patients?

Without being facetious, to feed lymphoma patients anything they will eat is the most important consideration. The availability of diets tailored to the needs of cancer patients in general is attractive and offers a theoretical advantage. However, it is more important that these patients continue to eat than it is that they get an ideally formulated ration. In fact, beside the theoretical consideration, the instances in which such diets have been shown to have clinical benefit are very limited. There is evidence that dogs with stage IIIa lymphoma do enjoy a survival advantage if fed a commercially available diet tailored to the needs of cancer patients.

42. Why does treatment fail?

The emergence of drug resistance, a process that may be stimulated by exposure to drugs but that also is part of the natural heterogeneity of cancer cells, is the primary reason treatment fails.

43. Is there a role for complementary or alternative treatments?

Many owners are interested in complementary or alternative treatments, but none of these approaches have been shown to be of benefit for dogs with lymphoma. It is likely, but not a certainty, that most of these treatments will be innocuous. Nonetheless, reports of adverse reactions are beginning to surface, and clinicians should be aware that there are no good data on possible interactions of the alternative compounds often suggested in varied combinations, either with each other or traditional cytotoxic agents. The most common downside of such approaches arises when an owner declines known effective therapy for unproven treatments of this type. Oncologists should have no argument with the use of natural substances because, in fact, many of the anticancer drugs are derived from plants and soil organisms. The question is rather one of subjecting complementary or alternative treatments to rigorous evaluation of efficacy, a criterion that has not been met to any degree.

44. What happens when treatment fails?

In almost every case, the disease will reappear where it was first noted or with the same clinical signs.

45. What should I do when a patient relapses?

Again, there is no simple answer. Relapse certainly demands renewed in-depth discussion with the owner about treatment strategies and prognosis. As at the outset, an array of options will be available, including humane euthanasia and no further therapy.

In almost every case, what was done first will be what works best, both in terms of likelihood of attaining a response and duration of response. There is even less consensus about second-line therapy than about first-line protocols. It does appear, however, that depending on circumstances including the time to initial relapse and current treatment interval, reinstituting the initial therapy may be helpful in a reasonable number of cases. Another theory is to use different drugs entirely.

BIBLIOGRAPHY

1. Keller ET, MacEwen EG, Rosenthal RC, et al: Evaluation of prognostic factors and sequential combination chemotherapy with doxorubicin for canine lymphoma. J Vet Intern Med 7(5):289–295, 1993
2. Madewell BR: Diagnosis, assessment of prognosis, and treatment of dogs with lymphoma: The sentinel changes (1973–1999) [editorial]. J Vet Intern Med 113:393–394, 1999.
3. Moore AS, London CA, Wood CA, et al: Lomustine (CCNU) for the treatment of resistant lymphoma in dogs. J Vet Intern Med 13:395–398, 1999.
4. Myers III MC, Moore AS, Rand WM, et al: Evaluation of a multidrug chemotherapy protocol (ACOPA II) in dogs with lymphoma. J Vet Intern Med 11(6):333–339, 1997.
5. Rosenthal RC, MacEwen EG: Treatment of lymphoma in dogs. J Am Vet Med Assoc 196(5):774–781, 1990.
6. Teske E, van Heerde P, Rutterman GR, et al: Prognostic factors for treatment of malignant lymphoma in dogs. J Am Vet Med Assoc 205(12):1722–1728, 1994.
7. Valerius KD, Ogilvie GK, Mallinckrodt CH, et al: Doxorubicin alone or in combination with asparaginase followed by cyclophosphamide, vincristine, and prednisone for treatment of multicentric lymphoma in dogs: 121 cases (1987–1995). J Am Vet Med Assoc 210(4):512–516, 1997.
8. Zemann BJ, Moore AS, Rand WM, et al: A combination chemotherapy protocol (VELCAP-L) for dogs with lymphoma. J Vet Intern Med 12:465–470, 1998.

30.2. MYELOPROLIFERATIVE DISEASE
Kevin A. Hahn, DVM, PhD, Dipl ACVIM

1. What is myeloproliferative disease?

Myeloproliferative disease (MPD) is uncommon in the dog and cat. It includes all of the nonlymphoid dysplastic and neoplastic conditions arising from the hematopoietic stem cell or its progeny. Thus, the chronic and acute myeloid leukemias, thrombocythemia, megakaryocytic myelosis, myelofibrosis, the myelodysplastic syndromes, and some cases of aplastic anemia may be viewed as variants of a single disease process.

2. What is the pathophysiology of MPD?

Myeloid cells arise from a common stem cell whose development is regulated by stimulatory and inhibitory growth factors. Pluripotential hematopoietic stem cells are most influenced by interleukin-3 (IL-3) granulocyte-macrophage colony-stimulating factor (GM-CSF), and stem cell factor, while committed progenitor cells are regulated by variable concentrations of GM-CSF, G-CSF, M-CSF, IL-5, erythropoietin, and thrombopoietin. As a result of their common origin, a key point to remember about myeloproliferative disorders is the involvement of multiple cell lines in dysplastic and neoplastic conditions. Dysplastic changes may signal early neoplastic changes, with cases progressing to acute leukemia. Myelo-dysplastic syndrome is associated with anemia or multiple cytopenias, normal to hypercellular bone marrow, ineffective hematopoiesis, and fewer than 30% blast cells of all nucleated cells in the bone marrow. Chronic myeloid leukemias also have fewer than 30% blast cells of all nucleated cells in the bone marrow and are distinguished from myelodysplastic syndrome by elevated cell counts of one or more cell lines with mature forms predominating. Acute myeloid leukemias, often the end result of all myeloproliferative disorders, are recognized by 30% or more blast cells of all nucleated cells in the bone marrow.

3. What are the clinical signs of a dog or cat with MPD?

The MPDs may present with a variety of clinical signs, including pale mucous membranes, lethargy, weight loss, abdominal distension (hepatosplenomegaly), peripheral lymphadenomegaly (in a few patients), regenerative or nonregenerative anemias, bleeding diatheses, septicemia, or fever of unknown origin. These signs will raise suspicions of MPD, but such disease may also be an incidental finding on routine hematologic examination.

4. Have any underlying causes or risk factors been identified?

In cats, the syndrome is most commonly associated with a concurrent feline leukemia virus infection. Cats recovering from panleukopenia or hemobartonellosis may have a relatively higher risk of developing a mutant cell line induced by feline leukemia virus. In dogs, the cause is unknown.

5. What are some of the more common findings on a hemogram obtained from the dog or cat with MPD?

Neoplastic cells (e.g., acute lymphocytic leukemia which is usually differentiated by special staining techniques); eosinophilia (e.g., parasitism, allergic disease, and eosinophilic gastroenteritis), which must be differentiated from eosinophilic leukemia; and severe hemolytic anemia, which must be differentiated from acute erythroleukemia.

Other findings include severe, nonregenerative anemia; circulating nucleated red blood cells; megaloblastic erythrocytes; leukocytosis or leukopenia; and thrombocytopenia with abnormal platelet morphology.

6. How do you diagnose MPD?

Critical to diagnosis are complete blood and bone marrow evaluations, including observation for dysplastic changes and blast cell quantitation. In addition, evidence for tissue infiltration identified through cytologic or histologic evaluations of lymph nodes, the spleen, or liver is recommended. Additional diagnostic information from cytochemical stains, immunohistochemical staining, and cytogenetic analysis can influence the final diagnosis when morphology alone is equivocal.

7. What is the treatment for MPD?

Treatment of acute MPDs is presently impractical in veterinary medicine. Therapy of the chronic MPDs depends upon the suppression of the proliferation of the affected clones together with attention to the secondary effects of the disease and to the adverse effects of therapy. Supportive care consists of blood transfusions and fluid therapy to correct dehydration; antibiotics are indicated in some patients to combat secondary infection.

8. If the origin is neoplastic, what is the most appropriate chemotherapy protocol?

Several case reports throughout the veterinary literature describe short-term efficacy of single-agent chemotherapy. Survival times range from a few days to a few weeks.

9. What measures are necessary in following a patient with MPD?

A complete blood count and examination of bone marrow aspirate should be performed regularly to determine response to treatment and progression of disease.

10. What is the prognosis for MPD?

The prognosis for chronic MPD is guarded; for acute MPD it is grave. Accurate identification of these disorders in animals is important. Investigation and greater understanding of the pathophysiologic mechanisms may lead to more lasting therapeutic successes in the future.

BIBLIOGRAPHY

1. Evans RJ, Gorman NT: Myeloproliferative disease in the dog and cat: Definition, etiology and classification. Vet Rec 121:437–443, 1987.
2. Gorman NT, Evans RJ: Myeloproliferative disease in the dog and cat: Clinical presentations, diagnosis and treatment. Vet Rec 121:490–496, 1987.
3. Harvey JW: Myeloproliferative disorders in dogs and cats. Vet Clin North Am Small Anim Pract 11:349–381, 1981.
4. Raskin RE: Myelopoiesis and myeloproliferative disorders. Vet Clin North Am Small Anim Pract 26:1023–1042, 1996.
5. Young KM: Myeloproliferative disorders. Vet Clin North Am Small Anim Pract 15:769–781, 1985.

30.3. MULTIPLE MYELOMA
Robert C. Rosenthal, DVM, PhD, Dipl ACVIM, Dipl ACVR

---

1. What cell becomes malignant in multiple myeloma?

Multiple myeloma is a neoplastic proliferation of plasma cells, the end differentiation of B-lymphocytes. The role of B-lymphocytes is the production of immunoglobulins. Thus, unregulated production of immunoglobulins leads to the presence of a monoclonal gammopathy. Strictly speaking, multiple myeloma refers to the monoclonal production of IgG, IgA, or light chains.

2. Is a monoclonal gammopathy pathognomonic for multiple myeloma?

No, monoclonal gammopathies may also be noted in other conditions, including some lymphomas or infectious disease, most notably ehrlichiosis.

3. What is the cause of multiple myeloma?

As with most neoplasms, the cause of multiple myeloma is unknown. Exposure to various carcinogens, chronic stimulation of the immune system, genetic predisposition, and viral infection have all been suggested as possible causes, but no demonstrations of causation have been conclusive.

4. How common is multiple myeloma?

Multiple myeloma is rare overall—less than 1% of all malignancies; but among hematopoietic malignancies it represents about 8% of the cases.

5. What breed is most commonly affected?

German shepherd dogs have been identified as the breed most often affected, and purebred dogs seem to develop multiple myeloma more frequently than do mixed-breed dogs. Cats are less commonly diagnosed than dogs.

6. Is there an age or gender predilection?

There is no clear gender predilection although some investigators have suggested a male predisposition. Multiple myeloma is seem most commonly in dogs 8–9 years of age, but a wide age range has been reported.

7. In what ways does multiple myeloma affect patients?

Patients can be affected by either direct tissue invasion or as the result of high concentrations of circulating antibodies. A variety of organ systems may be affected, including the skeletal system, renal system, neurologic system, and cardiovascular system.

8. How does multiple myeloma affect bones?

Multiple lytic osseous lesions or diffuse osteopenia may be seen. Up to two-thirds of dogs may be so affected; bony involvement is rare in cats. Vertebra, ribs, proximal long bones, pelvis, and skull are frequently involved. Pathologic fracture is a potential complication, or the patient may be presented for signs of pain unrelated to fracture.

9. What is the hyperviscosity syndrome?

With the overproduction of large immunoglobulin molecules, increased serum viscosity can result in dysfunction of a number of different tissues, including the heart and retina; coagulation may also be adversely affected, resulting in a bleeding diathesis. The overproduction of IgM molecules, the largest type of immunoglobulin, results most often in hyperviscosity. Hyperviscosity may be a problem in up to 20% of multiple myeloma patients.

10. How does hypercalcemia occur in multiple myeloma?

The hypercalcemia associated with multiple myeloma seems to be the result of the activation of osteoclast activating factors.

11. How are bone lesions best imaged?

The bony lesions of multiple myeloma are almost all lytic, not proliferative. Survey radiographs remain the preferred imaging modality compared to scintigraphic bone scans in this setting.

12. What criteria must be met to make a diagnosis of multiple myeloma?

Multiple myeloma is diagnosed if a patient exhibits at least two of the following four criteria:
• Monoclonal gammopathy
• Lytic bone lesions
• Bence-Jones proteinuria
• Neoplastic plasma cells or bone marrow plasmacytosis.

13. What are Bence-Jones proteins?

Bence-Jones proteins are light chains that are found in the urine. They are not detected by the usual dipstick methods. Bence-Jones proteins are detected by heat precipitation methods or by urine immunoelectrophoresis.

14. Are there useful prognostic factors to help predict outcome?

Hypercalcemia, Bence-Jones proteinuria, and extensive bony lysis have all been associated with shorter survival times compared to patients without these characteristics. Interestingly, azotemia, the immunoglobulin class, and hyperviscosity have not been shown to be negative prognostic factors.

15. What therapy is best for patients with multiple myeloma?

The mainstay of therapy for patients with multiple myeloma has been the combined use of **prednisone and an alkylating agent**, melphalan most commonly. This combination has offered better outcomes (median survival 540 days) than the use of prednisone as a single agent (median survival 220 days). The addition of either another alkylating agent (cyclophosphamide) or vincristine has not been shown to improve outcomes materially.

Throughout therapy, complete blood counts should be monitored regularly to help avoid problems associated with myelosuppression. Dose and schedule adjustments may be needed based on the patient's response, both positive and negative. Because multiple myeloma patients are immunocompromised, the use of antibiotics is especially warranted in the presence of fever or other signs suggestive of infection. Hypercalcemic patients should receive saline diruesis, but the best therapy for hypercalcemia is the proper management of the underlying malignancy.

16. What is seen with a good response to treatment?

Improvement in clinical signs, clincio-pathologic abnormalities, and radiographs have all been cited as evaluable parameters in multiple myeloma. Clinical signs usually improve first, often within 3–4 weeks. Bence-Jones proteinuria may lessen within 3–6 weeks. The response in bones is slower still and may take months to be recognizable. As with most malignancies, cure remains elusive, but a good quality of life can surely be attained. A reasonable goal of therapy is to reduce the abnormal proteins (serum or urine) by at least 50%. Serum proteins have a much longer half-life than Bence-Jones proteins and, therefore, take longer to normalize.

BIBLIOGRAPHY

1. Clark GN, Berg J, Engler SJ, et al: Extramedullary plasmacytomas in dogs: Results of surgical excision in 131 cases. J Am Anim Hosp Assoc 28(2):105–111, 1992.
2. Dorfman M, Dimski DS: Paraproteinemias in small animal medicine. Comp Small Anim Med 14(5):621–632, 1992.
3. Hammer AS, Couto CG: Complication of multiple myeloma. J Am Anim Hosp Assoc 30(1):9–14, 1994.
4. Matus RE, Leifer CE, MacEwen EG, et al: Prognostic factors for multiple myeloma in the dog. J Am Vet Med Assoc 188(11):1288–1292, 1986.
5. Rakich RM, Latimer KS, Weiss R, et al: Mucocutaneous plasmacytomas in dogs: 75 cases (1980-1987). J Am Vet Med Assoc 194(6):803–810, 1989.
6. Rusbridge C. Wheeler SJ, Lamb CR, et al: Vertebral plasma cell tumors in 8 dogs. J Vet Intern Med 13:126–133, 1999.

31. ORAL TUMORS IN DOGS AND CATS

Linda S. Fineman, DVM, Dipl ACVIM

1. What are the most common oral tumors in dogs and cats?

Dogs
Epulides (fibromatous and acanthomatous)
Malignant melanoma
Squamous cell carcinoma
Fibrosarcoma

Cats
Squamous cell carcinoma
Fibrosarcoma

2. What is the clinical presentation in animals with oral tumors?

Dogs and cats most commonly are presented with halitosis, ptyalism, blood-tinged saliva, dysphagia, reluctance to groom themselves, and facial deformity.

3. Are there breed or age predispositions?

Oral neoplasia is much more common in older animals, although there are some exceptions. For example, epulides may occur in young dogs, and unusual tumors like papillary squamous cell carcinoma and granular cell myoblastoma of the tongue are primarily seen in dogs younger than 2 to 3 years of age. Malignant melanomas are reported to be most common in poodles, Scottish terriers, and golden retrievers. Golden retrievers have been reported to get an uncommon variant of oral fibrosarcoma, which is a biologically high-grade and histologically low-grade form of the disease.

4. What is the biologic behavior of epulides?

Epulides are benign in dogs and cats. Acanthomatous epulides are characterized by locally aggressive behavior despite being called benign.

5. What is the biologic behavior of malignant melanoma?

These are highly aggressive neoplasms with a very high potential to metastasize and recur locally after incomplete resection. The prognosis seems to depend on location within the mouth and mitotic index. Tumors originating from the rostral mandible or maxilla may be associated with a better prognosis. While a low mitotic index has been correlated with less aggressive biologic behavior, some oral melanomas considered to be histologically benign may behave in a malignant manner. Metastasis is usually to regional lymph nodes and later to the lungs. Less commonly, melanomas may metastasize to other organs, including the kidney or brain. Although micrometastasis is believed to occur very early in the course of disease, most dogs will not have gross metastasis at the time of diagnosis. Because the growth rate of the metastatic cells is variable, a fairly long interval (1 to 2 years) between diagnosis and death due to metastasis may exist in some cases.

Little has been published about oral malignant melanomas in cats but, in the small number of reported cases, an aggressive biologic behavior similar to the disease in dogs has been observed.

6. What is the biologic behavior of squamous cell carcinoma?

There are several forms of oral squamous cell carcinoma in dogs. Gingival tumors are most common and are characterized by locally invasive disease with a low risk of metastasis. When metastasis does occur, it is usually to the regional lymph nodes. Pulmonary involvement is rare. Gingival tumors often extend into underlying bone, making surgical resection difficult. Lingual tumors are fairly common and are associated with a higher likelihood of regional lymph node metastasis. Papillary squamous cell carcinoma is seen in very young dogs and puppies. Metastasis is rare, but local control can be difficult. Tonsillar squamous cell carcinomas are highly malignant neoplasms with a tendency to infiltrate into surrounding tissues and metastasize to the regional lymph nodes early in the course of the disease. Distant metastasis to the lungs, liver, spleen, and bone has been reported.

In cats, squamous cell carcinomas are most commonly at the base of the tongue or in the gingiva with underlying bony lysis. Metastasis is uncommon and is usually to the mandibular lymph nodes. Regional lymph nodes may also be enlarged because of the significant inflammatory component associated with secondary bacteria infection and tumor necrosis.

7. What is the biologic behavior of fibrosarcoma?

In dogs and cats, this tumor behaves by extensive infiltration locally but has a low risk of metastasis. The exception to this may be in young dogs, where oral fibrosarcoma is more likely to metastasize. Histologically low-grade, biologically high-grade fibrosarcoma in the mouth of golden retrievers has been described as an extremely aggressive tumor that grows rapidly despite a very low mitotic index. Biopsies from these lesions may have a benign appearance, and often the pathologic diagnosis will be exuberant connective tissue or fibroma.

8. How are oral neoplasms treated?

As a general rule, oral tumors are best treated by wide surgical excision. Computed tomography is useful to help determine the best surgical approach as well as to help plan radiotherapy.

9. How are epulides treated?

Fibromatous and ossifying epulides are best treated with surgery. Because the tumors arise from the dental ligament, local recurrence is common with incomplete excision. These tumor types are slowly growing, justifying a less aggressive approach than the acanthomatous form. Acanthomatous epulides are best treated by wide local resection, usually a partial mandibulectomy or maxillectomy. Radiation therapy is also an excellent option, with about a 95% long-term local control rate, equal to that attained with aggressive surgery. (See Controversies for further discussion.)

10. How are oral malignant melanomas best treated?

Classically, malignant melanoma has been treated with wide local resection and follow-up chemotherapy. The role of chemotherapy is still not clear. Platinum-based drugs are believed to be the most efficacious, but overall response rates are still low, probably less than 25%. Whether the use of chemotherapy actually prolongs survival times or tumor-free intervals remains to be seen. Recently, interest in radiation therapy has been revived following reports that melanomas respond to radiation delivered in coarse fractions. Radiation therapy may be used as an adjuvant following surgical resection, but also is useful in palliation of large nonresectable tumors. Immunotherapy has been studied extensively in melanomas because these tumors are believed to be immunogenic. Cimetidine is used in horses with melanoma, but its efficacy in dogs is unknown. A combination of tumor necrosis factor and interleukin-2 was used in a group of 13 dogs with oral melanoma, but durable responses were seen only in two. Immunotherapy with heat-inactivated *Corynebacterium parvum* was found to be beneficial in dogs with very small tumors. Finally, L-MTP-PE (liposome-encapsulated muramyltripeptide-phosphatidyl ethanolamine) improved the likelihood of survival in dogs treated with surgery first. Unfortunately, many of the immunotherapeutics that have been studied are either not available or associated with unacceptable adverse effects. In the future, immunotherapy may play an important role in treating melanomas.

Very little clinical data have been published describing treatment of oral melanoma in cats.

11. How is oral squamous cell carcinoma treated?

Squamous cell carcinoma in dogs is best treated by wide local excision because the risk of metastasis is low with gingival tumors. Radiation therapy is recommended postoperatively for dogs with large tumors or where only incomplete resection was obtained. The optimal protocol and modality is unknown currently. Lingual and tonsillar squamous cell carcinomas in dogs are more difficult to manage. Wide surgical excision is rarely possible in either location. Radiation therapy may be used in a palliative attempt, but the relatively high risk of metastasis makes local therapy alone unlikely to be curative. The role of chemotherapy is not fully known currently. Chemotherapy is probably appropriate in dogs with tonsillar, lingual, or large caudal oral squamous cell carcinoma. Cisplatin and mitoxantrone have not been fully evaluated, but both have been reported to cause objective responses in dogs. Piroxicam was shown to have some activity against oral squamous cell carcinoma in dogs, presumably via its role as an immunomodulator. Further studies are needed to evaluate its efficacy.

Squamous cell carcinoma in cats is a very frustrating disease to treat. The best treatment approach is not known, but it is clear that surgery or radiation alone is unlikely to be curative in most cases. Local recurrence remains the biggest obstacle to long-term survival. The most promising approach currently is a combination of chemotherapy either with mitoxantrone or carboplatin with radiation therapy. Some oncologists feel that the only treatment that seems to prolong survival in cats with oral squamous cell carcinoma is placement of a gastrotomy tube. Certainly a gastrotomy tube can help maintain a good plane of nutrition while definitive treatment modalities are in progress.

12. How is oral fibrosarcoma treated?

Fibrosarcoma is best treated by wide surgical excision in cats and dogs. Radiation therapy may be a useful adjuvant to surgery but is unlikely to be curative when used as a single modality. The role of radiation therapy has not yet been clearly defined for this disease. Chemotherapy is generally not recommended because these tumors are not believed to be particularly chemosensitive.

13. How long do dogs live after they are diagnosed with a malignancy in the mouth?

It depends on the histologic type, the location in the mouth, the grade or growth rate of the tumor, and the owner's geographic and financial access to specialized care. Quality of life issues are the most important consideration.

14. What is the prognosis for dogs and cats with oral malignant melanoma?

Dogs treated with aggressive surgery alone (i.e., mandibulectomy or maxillectomy) have a reported median survival time of 7.3 to 9.1 months. Whether these survival times are improved with the addition of radiation therapy, chemotherapy, or immunotherapy has not been fully elucidated. Experience with cats is far less, but they are not expected to do well for any extended period.

Little data are available to determine which treatment modalities may improve survival rates.

15. What is the prognosis for dogs and cats with oral squamous cell carcinoma?

In dogs treated with aggressive surgery, median survival times varied from 9 to 18 months. Local recurrence was the biggest issue affecting survival. In one series of dogs treated with megavoltage radiation therapy, the median progression-free survival interval was about 17 months. Radiation therapy was also helpful in achieving long-term tumor control in three dogs with papillary squamous cell carcinoma, with no evidence of tumor recurrence 39, 32, and 10 months after treatment.

The prognosis for cats with oral squamous cell carcinoma is poor. Cats treated with surgery alone have a high rate of local recurrence. Radiation therapy used as a single modality has not been promising and has not been shown to prolong survival. The most promising protocol to date has been a combination of surgery and postoperative radiation therapy. In one study of seven cats, the median survival time was 12.5 months, but six cats had local recurrence. Mitoxantrone and radiation therapy were used in combination in one study, resulting in median survival times of 180 days and a 30% 1-year survival rate.

16. What is the prognosis for dogs and cats with oral fibrosarcoma?

Dogs have been reported to have a 50% 1-year survival rate in one study using mandibulectomy or maxillectomy to treat fibrosarcoma. Local recurrence remains the biggest problem, with rates of tumor recurrence varying depending on the surgeon and the location of the tumor. The role of radiation therapy has not been fully defined for this disease. In one study where dogs were treated with megavoltage radiation to a total dose of 48 Gy, the median progression-free interval was estimated to be 23 months, but this figure may be too optimistic.

Because few reports describe treatment of cats with oral fibrosarcoma, the prognosis is difficult to determine.

CONTROVERSIES

17. Does World Health Organization staging predict prognosis in dogs and cats with oral tumors?

Some studies suggest that stage is a good predictor, while others dispute this point. Common sense would suggest that small tumors located in surgically accessible parts of the oral cavity should have the best prognoses.

18. Does orthovoltage radiation therapy cause malignant transformation of acanthomatous epulides into squamous cell carcinomas?

While there are reports of malignant transformation from earlier literature, this has not been confirmed in more recent studies. Some authors suggest that the original diagnosis may have been incorrect in some reported cases of malignant transformation. Until proven otherwise, surgery should probably remain the treatment of choice, with radiation therapy a very acceptable alternative.

BIBLIOGRAPHY

1. Blackwood L, Dobson JM: Radiotherapy of oral malignant melanomas in dogs. J Am Vet Med Assoc 209:98–102, 1996.
2. Dhaliwal RS, Kitchell BE, Manfra Marretta S: Oral tumors in dogs and cats. Part II. Prognosis and treatment. Compend Contin Educ Vet 20(10):1109–1119, 1998.
3. Hutson CA, Willauer CC, Walder EJ, et al: Treatment of mandibular squamous cell carcinoma in cats by use of mandibulectomy and radiotherapy: Seven cases (1987–1989). J Am Vet Med Assoc 201:777–781, 1992.
4. Morrison WB: Cancers of the head and neck. In Morrison WB (ed): Cancer in Dogs and Cats: Medical and Surgical Management. Baltimore, Lippincott Williams and Wilkins, 1998, pp 511–519.
5. Oakes MG, Lewis DD, Hedlund CS, et al: Canine oral neoplasia. Comp Cont Educ Small Anim. January 15–30, 1993.
6. Ogilvie GK, Sundberg JP, O'Banion K, et al: Papillary squamous cell carcinoma in three young dogs. J Am Vet Med Assoc 192:933–936, 1988.
7. Postorino Reeves NC, Turrel JM, Withrow SJ: Oral squamous cell carcinoma in the cat. J Am Anim Hosp Assoc 29:438–441, 1993.
8. Salisbury SK, Lantz GC: Long-term results of partial mandibulectomy for treatment of oral tumors in 30 dogs. J Am Anim Hosp Assoc 24:285–294, 1988.
9. Schwarz PD, Withrow SJ, Curtis CR, et al: Mandibular resection as a treatment for oral cancer in 81 dogs. J Am Anim Hosp Assoc 27:601–610, 1991.
10. Theon AP, Rodriguez C, Griffey S, et al: Analysis of prognostic factors and patterns of failure in dogs with periodontal tumors treated with megavoltage irradiation. J Am Vet Med Assoc 210:785–788, 1997.
11. Withrow SJ: Tumors of the gastrointestinal tract. A. Cancer of the oral cavity. In Withrow SJ, MacEwan EG (eds): Small Animal Clinical Oncology, 2nd ed. Philadelphia, WB Saunders, 1996, pp 227–239.

32. MAST CELL DISEASE

Kevin A. Hahn, DVM, PhD, Dipl ACVIM

1. What is mast cell disease?

The overproliferation of mast cells.

2. What is the pathophysiology of mast cell neoplasia?

Histamine and other vasoactive substances within the cytoplasmic granules of mast cell tumors can cause erythema and edema. Heparin within the cytoplasmic granules increases the likelihood of bleeding.

3. What systems are commonly affected?

The skin and subcutaneous tissues are the most common location in dogs and cats. The spleen is a common primary location in cats but an uncommon primary location in dogs. Intestinal mast cell tumors are uncommon in cats and rare in dogs. In dogs, mast cell tumors located in the inguinal region tend to behave more aggressively than similarly graded tumors in other locations.

4. Are any predispositions known for this disease?

No genetic or geographic predisposition has been reported. Mast cell tumors represent 20% to 25% of all skin and subcutaneous tumors in dogs. Cutaneous mast cell tumor is the fourth most common skin tumor in cats after basal cell tumor, squamous cell carcinoma, and fibrosarcoma. Boxers and Boston terriers are predisposed. Siamese cats are predisposed to histiocytic cutaneous mast cell tumors.

5. What is the typical signalment of a dog or cat with mast cell disease?

In dogs the mean age is 8 years; in cats, 10 years. The disease can occur in all ages and has been reported in animals younger than 1 year old and in cats as old as 18 years. There is no known sex predilection in dogs; however, in cats, male cats may be affected more often than females.

6. What are the signs of a dog or cat with mast cell disease?

Clinical signs depend on the location and grade of the tumor. The animal may have had a skin or subcutaneous mast cell tumor for days to months at the time of examination. Recent rapid growth after months of quiescence is common. Recent onset of erythema and edema are more common with high-grade skin and subcutaneous tumors. Anorexia is the most common complaint in cats with a splenic mast cell tumor. Vomiting can occur secondary to both splenic and gastrointestinal mast cell tumors in cats.

7. What are some of the physical examination findings?

In dogs, findings are extremely variable; tumors can resemble any other type of skin or subcutaneous tumor, both benign and malignant. It can be primarily a skin or subcutaneous mass. Most tumors are solitary but can be multifocal. Approximately 50% are located on the trunk and perineum, 40% on the extremities, and 10% on the head and neck region. Regional lymphadenopathy may develop when a high-grade tumor metastasizes to draining lymph nodes. Hepatomegaly and splenomegaly are features of disseminated mast cell neoplasia.

In cats, cutaneous mast cell tumors develop primarily in the subcutaneous tissue or dermis. They can be papular or nodular, solitary or multiple, and hairy, alopecic, or have an ulcerated surface. There is a slight predilection for the head and neck regions. Cats with solitary dermal masses have a 15% to 45% metastatic rate.

Feline splenic mast cell tumors commonly present with splenomegaly as the only consistent physical finding. Cats may also have gastric or duodenal ulcers, presumably because of the release of histamine by the tumor. Mastocythemia and anemia develop in some cats; the latter is caused by erythrophagocytosis by the tumor, splenic sequestration, hemorrhage at the site of gastrointestinal ulceration, or splenic rupture.

In cats with primary gastrointestinal origin mast cell neoplasia, a firm, segmental thickening of the small intestinal wall measuring 1 to 7 cm in diameter may be present. Metastasis to mesenteric lymph nodes, spleen, liver and, rarely, the lungs occurs.

8. What causes mast cell neoplasms?

The exact cause is unknown; however, a hereditary predisposition has been postulated as well as sites of previous inflammation.

9. What are some differential diagnoses for mast cell disease?

Because the clinical findings on examination of dogs with a mast cell tumor are extremely variable, the tumor can resemble any other skin or subcutaneous tumor. A splenic mast cell tumor is the most common cause of splenomegaly in cats. An intestinal mast cell tumor in cats can resemble any primary gastrointestinal disorder (i.e., inflammatory and neoplasia).

10. What are some common diagnostic findings in a patient with mast cell disease?

Anemia and mastocythemia can be observed in some cats with a splenic mast cell tumor and some dogs with systemic mastocytosis. Most routine laboratory tests are unremarkable. Abdominal radiography may reveal splenomegaly in some cats with a splenic mast cell tumor and some dogs with systemic mastocytosis.

Cytologic examination of a fine-needle aspirate is the most important preliminary diagnostic test, revealing round cells with basophilic cytoplasmic granules that do not form sheets or clumps. If the malignant mast cells are agranular, the presence of a large eosinophilic infiltrate may suggest a mast cell tumor.

Tissue biopsy is necessary for definitive diagnosis and tumor grading. Staging the mast cell tumor allows one to determine the extent of disease and determine appropriate treatment. Diagnostic tests, in addition to those listed above to achieve complete staging, may include cytologic examination of a bone marrow aspirate, cytologic examination or biopsy of a local lymph node, thoracic radiography, abdominal ultrasonography, and hepatic or splenic aspiration.

Histopathologic examination allows grading of the tumor to predict biologic behavior. Mast cell tumors in dogs are graded I to III, with grade III being the most aggressive type.

11. How are mast cell tumors treated?

Aggressive surgical excision is the treatment of choice for a mast cell tumor in dogs. When histopathologic examination reveals that mast cell tumor cells extend close to surgical margins, a second aggressive surgery should be performed as soon as possible. It is impossible to comment on completeness of surgical excision and predict biologic behavior of mast cell tumors without histopathologic evaluation of the entire surgically excised tissue. A cutaneous mast cell tumor in cats tends to be somewhat less invasive than in dogs. At least 2-cm surgical margins should be obtained.

Splenectomy is the treatment of choice in cats with a splenic mast cell tumor. Biopsy of lymph nodes and other suspicious visceral organs is appropriate.

Radiotherapy is a good treatment option for a patient with a cutaneous mast cell tumor in a location that does not allow aggressive surgical excision. If possible, surgery should be performed before radiotherapy to reduce the tumor to a microscopic volume. A mast cell tumor located on an extremity responds better to radiotherapy than do tumors located on the trunk.

Median disease-free intervals following localized irradiation, regardless of grade, range from 8 to 125 months (median 60 months). In one study using an alternating-day fractionation scheme, median disease-free interval for dogs with grade I tumors was 123.5 months (n = 18 dogs); grade II tumors, 21.6 months (n = 89 dogs); and grade III tumors, 9.8 months (n = 27 dogs).

12. What is appropriate follow-up for a patient who has a mast cell tumor excised or irradiated?

A patient that has had more than one cutaneous mast cell tumor is predisposed to developing new mast cell tumors. Fine-needle aspiration and cytologic examination should be performed as soon as possible on any new mass. Appropriate surgical excision should be done as soon as possible. Regional lymph nodes should be evaluated at regular intervals to detect metastasis of grades II to III mast cell tumors.

13. Can mast cell tumors be treated with chemotherapy?

Yes. When a cutaneous mast cell tumor cannot be controlled by surgery or radiotherapy, medical treatment is appropriate. Prednisone has been the mainstay of treatment, but recent evidence suggests that prednisone alone achieves very short-term remission. Single-agent chemotherapy protocols such as with vinblastine, vincristine, CCNU, and cyclophosphamide can be added to the protocol to lengthen the remission of prednisone-sensitive mast cell tumors from 3 to 9 months. Single-agent chemotherapy does not appear to be as beneficial in the treatment of mast cell tumors than when combination protocols are used.

Prednisone and chemotherapy are indicated in cats with evidence of systemic mastocytosis after splenectomy. All cats with an intestinal mast cell tumor should be treated with prednisone and chemotherapy after surgery.

Histamine-blocking agents (e.g., cimetidine and ranitidine) are helpful, particularly in patients with systemic mastocytosis or when massive histamine release is a concern.

14. What is the expected prognosis for a dog with mast cell disease?

Survival may be prolonged if prednisone and chemotherapy are used in patients in which complete surgical excision or localized irradiation is not possible or that have evidence of metastasis to local lymph nodes.

15. What is the expected prognosis for a cat with mast cell disease?

Survival times of more than 1 year have been reported after splenectomy for a splenic mast cell tumor. Prognosis is poor if mastocythemia occurs concurrently, although prednisone and chemotherapy may achieve short-term remission. The prognosis for an intestinal mast cell tumor is poor, with survival times rarely longer than 4 months after surgery.

CONTROVERSIES

16. What is the diagnostic and prognostic value of a bone marrow aspirate or buffy coat smear?

Apparently very little. Although buffy coat evaluation has been suggested as a test with diagnostic and prognostic value, during a review of more than 50 dogs with mast cells detected on blood or buffy coat smears during a 2-year period, 95.5% of blood smears with mast cells detected during complete blood count determination were from dogs without mast cell tumors. For these dogs, diagnoses included inflammatory disease (28.2%), regenerative anemia (27%), neoplasia other than a mast cell tumor (25.9%), and trauma (11.8%). The two highest counts of mast cells or buffy coat smear were for dogs without mast cell tumors. Random detection of mast cells in blood smears during complete blood count determination in dogs is thus not secondary to mast cell disease.

In yet another review of 88 dogs presenting with incompletely excised mast cell tumors in which a bone marrow aspirate and buffy coat smear were reviewed, only two dogs (2.3%) had mast cells detected on bone marrow aspiration and, of these, only one dog (1.1%) had mast cells detected on a buffy coat smear.

17. Is abdominal ultrasonography useful?

In a review of 88 dogs with incompletely excised mast cell tumors, all 11 dogs with a grade I mast cell tumor had a normal-appearing abdominal ultrasound and were negative for the presence of mast cells on hepatic and splenic fine-needle aspiration cytology, buffy coat cytology smear, and bone marrow aspiration biopsy. Two of the 56 dogs with grade II mast cell tumors had an abnormal abdominal ultrasound (liver/spleen abnormal in appearance but negative for the presence of mast cells), and one of these dogs was positive for the presence of mast cells on a buffy coat cytology smear. Four of the 21 dogs with a grade III mast cell tumor had an abnormal abdominal ultrasonographic examination (liver/spleen). All four of these dogs were positive for the presence of mast cells on cytologic evaluation of hepatic and splenic fine-needle aspirates. Two of the four dogs had positive evidence of mast cells on bone marrow aspiration cytology. One of the four dogs was positive on buffy coat smear evaluation. None of the remaining 82 dogs having a normal abdominal ultrasound had abnormal cytologic findings.

The results of this study suggest that in dogs with grades II and III cutaneous mast cell tumors, abdominal ultrasonography is indicated and, when the liver or spleen has an abnormal ultrasonographic appearance, fine-needle aspiration biopsy is warranted.

BIBLIOGRAPHY

1. Bostock DC: The prognosis following surgical removal of mastocytomas in dogs. J Small Anim Pract 14:27–40, 1973.
2. Buerger RG, Scott DW: Cutaneous mast cell neoplasia in cats: 14 cases (1975–1985). J Am Vet Med Assoc 190:1440–1444, 1987.
3. Frimberger AE, Moore AS, LaRue SM, et al: Radiotherapy of incompletely resected, moderately differentiated mast cell tumors in the dog: 37 cases (1989–1993). J Am Anim Hosp Assoc 33:320–324, 1997.
4. King GK, Harris FD, Hahn KA, et al: Efficacy of an alternating day radiation therapy protocol in 133 dogs with incompletely resected mast cell tumors. Proc Vet Cancer Soc 2000.
5. LaDue T, Price GS, Dodge R, et al: Radiation therapy for incompletely resected canine mast cell tumors. Vet Radiol Ultrasound 39:57–62, 1998.
6. Liska WD, MacEwen EG, Zaki FA, et al: Feline systemic mastocytosis: A review and results of splenectomy in seven cases. J Am Anim Hosp Assoc 15:589–597, 1979.
7. McCaw DL, Miller MA, Bergman PJ, et al: Vincristine therapy for mast cell tumors in dogs. J Vet Intern Med 11:375–378, 1997.
8. McManus PM: Frequency and severity of mastocytemia in dogs with and without mast cell tumors: 120 cases (1995–1997). J Am Vet Med Assoc 215:355–357, 1999.
9. Molander-McCrary H, Henry CJ, Potter K, et al: Cutaneous mast cell tumors in cats: 32 cases (1991–1994). J Am Anim Hosp Assoc 34:281–284, 1998.
10. Patnaik AK, Ehler WN, MacEwen EG: Canine cutaneous mast cell tumors: Morphologic grading and survival time in 83 dogs. Vet Pathol 21:469–474, 1984.
11. Ramirez O, Poteet BA, Hahn KA, et al: The usefulness of hepatic and splenic fine needle aspiration cytology in the clinical staging of canine cutaneous mast cell tumors. An evaluation of 88 dogs (1987–1988). Proc Vet Cancer Soc 2000.
12. Rassnick KM, Moore AS, Williams LE, et al: Treatment of canine mast cell tumors with CCNU (lomustine). J Vet Intern Med 13:601–605, 1999.
13. Thamm DH, Mauldin EA, Vail DM: Prednisone and vinblastine chemotherapy for canine mast cell tumor—41 cases (1992–1997). J Vet Intern Med 13:491–497, 1999.
14. Turrel JM, Kitchell BE, Miller LM, et al: Prognostic factors for radiation treatment of mast cell tumor in 85 dogs. J Am Vet Med Assoc 193:936–940, 1988.

33. HEMANGIOSARCOMA

Alan Hammer, DVM, Dipl ACVIM

1. What breeds of dog are predisposed to developing hemangiosarcoma?

While hemangiosarcoma is a common neoplasm in the dog and may occur in any breed, the following breeds have been shown to be predisposed to developing hemangiosarcoma: German shepherd, golden retriever, English setter, bullmastiff, Great Dane, and the boxer.

2. What is the youngest dog reported with hemangiosarcoma?

The average age of dogs with hemangiosarcoma is 8 to 10 years; the youngest dog I have seen with hemangiosarcoma was a 5-month-old yellow Labrador retriever. Hemangiosarcoma is the second most common histologic tumor type in immature dogs; the most common type is lymphoma.

3. Is the ultrasonogram depicted below typical of splenic hemangiosarcoma?

Yes. This ultrasonogram displays the large size these tumors may achieve along with the typical mixed echogenicity associated with hemangiosarcoma. The hypoechoic areas usually represent hemorrhagic or necrotic regions in the tumor. While other neoplasms may have similar ultrasonographic appearance, the finding of this sort of mass arising from the spleen should raise the index of suspicion for hemangiosarcoma.

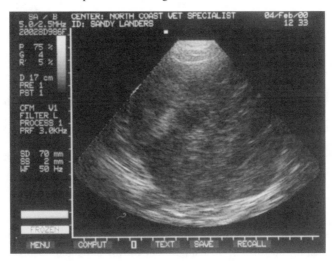

Abdominal ultrasound of the spleen in a 12-year-old spayed female German shepherd.

4. Where else do hemangiosarcomas arise besides the spleen?

Hemangiosarcoma is a neoplasm arising from the vascular endothelial cells. Therefore, it may arise from any tissue with blood vessels. Common sites include the spleen, right atrium, liver, subcutaneous tissues, and kidneys.

5. What is the cause of hemangiosarcoma?

Most hemangiosarcomas arising in dogs appear to be spontaneous in nature and do not have an identifiable etiology. Some known causes include strontium-90, ultraviolet radiation (associated with dermal hemangiosarcomas), and diethylnitrosamine. Thorium dioxide and vinyl chloride monomer have been associated with hemangiosarcomas in humans.

6. Why are dogs with hemangiosarcoma presented?

The most frequent presentation is weakness and acute collapse. These signs are the result of tumor rupture and acute intraabdominal hemorrhage. Dogs with right atrial hemangiosarcoma also may be presented with acute collapse secondary to either cardiac arrhythmias or pericardial tamponade. Dogs with subcutaneous hemangiosarcoma are presented when the owners palpate the mass. These are often bruised in appearance.

7. What is microangiopathic hemolysis?

The tortuous neoplastic vessels and fibrin strands in tumors may cause erythrocyte fragmentation. Microangiopathic hemolysis is characterized by fragmented red blood cells and usually results in a regenerative anemia. Disseminated intravascular coagulation (DIC) is another cause of microangiopathic hemolysis.

8. What is leukoerythroblastic reaction?

The presence of immature neutrophils (bands or metamyelocytes) and nucleated red blood cells in the peripheral blood. Leukoerythroblastosis is most commonly observed in dogs with hemangiosarcoma or immune-mediated hemolytic anemia. It may occur because of hemorrhage or necrosis within the tumor, intravascular hemolysis, or inflammation associated with the neoplasm.

9. Which erythrocyte morphologic changes are associated with hemangiosarcoma?

Fragmented erythrocytes (schistocytes), acanthocytes, and nucleated red blood cells.

10. What percentage of dogs with splenic hemangiosarcoma have a platelet count below 50,000/μl prior to surgery?

While the median platelet count in dogs with hemangiosarcoma is 137,000/μl, almost 30% of dogs have platelet counts below 50,000/μl. This is an important fact for the surgeon.

11. Why do many of the dogs on which I perform splenectomies develop ventricular arrhythmias postoperatively?

Arrhythmias may arise for a variety of reasons, including myocardial tissue hypoxia secondary to anemia and hypovolemia, myocardial metastases, and catecholamine release. An additional cause may involve the release of various cytokines (e.g., tumor necrosis factor and interleukin-1) from the tumor; these cytokines can have a negative impact on myocardial function.

12. I recently diagnosed systemic fungal disease in a dog based on the thoracic radiographs. When the dog died, it turned out to be diffuse pulmonary hemangiosarcoma. What are the thoracic radiographic findings in dogs with hemangiosarcoma?

The most common radiographic pattern in dogs with pulmonary metastases is poorly defined coalescing nodules. Well-circumscribed nodules are less common. Occasionally, alveolar patterns may be noted secondary to hemorrhage. Thoracic radiography has almost an 80% sensitivity in detecting metastatic hemangiosarcoma.

13. Is it true that hemangiosarcoma commonly metastasizes to the brain and spinal cord?

Yes. Hemangiosarcoma is the mesenchymal tumor most commonly metastasizing to the central nervous system. In one report, 14% of dogs with hemangiosarcoma had metastases to the central nervous system, and half of those had clinical signs referable to that process. Lesions are usually located in the cerebrum, predominantly in the gray matter. More than

90% of dogs with central nervous system metastasis have concurrent pulmonary involvement; therefore, thoracic radiographs can be very helpful.

14. How do I treat a dog with DIC due to hemangiosarcoma?

DIC is a syndrome secondary to another primary problem. Removing the underlying cause (in this case, the neoplasm) is the most important step. It is also important to correct any acid-base or electrolyte abnormalities, hypovolemia, and tissue hypoxia. Replacing missing coagulation factors with either fresh, whole blood or fresh frozen plasma is vital. Heparin should be administered at 10 to 100 units/kg subcutaneously every 6 hours to enhance antithrombin III activity. The initial dose of heparin may be incubated with the blood or plasma at 37° C for 30 minutes prior to administration. Unfortunately, the prognosis is still grave. It is difficult to monitor heparin therapy because of the need for frequent coagulation studies. Various doses and schedules have been proposed, and there is no consensus regarding the use of heparin.

15. I recently sent portions of a large splenic mass to the pathologist, who diagnosed splenic hematoma, but I was convinced that it was a hemangiosarcoma. Is this a common problem?

Unfortunately, this is a common situation. Even at universities, where the entire spleen is submitted, this can be a problem. Hematomas and necrotic or hemorrhagic areas may compose much of the actual tumor volume. It is difficult to select representative areas that will fit in the small formalin jars used to transport specimens. I recommend collecting specimens at the juncture of the tumor and normal tissue and collecting at least three samples. You may wish to consider collecting other samples and submitting them later if there is a discrepancy between the histopathology results and your clinical impression. In one study, hematomas constituted 12% of lesions in spleens. That study correlated survival times with pathology findings and clinical impression.

16. What is the expected survival time in a dog with splenic hemangiosarcoma treated only by splenectomy?

The median survival is only 60 to 90 days. Another way to look at these data is that only 6–7% of dogs treated by splenectomy alone will be alive 1 year later.

17. Is staging dogs with hemangiosarcoma of any clinical significance?

Dogs with splenic hemangiosarcoma are staged as follows:

Stage I—tumor confined to spleen

Stage II—ruptured spleen but no gross metastases

Stage III—metastatic disease present.

A recent study did not find any difference in survival following splenectomy based on stage I or stage II disease. The median survival was only 86 days. However, other studies using adjuvant therapy after splenectomy have found that dogs with early-stage disease do better than those with advanced-stage disease.

18. How do I manage a dog with right atrial hemangiosarcoma?

Initially, the goal is to stabilize the patient. This may require pericardiocentesis to correct pericardial effusion and tamponade or antiarrhythmic agents if arrhythmias are present. Long-term management may involve multiple pericardiocentesis, pericardectomy (which can now be performed thoracoscopically), or resection of the right auricular appendage if the tumor is confined to that location. Adjuvant chemotherapy using a doxorubicin-based protocol can reduce the tumor volume and, in some cases, result in complete remission with resolution of the pericardial effusion. Unfortunately, partial and complete remissions are not durable and at best last only 6 to 8 months.

19. I recently excised a mass that the pathologist diagnosed as an undifferentiated sarcoma. The differential diagnosis included poorly differentiated hemangiosarcoma. Are there special stains that would indicate this tumor as arising from endothelial cells?

Yes. Immunohistochemistry can be used to detect factor VIII-related antigen (von Willebrand factor) on the surface of the tumor cells. Antibodies directed against CD31 may also be helpful, as can the *Ulex europaeus* agglutinin I.

20. The following electrocardiogram was obtained from a dog postsplenectomy. How would you manage this patient?

This dog has ventricular tachycardia. I would correct any acid-base, electrolyte (including magnesium), hypovolemia, and decreased oxygen-carrying capacity problems that are present. I would start lidocaine at 50 μcg/kg/min after a bolus of 2 mg/kg and increase it to 75 μcg/kg/min. If that were insufficient to control the arrhythmia, I would add procainamide at 8 mg/kg intravenously or intramuscularly every 6 hours. Postoperative arrhythmias usually resolve within 72 to 96 hours. If oral maintenance therapy is deemed necessary, mexilitine at 4 to 8 mg/kg every 8 hours or procainamide at 8 to 20 mg/kg every 8 hours can be used.

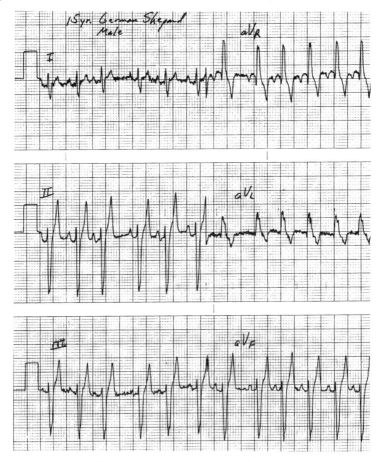

Six-lead electrocardiogram from a 15-year-old neutered male German shepherd with splenic hemangiosarcoma. Paper speed = 25 mm/sec, standard calibration (1 cm = 1mV).

21. Do cats get hemangiosarcoma?

Yes. The most common sites are cutaneous and subcutaneous, spleen, liver, and lung. The metastatic rate is very high in cats, and survival times are usually shorter than in dogs treated with surgery alone.

22. What prognostic factors are there for dogs with hemangiosarcoma that are surgically reduced to stage 0 disease?

Stage 0 disease is when there is no gross tumor following surgery. In dogs in which stage 0 status has been achieved, the use of adjuvant chemotherapy may be helpful. The primary site (i.e., subcutaneous, splenic, or right atrial) is also prognostic, as is the presence or absence of arrhythmias. Small, low-grade, dermal hemangiosarcoma may do well, but the more deeply they are located, the more aggressive their behavior.

23. Of what value is radiotherapy in the management of hemangiosarcoma?

Radiation therapy provides good local control when dealing with cutaneous, subcutaneous, or soft tissue tumors. In the latter two forms, adjuvant chemotherapy will be necessary because the metastatic rate is high.

24. In addition to chemotherapy, radiotherapy, and surgery, are there any other modalities to consider in treating hemangiosarcoma?

Yes. Use of liposome-encapsulated muramyltripeptide phosphatidylethanolamine (LE-MTP-PE) following splenectomy and doxorubicin-cyclophosphamide chemotherapy resulted in improved disease-free interval and prolonged survival compared with controls treated with surgery and chemotherapy alone. LE-MTP-PE is an immunotherapy agent that stimulates macrophage activity and is associated with increased tumor necrosis factor-α and interleukin-6 production. Unfortunately, this agent is not yet commercially available.

25. Which chemotherapy agent is believed to be most active in treating hemangiosarcomas in dogs?

Doxorubicin (Adriamycin) is the agent thought to be most active in treating hemangiosarcomas. Its use as a single agent gives results comparable to those seen when cyclophosphamide and vincristine are also used. There is less toxicity with single-agent doxorubicin (see below).

26. Suppose I have a dog with a splenic mass and the owners are unsure about what to do. If it is benign, they will proceed with surgery. If it is hemangiosarcoma, they will not pursue treatment. Are there any predictive factors that can help the owners with this decision?

Yes. Anemia, splenic rupture, nucleated red blood cells, and abnormal erythrocyte morphology are predictive of splenic neoplasia. A good review of the blood smear can be very helpful.

27. What percentage of dogs have hemangiosarcoma confined solely to their spleen at the time of surgery?

Only 12%; this is a very aggressive tumor.

28. I recently saw a whippet with a cutaneous hemangiosarcoma in the inguinal region. The pathology report indicated complete excision, and the tumor did not extend into the subcutaneous tissue. Is adjuvant chemotherapy necessary?

No. Hemangiosarcomas limited to the skin have a lower metastatic rate. They often arise in thin-haired regions of the body such as the inguinal or preputial areas and may be solar radiation-induced. Clinically, they present as "strawberry-like" lesions that hemorrhage easily. Surgical excision is often all that is necessary.

29. What is considered an ideal evaluation of the dog with suspected hemangiosarcoma?
If patient stability and time permit, the ideal evaluation should include a complete blood count, biochemical profile, urinalysis, hemostasis screen, abdominal and thoracic radiographs, abdominal ultrasonography, and cardiac evaluation through echocardiography and electrocardiography.

30. What adjuvant chemotherapy protocols are available, and how long should chemotherapy be given?
The three most common protocols are based on doxorubicin. The simplest is single-agent doxorubicin at 30 mg/m^2 intravenously every 3 weeks for five treatments. Another protocol (AC) uses doxorubicin at 30 mg/m^2 intravenously on day 1 and oral cyclophosphamide at 50 to 75 mg/m^2 on days 3 to 6. The cycle is repeated every 3 weeks. Four to five cycles are recommended. The most aggressive protocol (VAC) uses doxorubicin at 30 mg/m^2 intravenously and cyclophosphamide at 100 mg/m^2 intravenously on day 1 and vincristine at 0.7 mg/m^2 intravenously on days 8 and 15. The cycle is repeated on day 22, and four to five cycles are recommended. The median survival for the first protocol using single-agent doxorubicin was 172 days; for the protocol using doxorubicin and oral cyclophosphamide, the median survival was 202 days. Finally, the median survival for the most aggressive protocol was 172 days.

31. What toxicities may be seen with VAC chemotherapy?
Toxicities may include myelosuppression (i.e., neutropenia and thrombocytopenia), gastroenterocolitis, anaphylactic reactions, cardiotoxicity, hemorrhagic cystitis, extravasation tissue slough, and dermatologic changes.

32. How can the gastrointestinal toxicities be avoided?
Bismuth subsalicylate (PeptoBismol) can ameliorate the enterocolitis associated with doxorubicin. The recommended dose is one caplet per 20 lb of body weight twice a day for 1 week following doxorubicin administration. If vomiting is a concern, metoclopramide at 0.2 mg/kg orally three times a day or prochlorperazine at 0.06 mg/kg orally twice a day can be used.

33. How should a febrile, neutropenic dog be managed?
Very aggressively. Administer fluids along with a combination of a first-generation cephalosporin (such as cefazolin 10 mg/lb intravenously every 8 hours) and an aminoglycoside (such as amikacin 3 mg/lb intravenously every 8 hours). If shock is present, methylprednisolone succinate (Solu-Cortef) should be administered. The average time to normal temperature is 14 hours, and the average time spent in the hospital is 2 days. Aggressive therapy results in a high recovery rate.

BIBLIOGRAPHY

1. Hammer AS, Bailey MQ, Sagartz JE: Retrospective assessment of thoracic radiographic findings in metastatic canine hemangiosarcoma. Vet Radiol Ultrasound 34:235–238, 1993.
2. Hammer AS, Couto CG, Filppi J, et al: Efficacy and toxicity of VAC chemotherapy (vincristine, doxorubicin, and cyclophosphamide) in dogs with hemangiosarcoma. J Vet Intern Med 5:160–166, 1991.
3. Hammer AS, Couto CG, Swardson C, et al: Hemostatic abnormalities in dogs with hemangiosarcoma. J Vet Intern Med 5:11–14, 1991.
4. Johnson KA, Powers BE, Withrow SJ, et al: Splenomegaly in dogs: Predictors of neoplasia and survival after splenectomy. J Vet Intern Med 3:160–166, 1989.
5. Keller ET, Madewell BR: Locations and types of neoplasms in immature dogs: 69 cases (1964–1989). J Am Vet Med Assoc 200:1530–1532, 1992.
6. Kraje AC, Mears EA, Hahn KA, et al: Unusual metastatic behavior and clinicopathologic findings in eight cats with cutaneous or visceral hemangiosarcoma. J Am Vet Med Assoc 214:670–672, 1999.
7. Ogilvie GK, Powers BE, Mallinckrodt CH, et al: Surgery and doxorubicin in dogs with hemangiosarcoma. J Vet Intern Med 10:379–384, 1996.

8. Sorenmo KU, Jeglum KA, Helfand SC: Chemotherapy of canine hemangiosarcoma with doxorubicin and cyclophosphamide. J Vet Intern Med 7:370–376, 1993.
9. Spangler WL, Kass PH: Pathologic factors affecting postsplenectomy survival in dogs. J Vet Intern Med 11:166–171, 1997.
10. Vail DM, MacEwen EG, Kurzman ID, et al: Liposome-encapsulated muramyl tripeptide phosphatidylethanolamine adjuvant immunotherapy for splenic hemangiosarcoma in the dog: a randomized multi-institutional clinical trial. Clin Cancer Res 1:1165–1170, 1995.
11. Ward H, Fox LE, Calderwood-Mays MB, et al: Cutaneous hemangiosarcoma in 25 dogs: A retrospective study. J Vet Intern Med 8:345–348, 1994.
12. Wood CA, Moore AS, Gliatto JM, et al: Prognosis for dogs with stage I or II splenic hemangiosarcoma treated by splenectomy alone: 32 cases (1991–1993). J Am Anim Hosp Assoc 34:417–421, 1998.
13. Wrigley RH, Park RD, Konde LJ, et al: Ultrasonographic features of splenic hemangiosarcoma in dogs: 18 cases (1980–1986). J Am Vet Med Assoc 192:1113–1117, 1988.

34. CANINE TRANSMISSIBLE VENEREAL TUMOR

Steven Susaneck, DVM, Dipl ACVIM

1. How are transmissible venereal tumors (TVT) transmitted?

TVT is most often transmitted during coitus by transfer of cells from the affected dog to the healthy dog. The tumor may also be transmitted to nongenital areas such as the nose, the eyes, and the oral cavity by social behaviors such as licking and sniffing. The tumor appears to be more easily transmitted if there are abrasions or breaks in the integrity of the mucosal surface.

2. List some factors that are unique to TVT.

• TVT appears to be unique to the dog in its natural form.
• The tumors are transmitted by direct transmission of cells from carrier to recipient.
• TVT is the only tumor that is transplantable to adult, immunocompetent, allogenic dogs
• The chromosomal compliment of this tumor is constant worldwide, with 58 ± 5 chromosomes found in the tumor. The normal canine chromosomal compliment is 78.

3. What environmental factors appear to influence the reported incidence of the tumor?

These tumors have been reported in all parts of the world, but most commonly in temperate areas. Enzootic areas for TVT include southern United States, southeastern Europe, Central and South America, Japan, the Far East and parts of Africa. Animals at highest risk are those living in areas of high concentration of free-roaming dogs, inadequately enforced leash laws, and poorly controlled breeding.

4. Describe the typical clinical presentation of a TVT.

Tumors are located primarily on the external genitalia of the male and female dog. In the male the tumor is most commonly located along the shaft of the penis in the area of the gland of the penis. In many cases extrusion of the penis is necessary to visualize the tumor.

In the bitch the tumor is most commonly located in the vestibule of the vagina and can usually be visualized protruding through the lips of the vagina. The tumors range in size from 0.5 mm to more than 10 cm in diameter. They are usually cauliflower-like in appearance and are often friable. They are red to flesh colored.

5. What are the most common presenting signs for dogs with TVT?

In the male the most common presenting complaint is a serosanguinous discharge from the prepuce. In the female the most common complaint is vaginal bleeding or the presence of a mass protruding through the lips of the vulva.

6. Is cytology usually diagnostic for this tumor?

Yes. TVT has a very unique cytological appearance that is diagnostic in most cases. Because of the friable nature of the tumor, cells are shed quite readily.

7. What is the cytological appearance of a typical TVT?

The cells appear round to oval; mitotic figures are common; and the nuclear to cytoplasmic ratio is less than one. Chromatin clumping is common, and most cells contain one to two prominent nucleoli. Most cells contain multiple clear, cytoplasmic vacuoles that often appear arranged in chains. Cytological preparations made from the discharge or by impression smears of the surface often contain a large numbers of inflammatory cells. When seen in atypical locations the cytology may resemble other round cell tumors.

8. Can TVTs metastasize?

Yes. Although metastasis is uncommon, it has been reported. The most common site of metastasis is regional lymph nodes. Other distant sites that have been reported include skin and subcutaneous tissue, eye, liver, spleen, kidney, peritoneum, lung, and central nervous system. Direct extension of the tumor may be seen in the oral cavity, tonsils and lips.

9. What factors indicate that the immune system is important in the development and progression of TVT?

The TVT possesses tumor-associated antigens as determined by both immunodiffusion and Elisa techniques. A humoral immune response has been described. Specific antitumor antibodies of the IgG class have been detected in the sera of affected dogs. Tumor progression and metastasis occur in immunologically incompetent and compromised hosts. Increased numbers of lymphocytes and macrophages are seen in regressing tumors. Regression of the tumors is associated with immunity to subsequent reinfections. Spontaneous regression of the tumor has been reported.

10. What treatments are available for dogs with TVT?

Treatment methods include surgical excision, radiation therapy, chemotherapy, and immunotherapy.

11. Of the available treatments, which treatment or treatments are the most effective?

The most effective treatments are chemotherapy and radiation therapy.

12. What chemotherapy protocols are used in the treatment of TVT?

Single-agent therapy with vincristine is efficacious and cost-effective therapy. Four to eight weekly injections of vincristine at a dose of 0.5–0.75 mg/m² body weight are recommended. Cure rates of well over 90% have been reported with this treatment. In one study of 41 dogs treated with single-agent vincristine, 39 were cured. In another study using vincristine at a dose of 0.6 mg/m², complete remission was seen in 138 of 140 dogs treated.

Doxorubicin is also quite effective in the treatment of TVT. The typical dose is 30 mg/m² for one to four treatments.

13. What is the role of radiation in the treatment of dogs with TVT?

Radiation therapy is also an effective method of treating TVT. In one study, 18 dogs were treated with a total dose ranging from 10 to 30 Gy. Seven of eight dogs were cured with a single dose of 10 Gy. The other 10 dogs received multiple doses.

In another study, 15 of 15 dogs were cured with cobalt therapy.

14. What are the major disadvantages of surgery?

In most cases the tumor is too large and in a location that prevents adequate complete surgical excision. Recurrence rates after surgery are 20–60%.

15. Have biological response modifiers been effective in the treatment of TVT?

No. To date, treatments using biological response modifiers have not resulted in response rates comparable to those obtained using chemotherapy and radiation therapy.

BIBLIOGRAPHY

1. Rogers K: Transmissible venereal tumor. Compend Contin Educ 19(9):1036–1045,1997.

2. Calvert CA, Leifer CE, MacEwen EG: Vincristine for treatment of transmissible venereal tumor in the dog. J Am Vet Med Assoc 176:983–986, 1993.
3. Ogilvie GK, Moore AS: Tumors of the reproductive system. In Ogilvie GK, Moore AS (eds): Managing the Veterinary Cancer Patient. Trenton NJ, Veterinary Learning Systems, 1995, pp 415–429.
4. Madewell BR, Theilen GH: Skin tumors of mesenchymal origin. In Theilen GH, Madewell BR (eds): Veterinary Cancer Medicine, 2nd ed. Philadelphia, Lea & Febiger, 1987, pp 282–309.

35. THYMOMA

Karelle A. Meleo, DVM, Dipl ACVIM, Dipl ACVR

1. What is the most common presenting clinical sign in dogs with thymoma?

Coughing. Other signs related to the respiratory tract such as dyspnea, decreased exercise tolerance, and listlessness may be seen. Nonspecific signs such as decreased appetite and weight loss have also been reported.

2. Patients with thymoma may have Horner's syndrome due to tumor encroaching on what anatomic structure?

The vagosympathetic trunk.

3. What two mechanisms can lead to dysphagia or regurgitation in dogs or cats with thymoma?

The mechanical obstruction caused by a large intrathoracic mass can lead to these signs. In addition, megaesophagus may be seen secondary to myasthenia gravis.

4. Is there a gender predisposition for thymoma in dogs?

Yes; 40 of 61 reported dogs (65%) were female.

5. List paraneoplastic syndromes associated with thymomas in dogs and cats.

Myasthenia gravis
Hypercalcemia
Pure red cell aplasia
Polymyositis
Atrioventricular block

Paraneoplastic syndromes are less common in cats than in dogs.

6. What is the most specific test available for myasthenia gravis?

The presence of serum acetylcholine-receptor antibody.

7. In a cat with a cranial mediastinal mass, what is the main differential diagnosis other than thymoma?

Lymphoma.

8. Why can it be difficult to differentiate between lymphoma and thymoma on the basis of cytologic evaluation of an aspirate of a mediastinal mass?

Although thymomas originate from the thymic epithelium, they may contain a significant number of mature lymphocytes.

Differentiating between lymphoma and thymoma seems to be an especially common problem in cats. This differentiation can even be difficult on the basis of small biopsy samples (such as core needle biopsies). It is very important to keep both differentials in mind when evaluating a patient with a mediastinal mass. Signalment may be helpful with this. Thymoma generally affects cats that average 9 to 10 years of age, although cats as young as 3 years of age may be affected. The median age of cats with mediastinal lymphoma has been reported to be 2 years (mean 3.4 years), with most being feline leukemia positive.

9. How can ultrasound be used to help differentiate between lymphoma and thymoma in dogs?

Thymomas are often cystic, while lymphomas in the mediastinum are usually poorly echogenic.

10. Despite three aspiration cytology samples in a cat with a cranial mediastinal mass, you have been unable to definitively differentiate the tumor as lymphoma or thymoma. You have recommended core needle biopsy as your next step but have warned the owners that this procedure also may not be definitive. The owners want to know why you do not just use surgery to try to remove the mass, submitting the excised tissue to histopathology, especially because you have told them that if this is a thymoma, it should be removed. Justify your diagnostic recommendation.

Core needle biopsy is less invasive for the patient. The most important considerations are wound healing and the possibility of infection. Chemotherapy rather than surgical resection is recommended for the treatment of lymphoma. If the patient is ultimately diagnosed with lymphoma, chemotherapy would likely need to be delayed following a thoracotomy, or you will need to take the risk of immunosuppression in a patient in the perioperative period. Also, the patient will have gone through a painful procedure unnecessarily.

11. In addition to epithelial cells and lymphocytes, what cell type is frequently seen on cytologic evaluation of thymomas?

Mast cells. The presence of mast cells is another factor that can be used to help differentiate between lymphoma and thymoma.

12. In general, what treatment options can be considered for dogs and cats with thymoma?

Surgery, radiation therapy, chemotherapy, or a combination of these.

13. Surgery is considered the treatment of choice in which species: dogs or cats?

Cats.

In one study of 12 cats, two died in the postoperative period, four died of unrelated causes with no evidence of thymoma, and the other six cats survived 3 to 36 months following surgery, with a median survival of 16 months.

14. What is the reported median survival time for dogs with thymoma that undergo surgery?

Seven days.

15. What is the most significant prognostic factor for dogs with thymoma?

The absence of megaesophagus. In one study, the median survival for dogs with thymoma and megaesophagus was 4 days, with none surviving more than 71 days. The 1-year survival rate for dogs without megaesophagus was 83%.

16. What is a common life-threatening complication in dogs with thymoma and megaesophagus?

Aspiration pneumonia. This is an especially common postoperative complication and one reason why the survival time for dogs with thymoma that undergo surgery is so short.

17. Give two ways in which prednisone can play a role in the treatment of patients with thymoma.

Prednisone can act as a chemotherapeutic agent in lymphoid malignancies, and prednisone therefore may result in a decrease in the size of a thymoma due to activity against the lymphoid component of the tumor.

Prednisone may reduce acetylcholine-receptor antibody levels and therefore can decrease clinical signs associated with myasthenia gravis.

18. Why should a clinician use caution in prescribing prednisone for patients with thymoma?

Aspiration pneumonia is a common complication, and the immunosuppressive effects of glucocorticoids can increase the severity of infection.

19. In irradiating a patient with a thymoma using parallel opposed dorsal and ventral fields, which organs or tissues are at risk for late-term (several months or longer after treatment) radiation toxicity? What signs might be seen if this toxicity occurs?

The heart, lungs, and spinal cord are at risk. Heart pericarditis, pericardial effusion, myocarditis, and fibrosis; lung fibrosis, and pneumonitis; and spinal cord paralysis or paresis may be seen.

Custom field-shaping devices are recommended to minimize the volume of lung that is exposed to radiation.

20. How successful is radiation therapy in treating dogs with thymoma?

Orthovoltage radiation in combination with prednisone has been reported for the treatment of thymoma in one dog. A 60% reduction in tumor size and reversal of clinical signs of myasthenia was seen when a total dose of 54 Gy in 9 weekly fractions was delivered. The dog remained free of clinical signs for 6 months. In the author's experience of treating a limited number of dogs with thymoma with radiation therapy, complete responses and survival greater than 1 year are rare.

21. Can radiation therapy be used to treat cats with thymoma?

In the author's experience, the prognosis for cats with thymoma treated with surgery and radiation therapy is excellent. Radiation therapy alone can also be effective for the treatment of cats with thymoma, but surgery is still likely the treatment of choice in this species. Because the long-term prognosis for these cats is excellent, dose-fractionation protocols that minimize long-term adverse effects should be used.

22. Can chemotherapy ever be used successfully to treat thymoma?

In some cases, yes. There is a report of one dog that was treated with a combination of cyclophosphamide, vincristine, and prednisone following surgical resection of a thymoma that was still in clinical remission at 29 months. Other patients treated with this protocol have not responded as well; more work needs to be done in this area. The most effective chemotherapy protocols in treating people with thymoma include the drug cisplatin.

Chemotherapy has not been reported for the treatment of cats with thymoma, although prednisone can be used as part of the therapy especially if myasthenia gravis is present.

CONTROVERSIES

23. If chemotherapy and radiation are not particularly successful in treating thymoma in dogs, why not consider surgery and take special care in preventing aspiration pneumonia?

If megaesophagus is present, it is very difficult to prevent aspiration pneumonia in the perioperative period. In addition, because thymomas are often large and invasive, complete surgical resection may not be possible.

However, if the thymoma is small, surgery can be curative and should be considered. If megaesophagus is not present, the prognosis following surgical resection is fairly good. The reported mean and median survival time for this group is 19 and 16 months, respectively.

Ultrasonographic evaluation, computed tomography, or magnetic resonance imaging may be helpful in determining the size and invasiveness of the tumor and therefore may be helpful in determining if an individual patient may benefit from surgery.

24. Is histology a useful prognostic factor for dogs with thymoma?

While histologic type has not been shown to be an independent prognostic factor in dogs with thymoma that were treated with surgery alone, the influence of histology on prognosis for dogs treated with radiation therapy has yet to be determined. Because of the radiosensitivity of lymphocytes, dogs with thymomas that have a preponderance of lymphocytes may respond better to radiation therapy than those in which the epithelial component of the tumor predominates.

25. Do all dogs with thymoma need treatment?

Some may survive an acceptable time without therapy. Survival times of greater than 1 year have been reported. Obviously, a patient with dyspnea cannot have a good quality of life unless the tumor is decreased in size. If there are signs of myasthenia gravis, they must be managed, but there likely is a subpopulation of dogs that have slow-growing thymomas and can be long-term survivors with minimal or no intervention.

BIBLIOGRAPHY

1. Atwater SW, Powers BE, Park RD, et al: Canine thymoma: 23 cases (1980–1991). J Am Vet Med Assoc 205:1007–1013, 1994.
2. Cores BR, Berg J, Carpenter JL, et al: Surgical treatment of thymoma in cats: 12 cases (1987–1992). J Am Vet Med Assoc 204:1782–1785, 1994.
3. Hitt ME, Shaw DP, Hogan FM, et al: Radiation treatment for thymoma in a dog. J Am Vet Med Assoc 190:1187–1190, 1987.
4. Ogilvie GK, Moore AS: Managing the Veterinary Cancer Patient. Trenton, NJ, Veterinary Learning Systems, 1995, pp 445–449.

36. MESOTHELIOMA

Karelle A. Meleo, DVM, Dipl ACVIM, Dipl ACVR

1. What is the mean age at presentation for dogs with mesothelioma?

Eight years. The reported range is 4 to 15 years.

2. Is there a gender predisposition for dogs and cats with mesothelioma?

Yes. A female predisposition has been reported in dogs. Mesothelioma is less common in cats than in dogs, but three of four cats in the literature have been female.

3. Why does everyone always ask for common signalments? Does it matter if the patient is typical or unusual?

Such facts sometimes are easy to use to quiz students and residents, so they show up on exams. Sometimes it is just enjoyable to know some trivia. However, in diseases such as mesothelioma, which can be a diagnostic challenge, topics like age, gender, or an environmental history (indoor/outdoor) of the patient can help in ranking differentials, especially if one has to consider both neoplastic and nonneoplastic conditions in a patient with pleural or peritoneal effusion.

4. You are performing a cytologic examination on serosanguineous fluid obtained from a pleural effusion of a 7-year-old German shepherd. You see basophilic cells arranged mostly in clusters, with 5 to 10 cells per cluster. These cells have a high nuclear-to-cytoplasmic ratio, eccentrically placed nuclei, and prominent nucleoli. List three differentials to explain the cells you see.

Mesothelioma, carcinoma, and reactive mesothelial cells.

Differentiating between these three situations can be difficult. Normal mesothelial cells line the pleural, peritoneal, and pericardial cavities and the surface of the testes. When this lining becomes affected by neoplasia or other irritation, the mesothelial cells become reactive, and they cytologically are very difficult to distinguish from true neoplastic mesothelial cells as well as clusters of carcinoma cells.

5. How do I make a definitive diagnosis of mesothelioma?

Histologic evaluation of affected tissue is the only way to make a definitive diagnosis. Generally, surgical exploration is performed, but core needle biopsy guided via ultrasound or a computed tomography scan can occasionally be successful. Laparoscopy or thoracoscopy also can be used to obtain samples.

If an exploratory or a scoping procedure is done in a patient with body cavity effusion, biopsy of the pleura, peritoneum, or pericardium (as indicated) is important even if no gross lesions are present.

6. What is the typical gross appearance of sclerosing mesothelioma? In what gender and breed does it typically occur?

Sclerosing mesothelioma typically appears as thick fibrous linings of the pleural or abdominal cavities. It is seen primarily in males, and German shepherds have been reported to be overrepresented in the population of dogs with this unusual condition.

7. In people, mesothelioma is strongly linked to exposure to what carcinogen?

Aerosolized asbestos fibers.

8. Has there been any association between environmental carcinogens and mesothelioma in dogs?

Yes. Dogs belonging to owners who were exposed to asbestos have been reported to be at increased risk for mesothelioma. In addition, chrysotile asbestos fibers have been found in increased levels in the lungs of dogs with mesothelioma compared with normal dogs. Dogs in an urban environment overall seem to be at higher risk for mesothelioma.

9. Is visceral metastasis of mesothelioma common?

No. Although this neoplasm frequently implants on the surface of organs, it rarely exhibits true metastatic behavior in dogs or cats despite the presence of lymphatic invasion on tissue biopsy.

10. In what anatomic location can surgery be useful in the management of mesothelioma?

The pericardium. Pericardectomy can decrease the clinical signs associated with mesothelioma of the pericardium by preventing the effusion from causing cardiac tamponade.

11. Can chemotherapy be used to treat dogs or cats with mesothelioma?

Yes. There is a report of one dog treated with intravenous mitoxantrone (5 mg/m^2 intravenously every 21 days) that experienced a complete remission lasting 42 days. One dog has also been reported to have experienced a complete response to intravenous doxorubicin (30 mg/m^2). Intracavitary chemotherapy has also been reported to be successful in dogs with mesothelioma.

12. What is intracavitary chemotherapy?

Chemotherapy that is administered within a body cavity. Generally, it is given into the cavity that contains the neoplasm.

13. Which drug has been reported to be successful in the treatment of mesothelioma in dogs when it is delivered by an intracavitary route?

Success with cisplatin has been published. Success with carboplatin and mitoxantrone have been reported anecdotally.

14. What is the technique for delivering intracavitary cisplatin?

Diuresis with normal saline is required when cisplatin is given intravenously. One published protocol is 105 ml/m^2/hour for 14 hours prior and 6 hours postadministration of cisplatin. More compressed diuresis schedules can be considered (such as an 8-hour total diuresis schedule) but should be used with caution in patients with pleural or pericardial effusion.

After the initial diuresis, the cavity is drained of as much fluid as possible. Cisplatin at a dosage of 50 to 70 mg/m^2 is then mixed with the appropriate volume of saline, warmed to 37° C, and infused in to the cavity using a 16-gauge cannula over 15 minutes. A dose of 250 ml/m^2 is recommended for intrapleural administration and 1000 ml/m^2 for intraperitoneal administration. The cannula should be placed aseptically.

Unless there are signs of volume overload such as severe dyspnea, the fluid should not be removed. Mild dyspnea should be expected with the volume of saline recommended for pleural infusion.

Appropriate measures should be taken to ensure that all personnel are protected from accidental exposure to the chemotherapy during the procedure.

15. What do you do if the patient has both peritoneal and pleural involvement of mesothelioma?

The cisplatin dose should be divided between the two cavities, but otherwise the technique remains the same, including the volume of the intracavitary infusion.

16. How deep into the tissue can I expect cisplatin to penetrate?

Approximately 3 mm. This may not be an issue in the treatment of mesothelioma but should be taken in to consideration in deciding whether intracavitary treatment is an appropriate therapy in general. Intracavitary chemotherapy may not be successful in the treatment of sclerosing mesothelioma because of the thickness of the tissue.

17. What is the dose-limiting toxicity for intracavitary cisplatin in dogs?

Nephrotoxicity. This is why saline diuresis before and after the chemotherapy is essential.

18. Why might intravenous sodium thiosulfate be useful in treating dogs with intracavitary cisplatin?

It can potentially protect from the nephrotoxicity of cisplatin and thus might allow a higher dosage to be given.

Sodium thiosulfate given intravenously can neutralize cisplatin as it enters the circulation. The small amount of sodium thiosulfate that enters the pleural or peritoneal cavity has little overall effect on the efficacy of cisplatin within the cavity.

In people, the administration of sodium thiosulfate allows the intraperitoneal dosage of cisplatin to be safely increased to approximately three times the dosage that can be given in the absence of sodium thiosulfate. This potentially can increase the therapeutic index of intracavitary cisplatin.

In dogs treated with intracavitary cisplatin at a dosage of 50 mg/m^2 accompanied by saline diuresis, none developed renal failure. Some of the dogs received sodium thiosulfate, but because 50 to 70 mg/m^2 seems to be a safe dosage in dogs, the effect of sodium thiosulfate is not known. Escalating the dosage of cisplatin given into the body cavity, while giving sodium thiosulfate intravenously, remains to be studied.

19. What are the adverse effects of intracavitary cisplatin in dogs?

Vomiting is the most common adverse effect reported. Luekopenia can also be seen. Mild dyspnea should be expected with intrapleural administration. Disseminated intravascular coagulation was reported in one dog, but that patient also had experienced a recent surgery. Disseminated intravascular coagulation could have been associated with the tumor, the surgery, the chemotherapy, or a combination of these.

20. What is the dose-limiting toxicity for intracavitary cisplatin in cats?

Pulmonary edema. This is a usually fatal toxicity that can occur when cisplatin is given to cats at any dosage. Although it is possible that a low dosage of cisplatin could be used to treat cats with mesothelioma, this drug cannot be recommended in this species.

21. How do I treat cats with mesothelioma?

There are almost no data on the treatment of mesothelioma in cats. Intracavitary mitoxantrone (6 to 6.5 mg/m^2 intravenously every 3 to 4 weeks) can be considered. This should be a reasonably safe treatment, but the efficacy is unknown. Intracavitary carboplatin (200 to 210 mg/m^2 every 4 weeks) also can be used safely in cats.

Repeated centesis can be used to maintain the quality of life, although eventually this procedure may be required every few days.

22. Is intracavitary cisplatin successful in treating dogs with mesothelioma?

It seems to be a reasonably successful treatment. In one study, three dogs with pleural mesothelioma all had stable disease that lasted 129, 289, and more than 306 days.

Dogs that respond to treatment usually do so quickly, often within a few days. The volume of the effusion usually decreases in these patients. This can improve the dog's quality of life and increase the time it can remain comfortable between therapeutic taps. If there is no response after two treatments with intracavitary cisplatin, mitoxantrone (5 mg/m^2 every 3 to 4 weeks) can be considered as an alternative.

CONTROVERSIES

23. If the effusion due to a mesothelioma is obliterated after intracavitary treatment, should additional treatment be given?

Much depends on the owner's goals for the pet. Intracavitary cisplatin appears to be a reasonable method of palliation for dogs with mesothelioma. If palliation is the goal, therapy could be discontinued after the effusion is controlled.

Additional intravenous chemotherapy can be considered in hopes of prolonging a remission, but the efficacy of this approach is unknown.

24. What drugs should be used for additional intravenous treatments?

No one knows the ideal drug. In dogs, cisplatin, carboplatin, doxorubicin, or mitoxantrone could be considered. If there was a response to a platinum (cisplatin or carboplatin) drug delivered in to a body cavity, it seems logical to continue to use that agent intravenously. Historical responses of mesothelioma to the anthracyclines (doxorubicin and mitoxantrone) make a case for using one of these agents. A combination of a platinum drug and an anthracycline may be superior to single-agent therapy, but this has not been studied in dogs or cats.

25. Is intracavitary chemotherapy painful? If so, can we justify its use in a palliative setting?

In the author's experience, few dogs experience significant pain. The injection site is uncomfortable, but this can be alleviated with local anesthesia.

When given into the chest, chemotherapy may cause sclerosis. This can lead to obliteration of the pleural space and thus is ultimately a good method of palliation. The process of sclerosis can be painful. If there is evidence of pain, narcotics should be used as long as necessary. About 1 to 2 days of analgesic therapy is generally sufficient. Ideally, because of the potential for nephrotoxicity, nonsteroidal antiinflammatory medications should be avoided when giving cisplatin.

Intracavitary chemotherapy seems to be very well tolerated by cats. Significant pain has not been reported to be an adverse effect, but certainly the clinician should be aware that it could occur and be ready to treat it appropriately.

BIBLIOGRAPHY

1. Bergman PJ: Use of Carboplatin in Veterinary Oncology. American College of Veterinary Internal Medicine Annual Forum, May 1997.
2. Moore AS, Kirk C, Cardona A: Intracavitary cisplatin chemotherapy experience with six dogs. J Vet Intern Med 5:227–231, 1991.
3. Ogilvie GK, Moore AS: Managing the Veterinary Cancer Patient. Trenton, NJ, Veterinary Learning Systems, 1995, pp 442–445.

37. FELINE LEUKEMIA VIRUS (FeLV)

Dennis Macy, DVM, Dipl ACVIM

1. How common is feline leukemia virus infection?

Approximately 3% of the U.S. cat population carries feline leukemia virus (FeLV). It may be as low as 1% in single-cat households and as high as 33% in multiple-cat households. Approximately 20% of sick cats are infected with FeLV or feline immunodeficiency virus.

2. What clinical diseases are associated with FeLV?

- Neoplastic (three types of lymphosarcoma: thymic, alimentary, generalized)
- Myeloproliferative diseases and fibrosarcoma
- Degenerative (nonneoplastic diseases): anemia and immunopathologic diseases and diseases associated with immunodeficiency.

About 80% of cats dying of FeLV-related disease fall into the nonneoplastic or degenerative category.

3. How is the virus transmitted?

Mutual grooming and cat bites are considered the main route of transmission. However, iatrogenic transmission via blood transfusion has been documented, and testing all blood donors is recommended.

4. Which cats are most susceptible to acquiring the infection?

The young (85% of cats younger than 12 weeks of age) will become persistently infected if exposed. In cats older than 1 year of age, only 15% will become persistently infected with FeLV. Vaccination and testing should be used to reduce the chances of developing persistent FeLV infection.

5. What is the prognosis for a persistently infected cat?

The prognosis depends on a number of factors. Age has been shown to be an important prognostic indicator. Cats infected at younger than 1 year of age carry a poor prognosis. Cats that are infected as adults will carry a better prognosis. It has been published that 80% of infected cats die within 3 years of diagnosis, but this may be somewhat pessimistic. Cats with low lymphocyte counts (less than 1800/ml) 4 months from the time of diagnosis carry a less favorable prognosis. Cats with low CD4 and CD8 numbers carry a poor prognosis. Cats that are symptomatic for degenerative disease or have neoplastic diseases carry the poorest prognosis. Although cats may remain asymptomatic, when an FeLV-positive cat becomes ill, whatever the presentation, the prognosis is not favorable.

6. How do you diagnose FeLV-infected cats?

Two tests are readily available to the practitioner—enzyme-linked immunosorbent assay (ELISA) and the indirect immunofluorescence antibody (IFA) test. The former is available in a number of formats for in-house testing. This IFA procedure is done at reference laboratories. Both tests detect the presence of group-specific viral protein p27. The ELISA is the most sensitive and the IFA is the most specific test for FeLV antigens.

7. What samples do you submit for FeLV tests?

Viral protein p27 is contained within most body fluids—from blood to tears. Blood, saliva, and tears are the most frequent fluids used in ELISA testing. Buffy coat, blood smears, and bone marrow are used in the IFA procedure.

8. Can polymerase chain reaction be used for diagnosing FeLV in cats?

Polymerase chain reaction (PCR) is available through some reference laboratories and is indicated when the ELISA and IFA are negative but FeLV is still suspected. PCR-positive, ELISA-negative, IFA-negative cats carry FeLV encoded in their DNA but are not producing new virus or viral proteins. These cats are not generally contagious, but they are susceptible to developing FeLV-related disease.

9. Which tests are most sensitive?

PCR is most sensitive but does not necessarily mean the cat is shedding virus. ELISA is the next most sensitive and is 100 times more sensitive than the IFA. IFA correlates best with viremia and contagiousness.

10. What is a discordant cat?

A cat that tests positive on ELISA but negative on IFA is called discordant. Such cats usually have sequestered infection (one or two lymph nodes, bone marrow, or other tissues) but are not considered viremic. About 50% of discordant cats will become negative on both tests over time, 25% will remain discordant, and 25% will become positive on both tests. Discordant cats should not be stressed or given steroids.

11. What is a latently infected cat?

A cat that has been exposed to FeLV but whose immune system has eliminated infected cells that are producing virus or viral proteins. Thus, the cat tests negative by IFA and ELISA procedures. However, the cat is PCR-positive and has FeLV encoded in its DNA. A latently infected cat should not be stressed or given immunosuppressive drugs.

12. Can cats eliminate FeLV?

About 70% of cats exposed to FeLV are capable of eliminating these infections. However, after a cat has been determined to be persistently infected (i.e., IFA-positive), less than 3% will become negative.

13. How effective are antiviral agents?

Beyond supportive therapy, specific antiviral therapy is limited to a few agents. Parenteral interferon at 1.3 million U/m^2 subcutaneously three times per week has been shown to reduce virus load. Oral interferon therapy has not been shown to reduce viral load. Approximately 50% of cats treated with interferon will develop antibodies to the drug within 7 weeks. Zidovudine has also been shown to reduce viral load (5 to 10 mg/kg daily) but is associated with significant toxicity and is not recommended in asymptomatic cats.

14. When is antiviral treatment indicated?

In symptomatic cats. No one has demonstrated benefit of treatment on survival of asymptomatic cats.

15. How old should a cat be to be tested?

Because the tests detect viral protein as opposed to antibody, cats of virtually any age can be tested for FeLV. Most cats should first be tested at 8 to 16 weeks of age. At-risk cats should be tested yearly.

16. What is an "at-risk" cat?

Cats that roam, fight, or come in contact with other cats of unknown viral status are considered at risk.

17. What are major differential diagnoses in FeLV-infected cats?

FIV-infected cats mimic many of the same clinical signs as cats immunosuppressed due to FeLV infections. Cats tested for FeLV should also be tested for FIV. Coinfected cats carry a very guarded prognosis.

18. What are the potential outcomes after being exposed to FeLV?
- About 70% of cats do not become persistently infected with FeLV.
- Transient infection occurs followed by virus clearing.
- Latent infections occur.
- Persistent infections are seen in 30%.

19. What is the public health potential for exposure to FeLV-infected cats?

Several studies have addressed this question in various populations, and it appears that FeLV, when evaluated in a number of different settings, is not a public health threat. Two studies did suggest that children may, in fact, be at some additional risk, but the methodology of these studies and their true meaning was highly questionable.

20. In cats with lymphoma, what is the prognostic significance of the FeLV status? Are there other prognostic factors for treated cats?

Overall, FeLV-positive cats treated for lymphoma have a less favorable prognosis. Their median survival time is about $3\frac{1}{2}$ months compared with about 7 months for FeLV-negative cats. In addition, both the initial response to therapy and the clinical substage have been shown to be important in prognosis.

21. What is the most common site of lymphoma in cats?

Early studies from various centers pointed to different sites as the most common. With the advent of leukemia vaccination as a routine health care intervention, the most common clinical presentation seems to have changed over the years. Presently, the most common form of lymphoma in cats appears to be the gastrointestinal form.

22. Does the site of the lymphoma make a difference?

Over the years several studies have looked at different anatomic presentations specifically. In one study, in cats with gastrointestinal lymphoma, combination chemotherapy (vincristine, cyclophosphamide, prednisone) resulted in a median first remission in responding cats of about 20 weeks, but only 9 of 28 cats attained a complete remission; the overall median survival time was only 50 days when all cats were considered. In cats with gastrointestinal lymphoma treated with combination chemotherapy including asparaginase and doxorubicin as well, the median first remission overall was 20 weeks with a median survival time of twice that. Response in cats with either spinal or renal lymphoma have been reported to be shorter—14 weeks in cats with responding spinal lymphoma and 18 weeks in cats with responding renal lymphoma.

23. What chemotherapeutic agents should cats with lymphoma receive?

As in dogs, combination chemotherapy is preferable to single agent therapy. Combination protocols including doxorubicin have been reported to have median first remissions of approximately 280 days. At present, it appears that rational combinations of vincristine, cyclophosphamide, prednisone, and doxorubicin provide the best outcomes for cats with lymphoma.

BIBLIOGRAPHY

1. Lane SB, Kornegay JN, Duncan JR, et al: Feline spinal lymphosarcoma: A retrospective evaluation of 23 cats. J Vet Int Med 8(2):99–104, 1994.

2. Mahony OM, Moore AS, Cotter SM, et al: Alimentary lymphoma in cats: 28 cases (1988–1993). J Vet Med Assoc 207(12):1593–1598, 1995.
3. Mooney SC, Hayes AA, Matus RE, et al: Renal lymphoma in cats: 28 cases (1977–1984). J Vet Med Assoc 191(11):1473–1477, 1987.
4. Moore AS, Cotter, Frimbeger AE, et al: A comparison of doxorubicin and COP for the maintenance of remission in cats with lymphoma. J Vet Int Med 10(6)372–375, 1996.
5. Spodnick GL, Berg J, Moore FM, et al: Spinal lymphoma in cats: 21 cases (1976–1989). J Vet Med Assoc 200(3):373–376, 1992.
6. Vail DM, Moore AS, Ogilvie GK, et al: Feline lymphoma (145 cases): Proliferation indices, cluster of differentiation 3 immunoreactivity, and their association with prognosis in 90 cats. J Vet Int Med 12:349–354, 1998.
7. Zwahlen CH, Lucroy MD, Kragel SA, et al: Results of chemotherapy for cats with alimentary malignant lymphoma: 21 cases (1993–1997). J Vet Med Assoc 213:1144–1149, 1998.

38. VACCINE-ASSOCIATED SARCOMAS

Dennis Macy, DVM, Dipl ACVIM

1. How common are vaccine-associated sarcomas?

Studies indicate the incidence to be 1 in 1000 to 1 in 10,000 in animals receiving feline leukemia virus (FeLV) or rabies vaccination. Most experts believe the incidence to be 1 in 2000 and 1 in 4000 in cats receiving FeLV or rabies vaccination.

2. What vaccines have been most often associated with vaccine-associated sarcomas?

Adjuvanted feline vaccines have been most frequently reported to be associated with sarcoma development at injection sites. Killed adjuvanted FeLV and rabies vaccines are the vaccines that have been most frequently linked to injection-site sarcoma development.

3. Why adjuvanted vaccines?

Adjuvanted vaccines produce inflammation, stimulate fibroblasts to divide, and are responsible for free radical formation that results in oxidative damage to DNA.

4. Why don't the same rabies vaccines produce tumors in dogs?

Cats do appear unique in terms of their susceptibility to sarcoma development. It is believed that the cat's unique species susceptibility to oxidative injury (Heinz body anemia, Tylenol toxicity, steatitis) is one reason for the high vaccine-associated tumor rate.

5. If granulomas and inflammation occur in all cats receiving certain adjuvanted vaccines, why do only 1 to 5 in 10,000 develop a sarcoma?

It may depend on individual susceptibility to oxidative stress (reduced glutamine levels have been demonstrated in some cats with vaccine-associated sarcoma). Individual cats may have defects in their tumor suppressor gene, p53. Aberrations in these cats have been reported in some cats with vaccine-associated sarcomas.

6. Have these tumors been reported following administration of products other than vaccines?

Yes. Virtually anything that results in chronic inflammation, i.e., sutures, parenteral antibiotics, and injectable lufenuron. However, adjuvanted vaccines are the only substances that are consistently repeatedly injected in all cats.

7. What is the time from vaccine administration to subsequent tumor formation?

Reports indicate that tumors may develop 3 months to 11 years after vaccine administration. Tumors that occur sooner than 3 months after injection are probably due to previous vaccination or tissue injury.

8. What can be done to prevent vaccine-associated sarcomas?

- Do not overvaccinate.
- Limit the use of adjuvanted vaccines.
- Avoid using any medication that produces chronic inflammation.
- Use nonadjuvanted products when available.

9. How long do postvaccinal lumps remain?

Adjuvant vaccines produce granulomas that reach their maximum size 3 weeks after vaccination but disappear within 3 months after vaccination.

10. When should a postvaccinal lump be removed?

The Vaccine-Associated Sarcoma Task Force recommends that any lump at a vaccination site be biopsied and removed if it meets any of the following three criteria:
- Present 3 months after vaccination.
- Greater than 2 cm in size anytime after vaccination.
- Growing in size 4 weeks after vaccination.

11. What biopsy techniques should be used?

A wedge or Tru-Cut biopsy technique should be used. Fine-needle aspiration is considered unreliable.

12. Should granulomas be removed?

Yes. If a biopsy determines the postvaccinal lump to be a granuloma, simple marginal resection of the granuloma should be performed.

13. How should a vaccine-site sarcoma be managed?

Prior to treatment of a vaccine-associated sarcoma:
- Perform a computed tomography scan to determine the extent of the lesion.
- Perform a chest radiograph to determine if metastatic disease is present (usually 5% or less at the time of first diagnosis but may increase to 25% if the patient has received prior treatment).
- Perform an FeLV test to eliminate the possibility of a feline sarcoma virus–induced tumor. Sarcomas caused by the feline sarcoma virus do not benefit from surgery.

14. What treatment is best?

A combination of surgery, radiation therapy, and chemotherapy gives the best results.

15. Which treatment regimen should be used first?

Surgery followed by radiation therapy or radiation therapy followed by surgery have been recommended; chemotherapy usually follows radiation therapy and surgery treatment regimens.

16. How large a margin should be used?

The "dose" of surgery should be large. Margins between 2 to 5 cm are recommended.

17. Should I refer the surgery?

Significant improvement in disease-free interval has been shown if a referral institution does the initial or second surgery. No difference in disease-free interval is found if multiple surgeries have been done prior to referral.

18. What is the prognosis?

With surgery alone, 60% is the recurrence rate (86% of which recur within 6 months). Average survival is 1 to 1½ years. With radiation and surgery, 30% to 40% is the recurrence rate. Average survival is 700 to 800 days.

Some chemotherapeutic agents are active against vaccine-associated sarcomas but are marginally effective in adding to patient survival, perhaps adding 10% to survival time. Although a wide variety of drugs have been evaluated (including doxorubicin, carboplatin, mitoxantrone, cyclophosphamide, and vincristine), doxorubicin appears to be the most effective.

Reference

Macy D: Current understanding of vaccination site–associated sarcomas in the cat. J Feline Med Surg 1(1):15–21, 1999.

39. MALIGNANT HISTIOCYTOSIS

Alan Hammer, DVM, Dipl ACVIM

1. What is malignant histiocytosis?

Malignant histiocytosis is a progressive, neoplastic proliferation of atypical histiocytes and their precursors, which invade multiple organs.

2. How does *systemic* histiocytosis differ from *malignant* histiocytosis?

Systemic histiocytosis is a familial proliferative disorder diagnosed almost exclusively in the Bernese mountain dog. Nodular cutaneous lesions frequently involving the scrotum, nasal planum, eyelids, and face characterize systemic histiocytosis. Peripheral lymphadenopathy, hepatosplenomegaly, and other organ involvement may also be noted. Histologically, the histiocytes are angiocentrically located and lack the cellular atypia noted in malignant histiocytosis.

3. Is malignant fibrous *histiocytoma* the same as malignant *histiocytosis*?

No. Malignant fibrous histiocytoma is considered a soft tissue sarcoma arising from a primitive mesenchymal cell or fibroblast. Histologically, it consists of plump spindle cells arranged in a cartwheel (storiform) pattern. Pleomorphic areas consist of both the plump spindle cells and histiocytic cells. The cat often has a giant cell variant, with numerous multinucleated cells scattered throughout the tissue.

Recently, some dogs have been identified as having tumors with characteristics of both malignant fibrous histiocytoma and malignant histiocytosis. This blurs the classification of these tumors and indicates a spectrum ranging from cutaneous histiocytoma to systemic histiocytosis and malignant histiocytosis to malignant fibrous histiocytoma.

4. What dogs with malignant histiocytosis present to the veterinarian?

Dogs with malignant histiocytosis are presented with nonspecific complaints of weight loss, lethargy, and inappetence. Other clinical findings include dyspnea, neurologic abnormalities, ocular signs, lymphadenopathy, hepatosplenomegaly, and anemia.

5. Which dog breeds besides Bernese mountain dogs are reported to develop malignant histiocytosis?

While Bernese mountain dogs account for many of the reported cases, other breeds include rottweilers and golden retrievers. This may be a true breed predilection or simply reflect the current popular dog breeds. There is a higher frequency of malignant histiocytosis in males than in females.

6. I have heard about an unusual form of cancer in flat-coated retrievers. Is this malignant histiocytosis?

No. The tumor in question in flat-coated retrievers is called undifferentiated sarcoma of flat-coated retrievers. It has some histiocytic characteristics and has been diagnosed in the past as malignant histiocytosis, histiocytic sarcoma, malignant fibrous histiocytoma, or histiocytic lymphoma. This again illustrates the spectrum of pathology these tumor types are capable of displaying.

7. Which immunohistochemical stains may be used to confirm the diagnosis of malignant histiocytosis?

Lysozyme is the immunohistochemical stain most often used to confirm the diagnosis of malignant histiocytosis. Systemic histiocytosis will also stain positive, as will granulomatous panniculitis and some histiocytomas.

8. What characterizes the anemia found in dogs with malignant histiocytosis?

Dogs with malignant histiocytosis usually have a regenerative anemia secondary to ery-throphagocytosis by the neoplastic cells. Leukoerythrophagocytosis is also often noted. Other, less likely, underlying causes for anemia in these dogs include anemia of chronic disease and myelophthisis (infiltration of the bone marrow by the neoplastic histiocytes).

9. How often are neurologic signs found in dogs with malignant histiocytosis?

Neurologic signs are reported in approximately 25% of dogs with malignant histiocytosis. The findings range from seizures and nystagmus to peripheral neuropathies.

10. What are some of the thoracic radiographic findings in dogs with malignant histiocytosis?

Common radiographic findings in thoracic radiographs include sternal, hilar, and cranial mediastinal lymphadenopathy. Diffuse mixed pulmonary infiltrates are almost as common as nodular interstitial infiltrates.

11. Will dogs with cutaneous histiocytoma develop malignant histiocytosis at a later date?

Cutaneous histiocytoma is a common tumor in young dogs. There is no evidence linking histiocytoma with later development of malignant histiocytosis.

12. What is the best treatment for dogs with malignant histiocytosis?

Unfortunately, we have not identified a highly effective treatment for malignant histiocytosis. Current protocols include doxorubicin and prednisone. The CHOP (cyclophosphamide, doxorubicin, vincristine, and prednisone) protocol is commonly used. A drug with high ex-pectations is Doxil (liposome-encapsulated doxorubicin). The hope is that the malignant histiocytes will phagocytize the liposomes and achieve high intracellular concentrations. While Doxil is expensive, it has decreased cardiotoxicity compared with doxorubicin. However, an unusual adverse effect is palmar-plantar erythrodysesthesia, a syndrome characterized by ery-throderma and hyperesthesia of the footpads.

13. What is the prognosis for dogs with malignant histiocytosis?

Poor. The clinical course is rapidly progressive, with many dogs dying or being eutha-nized within 1 month of diagnosis.

14. Do cats get malignant histiocytosis?

Yes. There are two reports of cats with malignant histiocytosis.

BIBLIOGRAPHY

1. Kerlin RL, Hendrick MJ: Malignant fibrous histiocytoma and malignant histiocytosis in the dog—convergent or divergent phenotypic differentiation. Vet Pathol 33:713–716, 1996.
2. Moore PF: Systemic histiocytosis of Bernese mountain dogs. Vet Pathol 21:554–563, 1984.
3. Moore PF: Utilization of cytoplasmic lysozyme immunoreactivity as a histiocytic marker in canine histiocytic disorders. Vet Pathol 23:757–762, 1986.
4. Moore PF, Rosin A: Malignant histiocytosis of Bernese mountain dogs. Vet Pathol 23:1–10, 1986.
5. Rosin A, Moore P, Dubielzig R: Malignant histiocytosis in Bernese mountain dogs. J Am Vet Med Assoc 188:1041–1045, 1986.
6. Shaiken LC, Evans SM, Goldschmidt MH: Radiographic findings in canine malignant histiocytosis. Vet Radiol 32:237–242, 1991.
7. Wellman ML, Davenport DJ, Morton D, et al: Malignant histiocytosis in four dogs. J Am Vet Med Assoc 187:919–921, 1985.

INDEX

Page numbers in **boldface type** indicate complete chapters.